SMOKING BEHAVIOUR
Physiological and Psychological Influences

SMOKING BEHAVIOUR

Physiological and Psychological Influences.

Edited by

RAYMOND E. THORNTON

Senior Scientist
Group Research and Development Centre
British-American Tobacco Company Limited

CHURCHILL LIVINGSTONE
EDINBURGH LONDON AND NEW YORK 1978

CHURCHILL LIVINGSTONE
Medical Division of Longman Group Limited

Distributed in the United States of America by
Longman Inc., 19 West 44th Street, New York,
N.Y. 10036 and by associated companies,
branches and representatives throughout
the world.

ISBN 0 443 01815 4

Printed in Great Britain

Preface

This book is the result of the International Smoking Behaviour Conference held at Chelwood Vachery, Sussex, England, in November 1977. The objectives of the conference were:

'To explore some of the physiological and psychological effects of smoking which may be important in smoking behaviour and motivation, and to relate these effects (where possible) to:

(a) differences between smokers and non-smokers;

(b) the smoker's intake of tar, nicotine and carbon monoxide, including the extent to which this intake can be influenced by changes in cigarette design'.

Fifty-five behavioural, biological, medical and physical scientists convened at Chelwood to discuss these issues, and the thirty-one papers presented are the refined views of many of the workers in the wide area of smoking behaviour. Some authors act as spokesmen for research teams, while other papers represent the personal views of people engaged in research in this field. The views expressed are, of course, entirely those of the authors and not necessarily those of British-American Tobacco Company Limited or the editor. Papers are given here in the order they were presented at the conference.

No simple or single answer will be found to the questions raised by the conference objectives, but among the papers will be found a 1977/78 view on topics such as the differences between smokers and non-smokers, the effects of smoking on the central nervous system and on performance, the difficulties in relating laboratory studies to the real-life situation, the format of league tables, and the importance of nicotine in smoking motivation.

The editor would like to thank all those delegates who were prepared to put aside their other duties and responsibilities and spend three days at Chelwood, as well as a number of his colleagues for their help with various aspects of the conference. Kay Comer, in addition to her contribution towards the conference planning, meticulously checked many of the papers and references in this book. David Creighton helped at all stages of the conference and in the preparation of papers. Joan Pressey also helped both in preparing for the conference and in the publication of this book. Barbara Stone prepared the index.

R.E. Thornton

Participants

P. Adams,
Imperial Tobacco Limited, Bristol, U.K.

Dr. F. Adlkofer,
Verband der Cigarettenindustrie, Hamburg, West Germany.

Dr. A.K. Armitage,
Hazleton Laboratories Europe Ltd., Harrogate, U.K.

Dr. C.H. Ashton,
Dept. of Clinical Pharmacology, Newcastle University, U.K.

Dr. C.I. Ayres,
British-American Tobacco Co. Ltd., Southampton, U.K.

Dr. H. Barkemeyer,
BAT Cigaretten-Fabriken GmbH, Hamburg, West Germany.

Professor K. Bättig,
Swiss Federal Institute of Technology, Zurich, Switzerland.

Dr. C.D. Binnie,
Instituut voor Epilsiebestrijding, Heemstede, Holland.

P.W. Brown,
Carreras Rothmans Limited, Basildon, U.K.

Miss N. Cherry,
London School of Economics, London, U.K.

Mrs. A.K. Comer,
British-American Tobacco Co. Ltd., Southampton, U.K.

D.E. Creighton,
British-American Tobacco Co. Ltd., Southampton, U.K.

Professor G. Cumming,
Midhurst Medical Research Institute, Midhurst, U.K.

Dr. C.J.P. de Siqueira,
Cia Cigarros Souza Cruz Industrie é Comercio, Brazil.

Dr. P.J. Dunn,
Imperial Tobacco Limited, Montreal, Canada.

Dr. W.L. Dunn, Jr.
Philip Morris, U.S.A., Richmond, U.S.A.,

Dr. J.G. Esterle,
Brown and Williamson Tobacco Corporation, Louisville, U.S.A.

Dr. D.G. Felton,
British-American Tobacco Co. Ltd., Southampton, U.K.

R. Ferris,
British-American Tobacco Co. Ltd., Southampton, U.K.

Dr. E.O. Field,
Gallaher Limited, London, U.K.

Professor A. Gale,
Dept. of Psychology, Southampton University, U.K.

J. Golding,
Dept. of Experimental Psychology, Oxford University, U.K.

Dr. S.J. Green,
British-American Tobacco Co. Ltd., London, U.K.

Dr. C. Izard,
S.E.I.T.A., Paris, France.

Professor M.E. Jarvik,
Brentwood Veterans' Administration Hospital, Los Angeles, U.S.A.

S.J. Kane,
Gallaher Limited, Belfast, N. Ireland.

Dr. V.J. Knott,
Addiction Unit, Royal Ottawa Hospital, Canada.

Dr. R. Kumar,
Institute of Psychiatry, London, U.K.

Dr. P.H. Lewis,
British-American Tobacco Co. Ltd., Southampton, U.K.

Professor J.H. Mills,
Dept. of Medicine, Cambridge University, U.K.

Dr. A-L. Myrsten,
Psychological Laboratories, Stockholm University, Sweden.

Dr. A.J. Nelmes,
Department of Health & Social Security, London, U.K.

Dr. M. Oldman,
British-American Tobacco Co. Ltd., Southampton, U.K.

W. Paige,
Imperial Tobacco Limited, Bristol, U.K.

Dr. E. Radziszewski,
CERTSM, DCAN, 83800 Toulon-Naval, France.

Dr. R.G. Rawbone,
Charing Cross Hospital, London, U.K.

T. Riehl,
Brown and Williamson Tobacco Corporation, Louisville, U.S.A.

Dr. F.J.C. Roe,
Wimbledon, London, U.K.

Dr. W.D. Rowland,
Carreras Rothmans Ltd., Basildon, U.K.

Dr. M.A.H. Russell,
Institute of Psychiatry, London, U.K.

Professor S. Schachter,
Dept. of Psychology, Columbia University, New York, U.S.A.

Prof. Dr. H. Schievelbein,
Deutsches Herzzentrum, München, West Germany.

Dr. F. Seehofer,
BAT Cigaretten-Fabriken GmbH, Hamburg, West Germany.

P.L. Short,
British-American Tobacco Co. Ltd., London, U.K.

R. Stepney,
Dept. of Clinical Pharmacology, Newcastle University, U.K.

Dr. I.P. Stolerman,
MRC Neuropharmacology Unit, Birmingham, U.K.

S. Sutton,
Institute of Psychiatry, London, U.K.

Dr. D.H. Taylor,
Dept. of Psychology, Southampton University, U.K.

Professor J.W. Thompson,
Dept. of Clinical Pharmacology, Newcastle University, U.K.

Dr. R.E. Thornton,
British-American Tobacco Co. Ltd., Southampton, U.K.

R.S. Wade,
Imperial Tobacco Limited, Montreal, Canada.

Dr. D.M. Warburton,
Dept. of Psychology, Reading University, U.K.

A*

K. Wesnes,
Dept. of Psychology, Reading University, U.K.

D.J. Wood,
British-American Tobacco Co. Ltd., Southampton, U.K.

Contributors

P. Adams,
Imperial Tobacco Limited, Research Department, Bristol, U.K.

Karin Andersson,
Psychological Laboratories, University of Stockholm, Sweden.

A.K. Armitage,
Hazleton Laboratories Europe Ltd., Harrogate, U.K.

C. Heather Ashton,
Dept. of Pharmacological Sciences, University of Newcastle upon Tyne, U.K.

C.D. Binnie,
Instituut voor Epilepsiebestrijding, Achterweg, Holland.

J.E. Caille,
CERPA, Toulon-Naval, France.

Nicola Cherry,
MRC Unit for the Study of Environmental Factors in Mental and Physical Illness, London School of Economics and Political Science, U.K.

P.V. Cole,
Anaesthetic Research Laboratory, St. Bartholomew's Hospital, London, U.K.

A. Kay Comer,
British-American Tobacco Company Limited, Group Research and Development Centre, Southampton, U.K.

E.C. Cooke,
Addiction Research Unit, Institute of Psychiatry, Bethlem and Maudsley Hospitals, London, U.K.

D.E. Creighton,
British-American Tobacco Company Limited, Group Research and Development Centre, Southampton, U.K.

G. Cumming,
Midhurst Medical Research Institute, West Sussex, U.K.

P.J. Dunn,
Imperial Tobacco Limited, Montreal, Canada.

C. Feyerabend,
Poisons Unit, New Cross Hospital, London, U.K.

E.R. Freiesleben,
Imperial Tobacco Limited, Montreal, Canada.

J. Golding,
Department of Experimental Psychology, University of Oxford, Oxford, U.K.

S.J. Green,
British-American Tobacco Company Limited, London, U.K.

R. Guillerm,
Centre d'Etudes et de Recherches Techniques Sous-Marines, Toulon-Naval, France.

A.R. Guyatt,
Midhurst Medical Research Institute, West Sussex, U.K.

G. Heinemann,
Vorstand des Instituts für Klinische Chemi, Deutsches Herzzentrum München, West Germany.

M.A. Holmes,
Midhurst Medical Research Institute, West Sussex.

C. Izard,
SEITA, Paris Cedex, France.

M.E. Jarvik,
Psychopharmacology Research Unit, Brentwood Veterans' Administration Hospital, Los Angeles, California, U.S.A.

S.J. Kane,
Gallaher Limited, Belfast, N. Ireland.

V.J. Knott,
Addiction Unit, Royal Ottawa Hospital, Canada.

R. Kumar,
Institute of Psychiatry, De Crespigny Park, London, U.K.

M.H. Lader,
Addiction Research Unit, Institute of Psychiatry, Bethlem and Maudsley Hospitals, London, U.K.

P.H. Lewis,
British-American Tobacco Company Limited, Group Research and Development Centre, Southampton, U.K.

Karin Loschenkohl,
Vorstand des Instituts für Klinische Chemi, Deutsches Herzzentrum München, West Germany.

V.R. Marsh,
Department of Pharmacological Sciences, University of Newcastle upon Tyne, U.K.

J.E. Millman,
Department of Pharmacological Sciences, University of Newcastle upon Tyne, U.K.

I.H. Mills,
Department of Medicine, University of Cambridge Clinical School, U.K.

K. Murphy,
Cardiopulmonary Laboratories, Department of Medicine, Charing Cross Hospital Medical School, London, U.K.

Anna-Lisa Myrsten,
Psychological Laboratories, University of Stockholm, Sweden.

M.J. Noble,
Projects. C.G.C. Limited, Cheltenham, U.K.

E. Radziszewski,
Centre d'Etudes et de Recherches Techniques Sous-Marines, Toulon-Naval, France.

R.G. Rawbone,
Cardiopulmonary Laboratories, Department of Medicine, Charing Cross Hospital. Medical School, London, U.K.

M.D. Rawlins,
Department of Clinical Pharmacology, University of Newcastle upon Tyne, U.K.

M.A.H. Russell,
Addiction Research Unit, Institute of Psychiatry, Bethlem and Maudsley Hospitals, London, U.K.

Y. Saloojee,
Addiction Research Unit, Institute of Psychiatry, Bethlem and Maudsley Hospitals, London, U.K.

S. Schachter,
Department of Psychology, Columbia University, New York, U.S.A.

J. Schlegel,
Vorstand des Instituts für Klinische Chemi, Deutsches Herzzentrum Müchen, West Germany.

H. Schievelbein,
Vorstand des Instituts für Klinische Chemi, Deutsches Herzzentrum München, West Germany.

W. Schulz,
B.A.T. Cigaretten-Fabriken G.m.b.H., Hamburg, West Germany

F. Seehofer,
B.A.T. Cigaretten-Fabriken G.m.b.H., Hamburg, West Germany.

R. Stepney,
Department of Pharmacological Sciences, University of Newcastle upon Tyne, U.K.

S. Sutton,
Addiction Research Unit, Institute of Psychiatry, Bethlem and Maudsley Hospitals, London, U.K.

Rosemary Telford,
Department of Pharmacological Sciences, University of Newcastle upon Tyne, U.K.

J.W. Thompson,
Department of Pharmacological Sciences, University of Newcastle upon Tyne, U.K.

C. Troll,
Vorstand des Instituts für Klinische Chemi, Deutsches Herzzentrum München, West Germany.

D.M. Warburton,
Department of Psychology, University of Reading, U.K.

K. Wesnes,
Department of Psychology, University of Reading, U.K.

R.T. Whewell,
Projects C.G.C. Limited, Cheltenham, U.K.

Contents

1. Coping mechanisms in the brain

IVOR H MILLS

Using our brains in everyday life, both for work and for relaxation, is a process that we take for granted. We do not as a rule ask ourselves what the mechanisms are in the brain which enable it to carry out what we ask of it. If the processes are mechanical, like lifting an arm to reach a book on a shelf, we know fairly clearly how this movement is effected. It has been shown that during such muscular work, the part of the brain related to the movement has an increase in its blood supply (Ingvar and Schwartz, 1974).

Thinking and solving problems are quite different processes in the brain from initiation and control of muscle movements. For problem solving, changes occur in the blood flow through the brain. These results have been obtained by using injections of radio-active xenon or krypton into one carotid artery and measuring the radiation emitted by means of a series of 32 radio-active counters arranged around the skull. When the injection is stopped the radio-active gas is washed out of the brain by the blood flow and the rate of washout is proportional to the rate of blood flow (Sveinsdottir *et al*, 1970).

By computer analysis of the radio-activity picked up by each counter, the distribution of the blood flow in different parts of the brain can be established. Attempting to solve reasoning problems increases the blood flow through the association areas of the brain (Risberg and Ingvar, 1973). At the same time a rise in blood pressure of 10 to 30 mmHg occurs while the problem-solving is going on (Sharpey-Schafer and Taylor, 1960; Ludbrook, Vincent and Walsh, 1975). When the solution is arrived at the blood pressure comes down. In some individuals the rise in blood pressure is greater than 30 mmHg and in some there may be an appreciable delay before the blood pressure returns to normal when the problem is solved.

Many of the events of daily life are akin to problem solving exercises and we may assume that similar changes in brain blood flow occur with these problems as with those which are studied in the laboratory. Studies have not been carried out over a long period of time, equivalent to a full day's work, and it may be important to obtain such information. The very nature of everyday life is that of a series of challenges and little is known about the neuronal mechanisms associated with continued problem solving.

Catecholamine release

Another technique which has been used to assess the response to challanging events is the measurement of adrenaline and noradrenaline in the urine. This type of technique gives results which are an integration over time since the urine collections are usually of at least one or two hours duration and sometimes much longer.

Almost anything which causes mental stimulation leads to an increased excretion of these catecholamines in the urine (Levi, 1972). The stimulus may be something which is pleasurable, such as an exciting film, or it may be something which produces excitement by generating fear. Films which portray frightening events or high suspense may produce exactly the same biochemical responses as in real life. Crudely sexual films excite male subjects and though many female subjects may be disturbed by the films, stimulation of adrenaline excretion still occurs.

The arousal mechanism

There is no doubt that, in general, some excitement in life is pleasurable. A day with nothing going on is less satisfying than one punctuated by a series of events. Raising the arousal level is something which most people enjoy unless it is associated with fear or it causes severe fatigue. Within a certain range, which varies from one individual to another, some challenging events in the day produce the elevations of arousal that lead to a sense of satisfaction. Such challenges would be expected to cause changes in brain blood flow and in the excretion of catecholamines in the urine.

Though we know what happens in the short term with such challanges we do not know much about the longer term. There is evidence that constant presentation of minor challenges leads to adaptation so that the mental and physiological responses eventually fail to occur each time. On the other hand some types of repeated challenge maintain a constant response. This was shown, for instance, when invoice clerks were changed from weekly wages to piece work rates. So long as they were on piece work their adrenaline excretion remained high (Levi, 1972).

The term arousal has been used in a variety of ways. The sense in which we are using it here is well-known in everyday life. If you are involved in something which is very exciting shortly before you go to bed, you may have difficulty getting to sleep. If what you are doing is tiring, or if, before the exciting evening, you had had demanding activity all day, you may sleep because the fatigue overcomes the effect of the mental excitement.

Arousal is sometimes using in the sense of what would happen if you were suddenly faced with an attack by a wild animal. You would produce a lot of adrenaline but other things would happen as well, such as, an increase in your pulse rate and blood pressure, constriction of blood vessels in skin, kidneys and intestines; your hair might stand on end and you might well come out in a cold sweat. This is what happens in the fright reaction but all these things do not normally occur if your mental arousal level goes up while having an enjoyable party. Measurements of skin sweating and heart rate may not, therefore, give a good indication of the level of excitement of your brain.

Challenges of life

Life for most of us is made up of a series of challenges. They may vary from a housewife on a limited budget trying to work out how to feed her young family, to a major disaster such as a large tree falling on your house when you have not increased your insurance to take care of the effect of inflation.

If the mother of two school children decides to go to work part-time she not only meets the additional challenge of the job but she also has to make plans for some unexpected happening to the children as well as fitting in all the chores of housework into her "non-working" hours each day. The result will almost certainly be greater elevation of her arousal level, either as she plans how to do everything, or as she is faced with the problems she had not reckoned on.

The young baby beginning to walk is faced with the difficulties of maintaining his balance, of risking exploring new places, of being frustrated by his inability to do all the things his older brother does, etc. The child just going to school has to cope with being separated from his mother, being faced with a large number of noisy children around him (probably rushing madly about) of having to accept discipline at a much higher standard than he had at home, and so on. It may all be too overwhelming and he comes home crying and is terrified of going to school next day. The mother then has to cope with the emotional trauma of getting the child to school and, perhaps, hearing him screaming as she walks back home.

Insecurity is a major challenge whose severity depends upon the person's personality as well as on the degree of separation from relatives or friends. The teenager who has difficulty in making friends and in making conversation may feel isolated at school and at home. At that age the busy parents rarely think that he or she needs a strong right arm around him or her and the child may be too proud to let the need be known. The truth comes out if she has to go into hospital and takes her teddy bear with her. Even in their late teens or their twenties they may feel the need to take their security symbol with them when they are away from home.

Moving house is both exciting and traumatic. Most of the family can rise to the occasion and help with packing and unpacking, but deciding what to keep and what to throw away presents innumerable challanges. Finding new shops or making new friends are much more demanding challenges. For the shy child at a new school the demands on the coping mechanism may well be too great. With no friends, new teachers, new rules and new expectations it may be impossible, even with high arousal, to succeed against all the odds.

Even those who do not move house may find the demands of school extremely challenging. There is not only the work to be mastered but examinations of all sorts to be worked for and tackled. The response in the child depends upon personality. Those who are anxious to succeed may try very hard whereas those who dislike the strain of effort will be inclined to give up at an early stage. Some will respond to exhortations by parents or teachers and raise their arousal level out of respect for one or fear of the other. Major examinations cast their shadows many months before and it is likely that the atmosphere in the classroom will become more charged as the teacher reminds the children that they are trying to master information for the specific purpose of passing examinations and the results of those examinations may determine the rest of their lives.

For many children the challenges of school work may not be their only problems: they may be teased or tormented in or out of school hours, especially in the case of a boy with delayed puberty. Communal showers after games reveal all and those who are more advanced in puberty commonly regard themselves as superior to their fellows. What starts with a few boys boasting may end with a few boys at the other extreme of normality being mocked for the failure of evidence of their rising masculinity.

The combination of stress from other children and the effort of working for examinations may become too great for some of them to cope with. Lack of sleep, progressive irritability and difficulties in family life may all herald the impending failure of the coping mechanism.

Competition between children at home may impose similar problems to the child's brain: some will thrive on the challenges of a brother or sister, some will be unable to meet the demands on their coping ability. Those who are slow to make friends may be intensely jealous of their more sociable brothers and sisters. Isolation becomes that much more intense if even the members of the family become estranged from the shy child. When such children leave school and try to make their way in the world the difficulties in being sociable may impose intolerable burdens upon them.

Love affairs to the teenagers are immensely exciting and mentally arousing events. They can so easily lead to shortage of sleep either by social events keeping them out late or by the mental excitement leading to day-dreaming in bed instead of going to sleep. Such romances may give immense support to those who feel normally insecure but similarly they will be very disturbing when the relationship is suddenly broken. For those who have difficulties at school (or work) or at home, the break-up of an affair may leave them exhausted of reserves of coping power. They may then take desperate steps when they suddenly feel quite bereft of ability to cope. It is at that stage that they may take a handful of tablets (anybody's tablets) in order to escape from an intolerable situation. They may well be aware of the risk of killing themselves but will be undaunted by it when they have no coping power left.

Interaction between arousal and depression

Observations indicate that life events which cause increased arousal, whether self-engendered or initiated by external forces, cannot be tolerated indefinitely without some breakdown in the coping process. Those who opt out and make no effort to meet the challenges, of course, remain largely unaffected by them but some stimuli are quite difficult to escape from, especially challenges within a family where the only way to escape may be to walk out of the house. That then generates the problem of being self-supporting.

The mechanisms whereby normal life becomes abnormal is demonstrated in figure 1.1, A and B. In 1.1 A is represented the effect of the events during a day on the arousal level. Both enjoyable and taxing episodes combine to raise the arousal level. By the end of the day fatigue sets in and sleep comes naturally.

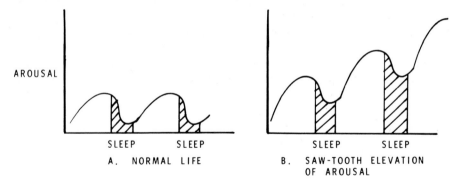

Fig. 1.1 A. The normal pattern of elevation of arousal level during waking hours and its decrease during sleep.
Fig. 1.1 B. What happens if arousal does not fall adequately during sleep but is still raised by the subsequent waking hours. Progressive elevation of arousal then occurs.

During sleep the arousal level falls and the next day begins as the previous one with the initial arousal level at the same point. Normal life goes in this fashion. In figure 1.1 B is shown what happens when the demands of the day raise the arousal level higher than usual. Although fatigue may be bad enough to bring sleep rapidly on going to bed, the high arousal level eventually breaks through and causes the person to wake part way through the night. If a few days like this follow each other the arousal level is pushed higher and higher.

The long term effects of this are shown in fugure 1.2. As arousal rises an increase

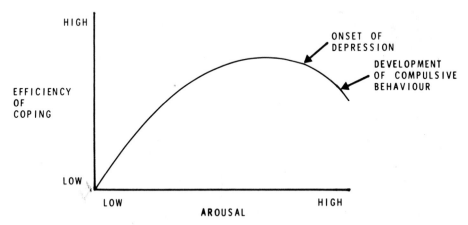

Fig. 1.2 Represents the bi-phasic relation between arousal and coping efficiency. Beyond a certain point, further elevation of arousal leads to depression which may remain masked. Still further elevation of arousal leads to the development of compulsive thought disorders and compulsive behaviour.

in efficiency occurs. The ease with which problems can be solved increases; the process of decision-making is facilitated; learning becomes more effective.

However, if the drive to raise arousal level becomes sustained, the elevation of mental efficiency flattens off and eventually falls. At this point the stimulation of arousal produces some degree of agitation; concentration on one thing at a time tends to be lost and this impairs efficient working.

At this point the underlying depression may break through, especially first thing in the morning when arousal has fallen during sleep, or when some frustration impairs the normal procedures of life. Stimulation of arousal may again camouflage the depression so that it becomes masked.

It requires a special type of personality to go on driving oneself to attempt achievement when the height of arousal is already impairing efficiency. The determined drive may carry the person to the point of generation of compulsive behaviour of various types. Some of these are well-known. Some people have an intense desire to eat, especially sweet things when under intense pressure raising their arousal level. Others may have to check their work over and over again so adding to the mental demands. However, when coping powers are stretched by non-work circumstances, as in disturbed family life, the effect tends to be different.

When husband and wife both go out to work, and especially if they each have very demanding occupations, their fatigue in the evenings makes them less tolerant of anything which irritates them. That soon leads to arguments either between themselves or with their children. As times goes on the strains within the family become too great. The children may not be able to stand hearing their parents arguing, or worse, being pulled first by one parent and then by the other. Not infrequently this is a major factor in interfering with their studying. In many cases the parents eventually decide to separate because they think it is no longer possible to live with each other. It always sounds so simple to split up but the challenges are vastly greater as a rule. Financially it is more difficult because the cost of running two homes are greater. Emotionally the effect on the children may well bring them to the limit of what their brains can cope with. The statistics show that the incidence of attempted suicide amongst those whose homes have been broken up is greater than among those in intact families (Greer and Gunn, 1966).

When constant strains are imposed for a long time depression almost invariably sets in. Arguments raise arousal level, sometimes to the point of loss of physical control. Meeting the constant challenges of a broken home imposes recurring demands upon the coping process - the financial difficulties, the lack of support to the single parent and to the children, the constant struggle to find solutions to new difficulties such as change of place of abode, change of school, loss of friends. Frequently the most acute situation is coped with because arousal level can be raised to solve the most demanding problems. It cannot be sustained for long periods of time without generating an underlying depression.

This situation explains the often mysterious breakdown of individuals when they have got past the worst of their problems. The time scale of the decrease in arousal is much longer than most people would suppose and is of the order of two to four weeks. This is most easily established among students where the end of examinations at the end of term gives a precise timing for the end of their drive to high arousal. About two or three weeks later the arousal level falls sufficiently to expose an under-lying depression. However, the masked depression may be exposed at any time by specific arousal-lowering mechanisms. The one which is familiar to many people is the effect of alcohol. If one goes to a party and consumes more alcohol than one is used to, the next morning it is not uncommon to feel intensely depressed. Indeed, this is a time when an attempt at suicide may well be made.

Arousal levels may be lowered by drugs, even by antidepressants. The arousal-lowering effect of the latter operates much faster than the anti-depressant action, especially if small doses are used. Lowering of arousal may occasionally be effected by various techniques of meditation and at times the underlying depression may be of suicidal intensity.

Another factor which plays an important part in our modern life is television. The almost instant transmission of pictures of events in one place to people in another may play an important part in the development of the sense of relative deprivation. The demonstration of availability of some of the luxuries of life to those without them may make them initiate steps to remedy their deficiencies. This may involve a man working more overtime or taking a second job.   Alternatively his wife may be enticed to go out to work in spite of having a young family to care for.   One of the favourite jobs for such a mother is to work the 'twilight shift' between 6 p.m. and 10 p.m. each evening.   This she can do when her husband looks after the children but it comes at the end of what is often a tiring day and many women find after a few months that they cannot cope with the strain. Irritability often heralds the onset of depression. This may be precipitated by her being away from it for a few weeks. Sometimes the family's summer holiday is spoilt as the masked depression emerges in the second week.

Another aspect of television is perhaps much more serious and very little appreciated. There are constant complaints that too much sex and violence are shown on television but these are but examples of a more widespread problem. Studies of what children prefer to watch on television have shown that they choose the most exciting programmes.   There is no reason to suppose that these programmes watched at home have any different effect from those shown in laboratories. The studies reported by Levi (1972), indicate that exciting films may be of violence, suspense or terror and these produce an increase in the excretion of adrenaline in the urine. Only overt sexual presentations do the same in adults. Since many children are allowed to look at television for several hours a day, the constant stimulation of suspense and fear-inspiring films will be exactly the same as those portraying violence even though no violence is shown. In this country it is doubtful if any sexual presentation on television is explicit enough or lasts long enough to have a comparable effect. Children under the age of sexual awareness seem to be very little affected by such sexuality as is shown on television. However, the constant stimulation, especially of children by television, night after night may well play a part in the development of arousal to the point where an underlying depression is engendered.

Watching sport on television is not usually classed as something which has dangers to the viewers. It is, however, well-known that the viewer may become so involved in supporting one side or the other that his arousal gets very high. In middle aged men with early coronary heart disease, attacks of angina pectoris may be precipitated by such excitement. With major events such as international boxing, a number of viewers actually sustain a heart attack while viewing.

Purposely stimulating arousal

There are circumstances in which the level of arousal is stimulated for a specific purpose. Sometimes the stimulation may be described as stressful although it is beneficial. This is discussed at length by Poulton (1976) when he points out that vigilance tasks are often helped by noise or vibration or heat which ordinarily would have been described as unpleasant. The very quality of being unpleasant can cause stimulation of the brain so that arousal is raised and this facilitates prolonged vigilance.

This fact, in this context, is not widely known but on the other hand the stimulating effect of the caffeine in coffee is not only well-known but often used when mental tasks demand high arousal for continued efficiency. However, as we have described in the previous sections, the maintainance of high arousal over a long period commonly leads to sleep disturbance and depression. The average individual may not be able to distinguish when the beneficial effect changes over to the deleterious one.

The mother with a baby knows that if the baby cries and she picks it up it often stops crying. If it is hungry it will soon start again although in her arms. After feeding it, she knows it will probably go to sleep. Suppose she has a friend with her for the evening while her husband is out. Unexpectedly the baby cries: she checks all the things she knows that may have caused it to cry but to no avail. She nurses the baby while talking to her friend. Then it goes on crying. She walks up and down with it, she jogs it, she pats it, she waves things in front of its eyes, she makes stimulating noises, she flashes a torch at it - and so it goes on for an hour or two. While stimulated the baby stops crying but when the stimulation stops the baby starts again. All these stimuli will act to raise the baby's arousal level. Though it may fall asleep from exhaustion when the woman goes to bed, she will be both surprised and annoyed when the baby starts again at 3 a.m. So it all starts all over again. The baby sleeps fitfully but can be made to stay quiet with constant stimulation. In this way babies can be made into hyperactive children making immense demands upon not only the mother but the whole family. Once the high arousal state as shown in figure 1.1 B has been established for a few weeks, it becomes extremely difficult to get it out of this state except with drugs which specifically lower arousal level throughout the sleeping hours.

Some individuals have learnt that sleep deprivation continued for several nights can produce a high arousal state. Under these conditions students may be able to work more effectively. If continued for too long, this type of stimulation will eventually cause exhaustion and intense depression becomes manifest as the arousal level is allowed to come down. It is hard to carry out sleep deprivation on anti-depressant drugs because they stimulate the normal sleep pattern.

It is fashionable, in the last ten to fifteen years, for young women to have a slim image. So great is the pressure of the peer group that many girls and young women are tempted to embark on dieting. Most of them give up in less than a week because they cannot stand being hungry. The more determined ones go on. They are self-selected for determination and end up with anorexia nervosa. They are more likely to persist with their dieting if they become aware that it raises their arousal level. As in most cases, the increased arousal level gives a satisfying feeling. If she is under pressure at this time she will sense that her brain copes better. The professional fasters at the beginning of the century first showed that the brain is more alert and more efficient during starvation. The speed and accuracy of mental arithmetic was found to reach a plateau at about fourteen days (Benedict, 1915).

When the girls are badgered and cajoled by the family to stop starving they may be persuaded to go back to eating. They soon find that mental efficiency falls if they have demanding tasks to cope with. The commonest mental demands on young women today are examinations and this accounts for the fact that we found that in 75% of girls with anorexia nervosa they started their crash dieting in the year in which they were working for a major examination (Mills *et al*, 1973).

In other cases the mental demands may be different and in yet another group they may find the elevated arousal caused by starvation or semi-starvation masks their depression. When made to eat, they may suddenly become aware of depression and then return to crash dieting again.

Children at school not infrequently find that causing some disturbance in the class-room causes excitement. When one or two start it, the others will often join in. It makes great demands on a teacher to control this type of disturbance once it becomes a frequent occurence. Some children rapidly sense that the excitement produced will mask their depression. For this reason they repeat it as often as it is necessary to maintain their arousal level high enough to make them unaware of the underlying depression. As the frequency of the disturbances increases so usually does some form of retribution. The combination imposes a greater strain on the child, which is made worse once the parents are made aware of the child's behaviour. Eventually the depression becomes intense enough that no level of stimulation will mask the depression. It is at this point that the child is likely to attempt suicide. The coping power is totally exhausted in these children and they often feel that no-one is on their side. The final straw may be a trivial affair but it is only the trigger which is released because of some months of erosion of coping ability by the repeated sequence, depression, excitement, raised arousal, retribution, depression, excitement, ...

It commonly takes many months to treat these children and not infrequently problems at home have played a part in initiating the depression. With help and discussion all round it may be possible to cure the child and if she is the ring-leader the rest of the class may work in peace when no-one starts the commotion.

Some of the problems at home are initiated by one of the family using stimulation of arousal to camouflage their own depression. This may present as constant disobedience in a child or recurrent rows between one child and anyone near at hand, stealing, running away from home, etc. If the problem originates in the mother it may be because she has started a part-time job to provide extra money for the family As she gets worn out and irritable she make take on extra things to add to her mental stimulation. It may be work at the church, helping to run a club for teenagers, working on the parish council or the works' social club. These things may well stimulate arousal for a time but eventually as exhaustion sets in the inevitable depression becomes uncontrollable without drugs. Even when treated, these people often return to their highly stimulating life because they have come to rely on the exhilaration of the high arousal state.

Drugs and the arousal level

Many of us are aware that the stimulants in tea and coffee facilitate mental tasks although too much coffee may lead to tremors and lack of sleep. Nevertheless these drinks and caffeine-containing cola drinks are commonly used as stimulants.

In some individuals they are aware that smoking serves the same purpose. There may be psychological effects besides the specific effect of nicotine but many people are able to adjust their nicotine intake according to the mental demands being made upon them (Schachter, 1977).

Alcohol is now more widely used than ever before and especially by the young (Mills and Eden, 1976). It is more commonly used to lower tension and remove social inhibitions than to improve mental performance. Most of the evidence indicates a deterioration in tests of mental and physical efficiency (Mills and Eden, 1976).

Patients who are tense, unable to sleep and with minor evidence of being under strain are most commonly prescribed drugs like diazepam (Valium) and chlordiazepoxide (Librium) but there is no evidence that these are of any value in those with over-stimulated arousal level. They may well help sleep but never seem to prevent the onset of depression which follows prolonged high arousal level.

The anti-depressants function in a variety of ways and not all their effects are properly understood. They frequently are the most effective drugs in those who complain of early morning waking. The less sedative ones may facilitate rather than impair use of machinery which requires speed of response. They are usually essential in those who are stimulating arousal to mask their depression but it may also be essential to find ways to decrease the numbers of challenges in their lives so that the need for future overstimulation of arousal is no longer there.

References

Benedict, F.G. (1915) *A Study of Prolonged Fasting.* Washington: Carnegie Institution of Washington.

Greer, S. & Gunn, J.C. (1966)   Attempted suicides from intact and broken parental homes. *British Medical Journal,* 2, 1355-1357.

Ingvar, D.H. & Schwartz, M.S. (1974) Blood flow patterns induced in the dominant hemisphere by speech and reading. *Brain,* 97, 273-288.

Levi, L. (1972) In *Stress and Distress in Response to Psychosocial Stimuli,* ed. Levi, L., pp. 106-118. Oxford: Pergamon.

Ludbrook, J., Vincent, A. & Walsh, J.A. (1975) Effects of mental arithmetic on arterial pressure and hand blood flow. *Clinical and Experimental Pharmacology and Physiology, Suppl. 2,* 67-70.

Mills, I.H. & Eden, M.A.M. (1976) Social disturbances affecting young people in modern society. In *Man in Urban Environments,* ed. Harrison, G.A. & Gibson, J.B. Ch. 12, pp. 217-246. Oxford: Oxford University Press.

Mills, I.H., Wilson, R.J., Eden, M.A.M. & Lines, J.G. (1973) Endocrine and social factors in self-starvation amenorrhoea. In *Symposium Anorexia Nervosa and Obesity.* ed. Robertson, R.F. pp. 31-43. Royal College of Physicians of Edinburgh, Publication No. 42.

Poulton, E.C. (1976) Arousing environmental stresses can improve performance whatever people say. *Aviation, Space, and Environmental Medicine,* **47**, 1193-1204.

Risberg, J. & Ingvar, D.H. (1973) Patterns of activation in the grey matter of the dominant hemisphere during memorizing and reasoning. A study of regional cerebral blood flow changes during psychological testing in a group of neurologically normal patients. *Brain,* **96**, 737-756.

Schachter, S. (1977) Nicotine regulation in heavy and light smokers. *Journal of Experimental Psychology: General,* **106**, 5-12.

Sharpey-Schafer, E.P. & Taylor, P.J. (1960) Absent circulatory reflexes in diabetic neuritis. *Lancet,* **1**, 559-562.

Sveinsdottir, E., Torloff, P., Risberg, J., Ingvar, D.H. & Lassen, N.A. (1970) Calculation of regional cerebral blood flow (rCBF): initial slope-index compared to height-over-total-area values. In *Brain and Blood Flow,* ed. Ross-Russel, R.W. pp. 85-93. London: Pitmans Publications.

2. A longitudinal study of smoking and personality

NICOLA CHERRY AND KATHLEEN E KIERNAN

This short paper reports on a study in which personality scores, collected in late adolescence, are related to changes in cigarette smoking during the next few years. The study has been reported in detail elsewhere (Cherry and Kiernan, 1976); the present concern is to point out those findings that illustrate most clearly the ways in which patterns of cigarette smoking are related to aspects of the survey member's personality.

The men and women included in the study are all members of the National Survey of Health and Development, a national sample of young people followed up since their birth. The members of the group formed a stratified sample of births in Britain from the 3rd to the 9th March 1946; they have been followed up at least every two years since birth, and in 1962/63 (at 16 years) they completed the short form of the Maudsley Personality Inventory (Eysenck, 1958). When survey members were twenty years old (in 1966) they completed a questionnaire asking for retrospective data on age at starting to smoke, the quantity presently smoked, and whether or not they inhaled. At 25 years (1971) further smoking information was collected, including whether they inhaled 'deeply', 'moderately', 'slightly' or 'not at all'. All information was by self report only and the brand smoked is not known. Both personality inventory data and smoking information were available for 2753 survey members, pipe and cigar smokers being excluded.

The sample has formed the basis for two earlier papers on smoking (Colley *et al,* 1973; Kiernan *et al,* 1976) but on this occasion the initial intent was to look at the general finding (Smith, 1970) that extraverts were more likely to smoke than introverts and to establish whether extraversion was manifest before the habit was taken up. The second aim was to investigate, using this large longitudinal sample, how far (if at all) neuroticism was related to smoking. Smith, in his review of this topic, reported conflicting findings on the relation of this personality dimension to smoking.

The first results of this inquiry are given in table 2.1. It is found that non-smokers are less extraverted and more stable than those who have ever been regular smokers (by the age of 25 years) and those who take up smoking early are more extraverted and more neurotic than those who start the habit after 16 years. It is not clear, from our data, whether the teenager with a high neuroticism or extraversion score is more likely to try the habit at an early age or whether early experimentation is common to all personality types and that the neurotic or extraverted youngster is more likely to persist. However this may be, the early smoker is found to be a heavier smoker (more cigarettes and deeper inhalation) at 25 years than the boy or girl who has taken up the habit at a later age.

Table 2.1 Mean personality scores and age at starting to smoke cigarettes

Age at starting to smoke	MEN				WOMEN			
	Neuroticism	Extraversion	Number in Sample		Neuroticism	Extraversion	Number in Sample	
Started by age 16	5.7	8.4	399		7.6	8.2	282	
Started after age 16	5.0	8.2	364		7.3	7.9	427	
Not Smoked by age 25	4.7	7.8	525		6.6	7.3	746	

Table 2.2 Likelihood of men in the sample taking up cigarette smoking by personality scores.

Extraversion	Neuroticism			Number in Sample
	Low	Medium	High	
Low	44%	55%	60%	382
Medium	48%	59%	64%	427
High	59%	69%	73%	489
Total Number in Sample	445	424	429	1298

The difference in means in table 2.1 can be tested statistically (the clear trends are all significant) but, in this form, the difference in smoking between personality groups is difficult to gauge. Table 2.2 shows the predicted proportions taking up smoking when a logistic model is fitted (Dyke and Patterson, 1952) to be observed proportions. It will be seen that 44% of male stable introverts would have been regular smokers by 25 years, compared with 73% of neurotic extraverts. Equivalent data for women are 32% for stable introverts and 62% neurotic extraverts. This analysis is presented in more detail in Cherry and Kiernan (1976) but it is clear even from the limited data presented here, that those who become smokers are both more neurotic and more extraverted than those who do not, and that the two personality dimensions are independent and additive in their effect on the likelihood of becoming a regular smoker.

The analysis so far is of interest in that it confirms the relationship between extraversion, neuroticism and smoking, and establishes that the position on the personality dimension pre-dated the smoking habit for those who took up smoking after 16 years. A question of even greater interest, perhaps, is whether personality scores are related to changes in smoking, once an individual is established as a regular smoker.

Table 2.3 gives the mean extraversion and neuroticism scores of past, present and non-smokers. It appears (although these differences are not statistically significant) that both male and female ex-smokers are more extraverted and less neurotic than those who, at 25 years, were still smoking cigarettes regularly.

Table 2.3 Mean personality scores for past, present and non-Smokers

| Smoking status | MEN | | | WOMEN | | |
	Neuroticism	Extraversion	Number in Sample	Neuroticism	Extraversion	Number in Sample
Never smoked	4.7	7.8	525	6.6	7.3	746
Present smoker	5.5	8.2	616	7.4	8.0	535
Ex-smoker	5.2	8.5	157	7.4	8.2	174
Whole sample	5.1	8.1	1298	7.0	7.7	1455

B

This finding, for the men at least, is paralleled by the relationship between personality and depth of inhalation. Men who report that they inhale slightly are no more neurotic (but much more extraverted) than the non-smoker (table 2.4). A rather similar result is found for women, although women who inhale deeply have the highest extraversion score of the female groups.

Table 2.4   Mean personality scores by depth of inhalation at 25 years - men only.

Depth of Inhalation	Neuroticism	Extraversion	Number in Sample
Slight	4.6	8.7	74
Moderate	5.1	8.3	347
Deep	6.7	7.9	172

It appears then that stable extraverts are more likely to be ex-smokers at 25 years and amongst those who are still smoking, it is the stable extraverts who are at least likely to inhale deeply. How far, it may be asked, is a break in the smoking habit related directly to personality and how far to differences in depth of inhalation found amongst those of different personality types?

The data so far available do not allow this question to be answered fully. Information on depth of inhalation was collected at twenty-five years but not at twenty years and it will need answers from the survey being undertaken at present (in November 1977) to establish whether personality has any power to predict changes in smoking behaviour, once full allowance has been made for (self reported) depth of inhalation.

The interest in this future study arises not only from the data presented in tables 2.3 and 2.4 but also from the limited analysis possible using the data available at twenty years.

On the basis of this information survey members were identified who (by their own report) inhaled, who had begun to smoke by sixteen years and who were still smoking at twenty years. This group, it was felt, could be regarded as established smokers and the likelihood of giving up the habit was related to the two personality dimensions and to the reported daily consumption of cigarettes. Neuroticism was not related to a change in smoking habits for women, but amongst the men, those who were emotionally stable were more likely to have given up the habit. For both men and women extraversion was related to a change in cigarette smoking, extraverts (who, it will be remembered, were more likely to have taken up smoking) being more likely to give up smoking cigarettes than introverts. Finally, as expected, it was observed that men and women with a high consumption at twenty years were less likely to have given up completely by twenty-five years than with those who smoked only a few cigarettes each day.

The likelihood of giving up smoking differs substantially between groups, predicted probabilities (on the method of Dyke and Patterson, 1952) are given for the men in table 2.5. The model fitted to the observed data suggested that only 2% of neurotic introverts with a daily consumption of greater than twenty cigarettes had given up by twenty-five years compared with 47% of those with a daily consumption of less than ten cigarettes, and who, at sixteen years, have recorded personality scores suggesting that they were stable extraverts. On the limited data available so far, it appears that different personality types do indeed have different patterns of giving up smoking, and that this cannot be entirely explained by differences in the way they use cigarettes.

Table 2.5 Likelihood of men giving up smoking between 20 and 25 years by number of cigarettes smoked at 20 years and personality scores.

Consumption At age 20 per day		Introverted	Extraverted
21+	Neurotic	2%	7%
	Stable	4%	13%
11 - 20	Neurotic	7%	22%
	Stable	13%	35%
1 - 10	Neurotic	12%	32%
	Stable	20%	47%

A longitudinal study has substantial advantages for research into smoking. In the present paper it has allowed the temporal relationship between personality and smoking behaviour to be explored: in future it will be possible to establish whether those (particularly the extraverts) who are no longer smoking at twenty-five years to go back to cigarettes and to investigate more generally the factors that mediate in the relation of personality to smoking. For the purpose of this conference on smoking behaviour, however, it is perhaps most relevant to end by restating the conclusion to be drawn from tables 2.1 and 2.2; extraverts and neurotics are more likely than other young people to have become regular smokers by the age of twenty-five years.

References

Cherry, N. & Kiernan, K. (1976) Personality scores and smoking behaviour - a longitudinal study. *British Journal of Preventive and Social Medicine,* **30**, 123-131.

Colley, J.R.T., Douglas, J.W.B., & Reid, D.D. (1973) Respiratory disease in young adults: influence of early childhood lower respiratory tract illness, social class, air pollution and smoking. *British Medical Journal,* **3**, 195-198.

Dyke, G.V. & Patterson, H.G. (1952) Analysis of Factorial arrangements when the data are proportions. *Biometrics,* **8**, 1-12.

Eysenck, H.J. (1958) A short questionnaire for the measurement of two dimensions of personality. *Journal of Applied Psychology,* **42**, 14-27.

Kiernan, K.E., Colley, J.R.T., Douglas, J.W.B. & Reid, D.D. (1976) Chronic cough in young adults in relation to smoking habits, childhood environment and chest illness. *Respiration,* **33**, 236-244.

Smith, G.M. (1970) Personality and smoking: a review of the empirical literature. In *Learning Mechanisms and Smoking,* ed. Hunt, W.G. Chicago: Aldine.

3. Individual differences in smoking and attentional performance

DAVID M WARBURTON AND KEITH WESNES

Introduction

In this chapter we will discuss the possible neurochemical mechanisms that underlie individual differences in smoking and attentional performance that we have observed consistently in our studies (see Wesnes and Warburton, 1978). In most studies in psychology and psychopharmacology inter-subject variability is considered as a problem and a great deal of effort is spent on minimising its effects so that the main treatment effects are not obscured. Sidman (1960) makes an important distinction between imposed and intrinsic variability. Imposed variability is a consequence of the experimenter's experimental operations and they may be eliminated by manipulation of the appropriate factors. In addition there is intrinsic variability due to differences in the subject's anatomy and the many aspects of internal function. Intrinsic variability does not imply indeterminism of behaviour, and ultimately we will be able to measure these variations in the organism's biochemistry especially the biochemistry of the brain.

Variation in the neurochemistry of the brain has been grossly neglected even though it is crucial to the explanation of an individual's behaviour. In his discussion of the importance of individual variability for medicine Williams (1956) pointed out that practically every human being is a deviate in some respects. His argument went as follows: an individual is considered a deviate for a particular biological measure if his value on that measure lies outside those possessed by 95 per cent of the population. If we considered a set of n uncorrelated measures then only 0.95^n would be normal with respect to these characteristics. For example, if we considered ten measures then only sixty per cent (0.95^{10}) will be normal and for forty measures only 12 per cent will be normal with respect to those measures, while 88 per cent are abnormal. If these measures are of neurochemical pathways that control behaviour then the majority of the population in a psychopharmacological experiment will not be composed of individuals with normal attributes but individuals who deviate from the normal range in several respects. At our present state of relative ignorance of the neurochemical pathways in the brain we cannot give an estimate of the percentage of normal subjects, but it seems likely to be small. Of course, if the drug is biochemically specific and is only influencing a small subset of the pathways then the percentage of normals will be larger. However, it must be remembered that we are not really talking about a uniform 'normal' population but a set of individuals with values along a continuum some close to the mean value for the population and others

19

close to the lines of demarcation between normal and abnormal. Thus there will be a whole range of biochemical variation and consequently a whole range of behavioural variation.

The major problem of the biochemical approach to behaviour is to determine the specific neurochemical variability that is correlated with behavioural variability. One method is to infer by analogy that if the behavioural changes produced by a drug of known biochemical properties resemble the normal variation in behaviour then both normal and drug-induced variation depend on changes in the same biochemical systems. This form of argument is common in psychopharmacology, but is a very risky form of inference and it depends on the number of relevant resemblances. However, it can be used to derive hypotheses for the second method. In this procedure subjects are assessed on some behavioural test, their behavioural responses to the drug measured and then the two behavioural measures are correlated. A significant positive or negative correlation can be used to infer that the biochemical system modified by the drug underlies the normal variability in behaviour. The form of argument is not without risk either and its strength will depend on the number of significant correlation that are obtained. The ultimate confirmation of a relation depends on the direct demonstration of biochemical variations in the brain that are correlated with individual variations in behaviour.   At the moment it is impossible to do this for the biochemical systems in the human brain.

One branch of psychology which has been concerned with individual variation is behavioural genetics. It is concerned with the interaction of genetic and non-inherited forces in determining behaviour and estimating their respective influences on behaviour. The inherited determinants are viewed as the resultant of a large number of genes and the non-inherited factors are the prenatal and postnatal environments. At the moment of conception the genetic complement of the individual is established and the neurochemical limits are set, but these limits will vary depending on the environment. The intrauterine environment is extremely important for the development of the neurochemical pathways as studies of maternal stress, and maternal undernutrition have shown (see Warburton, 1975a). Even after birth the organisation of the brain is still proceeding because the human neonate's brain is only a quarter of the solid matter of an adult brain. During maturation a two way interaction will be going on. The organism's behaviour will be determined by the unique characteristics of his neurochemical pathways at that moment and his experiences as a result of that behaviour will influence any further development of those pathways. In addition these experiences will shape his cognitive development so that adult behaviour will be a result of the neurochemical systems and cognitive structures that have developed. Thus, the biochemical characteristics of the individual have influenced an adult's behaviour, his life style, both directly and indirectly by their influence on the sorts of experiences the person encountered.

One influential theory of individual differences in life style was based on the traditional dichotomy between introverts and extraverts (Eysenck, 1957; 1967). The life-style of an introvert is quiet and retiring. He is introspective, reserved and distant except from intimate friends. He does not like uncertainty so that he prefers an orderly existence and plans ahead. He is reliable but pessimistic. He is not expressive and keeps his feelings under control. In contrast, the stereotype of the extravert is characterised by excitement. He is not introspective and likes to have many friends. He takes chances and often acts on the spur of the moment. Thus he tends to be optimistic and unreliable. He is expansive, but also loses his temper easily. Of course, these are ideal cases of each type and any individual will be a mixture of characteristics. A personality questionnaire such as the Eysenck Personality Inventory (Eysenck and Eysenck, 1964) can be used to assess the degree of behavioural extraversion based on questions about his modes of behaviour and his attitudes.

The same questionnaire has items that are designed to assess behavioural neuroticism, which is an independent dimension of personality. The stereotype of the neurotic is a person who displays much more labile emotional behaviour. He is more anxious, irritable, moody, restless, excitable, changeable - an unstable person. The contrasting type is the stable person who is calm, even tempered and reliable - the ideal leader.

From these personality scores it would be convenient if we could make inferences about the neurochemical differences which form a constitutional basis for individual differences in behavioural extraversion and neuroticism. One problem is that the questionnaire enquires about the person's life style and this will be influenced by the environment to which the person has been exposed. Two people with the similar biochemical constitution will have divergent life experiences. One aspect of life style which might be very revealing is drug taking because it is likely to reflect neurochemical differences in the brain. In particular the consumption of the commonly available drugs like alcohol and nicotine might be particularly revealing.

Another approach to this problem will be inferences from behavioural tests that are less likely to reflect environmental influences and more likely to reveal the underlying neural processes. These sorts of tests might include measures of perceptual performance, attentional performance and learning. All these tests have been used to examine differences between introverts and extraverts (Eysenck, 1967). In the second section we will consider studies of attention in vigilance situations but first we will discuss individual differences in smoking behaviour.

Individual differences and smoking

The largest surveys of smokers were made by Eysenck (Eysenck et al, 1960; Eysenck, 1963a). From these investigations a very highly significant positive correlation was found between cigarette smoking and extraversion. Heavy smokers were the most extraverted, medium smokers were less extraverted, light smokers were less extraverted still and non-smokers were the least extraverted. Ex-smokers scored in between light and medium on the extraversion scale. Subsequent studies on both sexes have confirmed this statistical relationship between smoking and extraversion.

There is less consistency in the evidence for a relationship between smoking and neuroticism. Eysenck's studies of men gave no evidence for a significant correlation (Eysenck et al, 1960; Eysenck, 1963a) and Rae's (1975) survey of 253 female education students revealed no differences in neuroticism between non-smokers, ex-smokers, light smokers or medium smokers. There were very few heavy smokers in the college. However, at least seven studies have suggested a positive relationship and one has found a negative correlation. The interesting pattern that emerges from these surveys is that there was more likely to be a significant trend between cigarette consumption and neuroticism for women than men (Meares *et al*, 1971; Waters, 1971; Dunnell and Cartwright, 1972). In agreement with the notion of sedative smoking Matarazzo and Saslow's (1960) survey shows clearly that young normal smokers have higher anxiety scores than non-smokers. In a study of older men, heavy smokers showed a greater number of signs of psychological tension than moderate smokers (Lawton and Phillips, 1956).

It could be argued from these data that it is smoking that is producing extraversion or neuroticism rather than smoking being adopted by individuals with one or other constitution. However, a logitudinal study of young people suggests that smoking is adopted by individuals with a certain constitution (see Cherry and Kiernan, 1976, 1978). Personality assessment was made at the age of 16 years, before smoking had been established, and information on smoking was collected at twenty years and twenty-five years. It was found that smokers of both sexes had a higher mean neuroticism score than non-smokers and that there was a significant relationship between daily consumption and neuroticism for women but not men. The mean neuroticism score increased for depth of inhalation in both men and women. Smokers also tended to be more extraverted than non-smokers. Thus, there was an increase in the proportion of smoking with increasing neuroticism and extraversion score *and* the very important finding that the two facts operated independently to produce smoking. It follows from this analysis that the stereotype of the smoker would correspond to the neurotic extravert which according to Eysenck (1957) is touchy, restless, aggressive, excitable, changeable, impulsive, optimistic and active. It is amazing how well these characteristics can be matched with the individual traits and life-style characteristics by which smokers can be distinguished from a group of non-smokers as listed by Dunn (1973).

Individual differences and vigilance performance

Studies of attention are plagued by marked individual differences in performance and these have been recorded in the literature. For example, Mackworth (1950) reported considerable variation in the amount of deterioration in vigilance performance. In his study this may have been related to the initial level of performance which depended on the experience of the subjects. However, Broadbent (1950) did find individual differences in performance decrement that could not be attributed to initial levels. In this study and later work Broadbent found that resistance to attentional lapses during a long and boring task correlated well with the subject's goal discrepancy score, but not with other measures like intelligence (Broadbent, 1951). A goal discrepancy score is the difference between a subject's estimate of his future performance and his past performance. A large goal discrepancy score is associated with a high introversion score on a personality scale (Eysenck, 1967).

Test of groups of introverts, extraverts and normals on attentional tasks have tended to show that introverts perform better overall and extraverts perform worst. In a digit test subjects were required to detect three successive odd digits from a series of digits repeated at a rate of one per second (Bakan, Belton and Roth, 1963). The data show that during the first 16 minutes, the introverts detected fewer than the extraverts but during the second 16 minute period the introverts improved, while the normals and extraverts showed a vigilance decrement. In the third 16 minute period all groups showed a decline in detections, but the introverts detected the same number of signals as in the first period i.e. more signals than the normals and the normals detected more signals than the extraverts.

In another digit checking task Davies and Hockey, (1966) asked introvert and extravert subjects to check discrepancies between a visually presented series of digits and a typed list. Extraverts showed a significant decrement in detections while introverts showed no significant performance decline. When extraneous noise was introduced the decrement in detections of the extraverts was prevented while the performance of the introverts was not affected. The vigilance decrement has been attributed to the decreased arousal that is induced by performing a long boring task alone in a dim room and subjective reports support this (Bakan, 1963). The introduction of noise improves performance in simple vigilance situations and this has been interpreted in terms of increased arousal facilitating performance (e.g. McGrath, 1963). From this interpretation we could hypothesise that extraverts are less aroused than introverts and so noise would improve their performance. At this stage the concept of arousal is being used in a very general way, but it will be considered in more detail later.

A related set of results were obtained by Bakan (1959) and Claridge (1960). Bakan used the digit test that we described previously, but in one condition there was a secondary task where the subject had to press a button when he heard the digit 6. Performance on the primary task was worse for extraverts than introverts. The addition of the second task did not detract from the main task since both were listening for digits. On the contrary, there was improved detection of the triple odd numbers for both introverts and extraverts, and the improvement for extraverts was greater than for introverts. The introduction of the secondary task was arousing and since it was compatible with the primary task it improved performance. In a complementary study with the same task, Claridge (1960) obtained improved performance for extraverts and a normal group when the secondary task was introduced after thirty minutes on the primary task. In this case the performance of introverts was impaired, perhaps because the second task was now distracting although the introverts in the single task study of Bakan et al, (1963) were also poorer initially than extraverts and normals.

Another explanation can be made in terms of an 'inverted-U' relationship between vigilance performance and arousal. This relationship has been used to explain the performance of introverts and extraverts by Colquhoun and Corcoran (1964) and Corcoran(1965) in a number of situations. Two subjects at the same height on the inverted-U but on opposite arms will show different effects of an equal increment in arousal. Thus an extravert at the low end of the arousal continuum (left arm of the curve) will show an increment in performance when arousal increases whereas the highly aroused introvert, on the right hand arm, will show a decrement in performance which is what Claridge (1960) found. In some cases a change in arousal may produce no change in performance if the arousal shift merely moves the subject to the same level on the other arm. This pattern of results fits exactly those obtained by Bakan et al (1963). In the Bakan (1959) and Claridge (1960) experiments the secondary task increases arousal and if both sets of subjects are on the left arm of the curve the lower aroused subjects (extraverts, on our hypothesis) will show greater improvements in performance than higher aroused subjects for the same increment in arousal.

Eysenck (1963b) has similar ideas and has suggested that the optimal level of arousal required for performance is lower for introverts so they can cope better with vigilance tasks, and has proposed that a person's position on this 'arousal' continuum can be manipulated by means of drugs. Drugs classed as stimulants will have an introverting effect on performance, while drugs described as depressant agents will have an extraverting effect. Thus amphetamine, a so-called 'stimulant' drug prevents a decrement in vigilance performance, while alcohol, a so-called 'depressant', impairs vigilance performance. Nicotine is a stimulant drug and it would be predicted that it would increase arousal i.e. have an introverting effect and improve vigilance performance. He has argued that the reason that extraverts smoke is for the introverting (normalising for the extravert) effects of nicotine (Eysenck, 1965). In order to be testable the concepts of 'stimulant drug' and 'arousal' must be specified more precisely.

A drug can act as a behavioural stimulant by stimulating a neural pathway (neural stimulant) or by depressing activity in an inhibitory pathway (neural depressant) and there are correspondingly two ways in which it could act as a behavioural depressant. In addition, drugs do not act on single behavioural systems in the brain because different forms of behaviour may be controlled by pathways with the same transmitter and because very few drugs are biochemically specific. Let us consider alcohol which is classified as a depressant drug by Eysenck (1963b; 1965). Alcohol elevates mood and activity initially in most people (i.e. behavioural stimulation) by increased release of catecholamines; it decreases cortical arousal and attention by blocking the acetylcholine pathways (i.e. behavioural depression by neural depression); and it tends to produce drowsiness and behavioural depression, by increased release of serotonin i.e. neural stimulation. In conclusion, the terms stimulant or depressant drug are virtually useless without specifying the system that is modified.

Arousal is another general term which is virtually useless without further description. Arousal is a theoretical construct that is inferred from various indices. Early neurophysiological measurements suggested that the behavioural arousal of an awake active animal was correlated with electrocortical arousal, low voltage fast activity of the electroencephalogram (Moruzzi and Magoun, 1949). However, research on sleep showed that during dreaming there was electrocortical arousal but obviously not behavioural arousal (Dement and Kleitman, 1957). Studies of cholinolytic drugs have demonstrated that electrocortical arousal could be reduced by these drugs, but there was no evidence of any decrease in behavioural arousal in man (e.g. Ostfeld, Machne and Unna, 1960). As well as electrocortical arousal research workers had associated behavioural arousal, for example the response to novel stimuli, with various autonomic measures like heart rate, blood pressure, palmar conductance, respiration. Once again, more extensive research (e.g. Lacey, 1967) showed a poor correlation between behavioural arousal and autonomic arousal or even between the different indices of autonomic arousal.

Eysenck (1967) hypothesised that extraverts and introverts differ in their cortical activity with extraverts having lower cortical arousal. In vigilance tests in which a subject is asked to respond to rare signals in a monotonous situation over a long period of time, extraverts show lower levels of cortical arousal (i.e. lower alpha frequencies and higher amplitudes) than introverts (Gottlober, 1938; Savage, 1964; Gale *et al*, 1971). However, if the situation is too boring then arousal seems to occur (Gale, 1973).

In a review of the psychophysiological literature Warburton (1978b) proposed that lower levels of cortical arousal resulted in impaired information processing so that as a person's cortical activity becomes more synchronised (i.e. higher amplitude, lower frequency) they attend less to external stimuli. For example, the monitoring efficiency in a vigilance situation was inversely related to the amount of theta activity (high amplitude, low frequency) of seven cycles per second (Beatty *et al*, 1974). As we mentioned earlier, drugs can also be used to modify electrocortical activity. Scopolamine and other cholinolytic drugs induce a shift in the spontaneous electro-encephalogram rhythm towards the slower frequencies (Grob, *et al*, 1947; White, Rinaldi and Himwich, 1956; Ostfeld *et al*, 1960) and alpha rhythm (10 - 12 cycles per sec.) occurred less frequently. Cholinolytic drugs produced marked changes in behaviour; subjects frequently report loss of awareness and difficulties in concentrating (White *et al*, 1956; Ostfeld *et al*, 1960). In experimental tests various attentional deficits have been demonstrated, including impaired vigilance (Wesnes and Warburton, 1978). There was a close relationship between the decreased desynchronisation and the onset and termination of the behavioural effects. The inescapable conclusion from these experiments and the other studies reviewed was that attentional performance was a function of the amount of cortical arousal. Desynchronisation represents the random spontaneous activity of some of the cells at the sensory cortex. Increased excitability of these cells would result in a greater number being activated by sensory input. As a consequence cortical evoked potentials will be larger and of longer duration, both of these changes have been found to be characteristics of the degree of attention (see Warburton, 1978b). The probability of a response will be related to the magnitude of the sensory evoked potential, and when the evoked potential size is small, weak stimuli from outside the person or inside the brain may control responding. In other words, the person will be distracted by outside events and his own thoughts.

We can now draw together the information on cortical arousal, vigilance and extraversion-introversion to formulate a hypothesis about the poorer vigilance performance of extraverts. Extraverts have lower cortical arousal than introverted subjects during a vigilance test, and we would expect a decrease in the size and duration of the evoked potential. Evidence consistent with this notion was obtained by Hendrickson (1972) who found that extraverts had smaller amplitude sensory evoked potentials compared with introverts. Consequently, extraverts are more distractable by stimuli from both the external world and internal world (thoughts, phantasies, daydreams) and miss experimental signals. A vigilance decrement will represent the increased occurrence of these lapses in attention.

Following from this hypothesis we would expect that the vigilance performance of extraverts might be improved by a drug which increased cortical arousal. Nicotine is one compound which has this property. However, nicotine has a biphasic action on the cortex which depends on the dose, rate of administration and the cortical state at the time of administration (Armitage, Hall and Morrison, 1968). Small doses of nicotine increased the release of acetylcholine and the amount of cortical arousal in cats. At higher doses there was an increase in acetylcholine release and increased cortical activity in some animals, but a decrease in release and arousal in others. These individual differences seemed to depend on the state of arousal when the drug was given. In other words, from the point of view of extraverts with low levels of cortical arousal, we would predict that nicotine would improve performance, but the performance of introverts might be impaired by the same dose. Thus the effect of the drug on subjects would depend on their position on the constitutional extraversion-introversion continuum. We would also expect that nicotine would have the most dramatic effects at the end of a vigilance session, especially on the performance of extraverts. If subjects were allowed to adjust the dose of nicotine by smoking we would expect that extraverts would take higher doses than introverts and that they would smoke more at the end of a session when arousal was lowest.

Experimental studies

Our experiments were based on the synergistic research model for smoking behaviour (Dunn, 1973). We were interested in the interaction between the constituents of the cigarette smoke and the biochemical constitution of the smoker as it is reflected in his performance in our experimental situation. In other words, we were looking for a significant personality trait-smoking relation. In order to do this we assessed the degree of extraversion and neuroticism of our subjects to give us measures which would reflect two aspects of their constitution and then tested them in a vigilance situation with cigarettes of varying nicotine contents.

Subject population

The experimental population in this study were undergraduate and postgraduate students at Reading University. In a campus-wide survey made in 1974, Brown and Gunn (1975) found that about 19% of the students smoke cigarettes while a further three per cent smoke pipe or cigars. This figure compares with an estimate of 56% for the age group 20 - 24 in the general population (Lee, 1976). Altogether we tested 48 students of whom 12 were non-smokers, 12 were light smokers (less than five per day) and 24 were heavy smokers (more than 15 per day). Eighteen of the group were female (six in each group). The personality characteristics of the group were assessed using Form B of the Eysenck Personality Inventory (Eysenck and Eysenck, 1964) which measures behavioural extraversion and behavioural neuroticism. Thirty-two of the subjects agreed to fill in the questionnaire. On this scale the means for a normal population are 14.148 on the extraversion scale and 10.523 on the neuroticism scale while the mean for a student population was 13.438 on extraversion and 11.037 for neuroticism. The student smokers in our study had a mean extraversion score of 16.188, and a mean neuroticism score of 10.656 which is more extraverted than the average student population but close to the neuroticism mean for the same group. It is difficult to compare these means with those of other smoking populations because most have used the Maudsley Personality Inventory, the parent questionnaire for the Eysenck Personality Inventory. Nevertheless, they do substantiate the common finding that smokers are more extraverted than the normal population (e.g. Eysenck *et al,* 1960).

Procedure

The subjects were tested using a version of the Mackworth Clock Test (Mackworth, 1950) in which subjects observed the second hand of a clock and were asked to report whenever they thought they saw the hand stop for 0.1 sec. Previous work in our laboratory (Wesnes and Warburton, 1978) had shown that detection performance on this task declined markedly in untreated subjects over an eighty minute session. In the drug conditions nicotine, in the form of tablets or cigarettes, was made available to the subject at twenty, forty and sixty minutes. Thus the performance on the first twenty minutes was not under the influence of the drug, and so we were able to assess the drug effects relative to a baseline score for each individual. The typical finding of the studies has been that nicotine tablets and cigarettes containing nicotine improved the performance of the group, although there were wide individual differences in baseline and the magnitude of the drug effect. In order to analyse the variability further we also gave our subjects a smoking motives questionnaire (Russell, Peto and Patel, 1974). The various performance and smoking measures were then correlated in order to discover the degree of association between the various characteristics of the individual and performance. The performance data were probabilities of responding and so were not normally distributed. Accordingly the degree of association was assessed by means of a Spearman's rho correlation coefficient (Siegel, 1956). With the correlation method of analysis we were looking for patterns of correlations and not too much emphasis was placed on single pieces of evidence.

Baseline performance

The first aspect of performance that was examined was twenty minute baseline scores. In order to minimise the effect of day-to-day variability in this measure of performance a mean value was calculated for the three drug sessions. This value was then correlated with the degree of extraversion score and the neuroticism scores. As one can see by inspection of Figure 3.1 there is very little relation between extraversion and the baseline scores and the correlation coefficient of +0.09 confirms this. However, it should be noted that there is a narrow range of scores, only two below 12, which decreases the likelihood of obtaining significant correlations with the extraversion scores. This problem occurred repeatedly in the analyses.

There appears to be a much more interesting relationship between the baseline scores, measured in terms of a probability of hit, and neuroticism (see Figure 3.2). There is a -0.82 correlation which is significant ($t = 8.56$, df $= 38$; p <0.01). This finding implies that lower hit rates are associated with higher degrees of neuroticism. However, the relationship between the two variables is not linear and it appears that the best baseline performance was produced by subjects with a moderate degree of neuroticism (6 - 11).

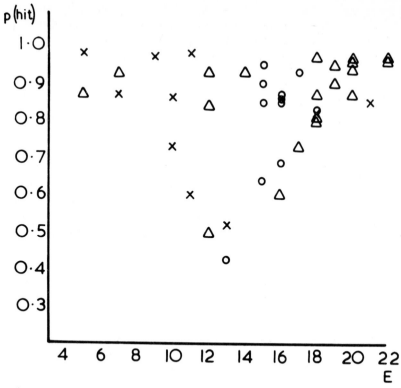

Fig. 3.1 A scattergram of the baseline vigilance scores of the subjects and their extraversion scores.

In this experiment it is assumed that scores on the neuroticism scale are in some manner reflecting emotional responsiveness which in turn seems to interact with performance in our situation.   There is very little data in the literature on neuroticism and performance but a great deal of work has been concerned with performance and scores on the Manifest Anxiety Scale (Taylor, 1953).   Scores on this scale correlate highly with neuroticism (Franks, 1956; Bendig, 1957) and it is believed that this scale is measuring other neurotic characteristics besides anxiety (Bendig, 1958).   Many of the studies have been devoted to conditioning performance but there have been some experiments using stress situations.   In one of these (Davidson, Andrews and Ross, 1956) subjects were asked to name colours presented to them rapidly.   Stress was manipulated by both the rate of stimulus presentation and feedback of failure rates to the subjects.   Complex interactions occurred between personality, and the two stress manipulations and subjects with higher MAS scores were most sensitive to experimental stress and showed decrements in performance.

There is also a large literature that has shown that highly 'emotional' subjects do perform worse than less 'emotional' subjects in a variety of tests (See Sarason, 1972). Sarason (1972) has published a number of studies which suggest that the highly anxious individual is preoccupied with thoughts of failure.   He is concerned with his inadequacies and thus his ability to cope with the problem.   These preoccupations

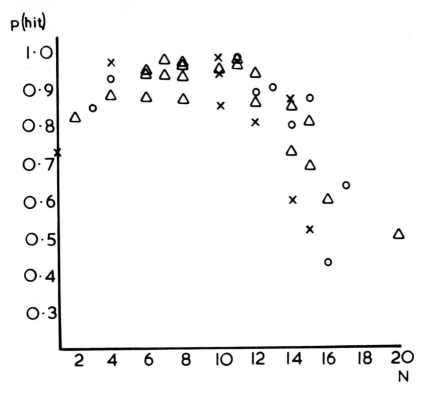

Fig. 3.2 A scattergram of the baseline vigilance scores of the subjects and their neuroticism scores.

have a detrimental effect on attentiveness to external cues. In our situation the decreased attention will be reflected in poorer vigilance performance initially until the subject is reassured by the simplicity of the task.

Smoking behaviour

In the first study a group of 12 male heavy smokers were tested in the vigilance task after 12 hours deprivation of cigarettes. They were allowed to smoke a cigarette at twenty, forty and sixty minutes during the session. Member companies of the Tobacco Research Council kindly supplied us with different types of cigarette which yielded 0.31 mg. (low), 0.71 mg. (medium) and 1.65 mg. (high) of nicotine using the Government analysis procedure. The subjects were tested on three separate occasions, and the cigarette butts were collected for each session.

The amount of nicotine each subject took into his mouth was estimated from the amount of nicotine retained in the butt (measured at British American Tobacco, Southampton) and the filtration efficiency of the tip. The accuracy of the estimation is a matter of some dispute, but it is thought that the error range is between $\pm$ 10% and $\pm$ 20% although if a smoker smokes in an unusual way it may be as much as $\pm$ 40% (Creighton and Lewis, 1978). We have assumed a figure of $\pm$ 15% to cover the possibility that there were a few unusual smokers in the group. It should be realised that these estimates do not tell us how much nicotine entered the blood stream. However, all our subjects were deep inhalers and so we might expect a good positive correlation between blood nicotine and the amount taken into the mouth (Kuhn, 1965).

In the Introduction it was predicted that subjects who had a high extraversion score would smoke more than less extraverted subjects. It was found that there was a strong positive correlation (rho = +0.92; p <0.01) between extraversion and intake on the first medium nicotine cigarette and a small positive correlation with the low nicotine cigarette (rho = +0.23; p >0.10) and the high nicotine (rho = +0.45; p >0.10). These coefficients give some support for the hypothesis that all subjects may have smoked the first experimental cigarette harder because they were deprived for at least 12 hours prior to testing and this was the first cigarette of the day.

Correlations were also made with the neuroticism scores for the smoke intake from the three cigarettes. For the low nicotine cigarette rho was +0.35 (p >0.10); for the medium nicotine cigarette rho was +0.55 (p <0.10); and rho was +0.57 (p <0.07) for the high nicotine cigarette. There is a suggestion that the more neurotic subjects smoke more than the more stable subjects on this first cigarette, but as we have pointed out already this cigarette may be smoked atypically and so any differences were masked.

One interesting aspect of the smoking behaviour of our subjects can be see in Figure 3.3. There is a compensation pattern in the intake so that smokers take

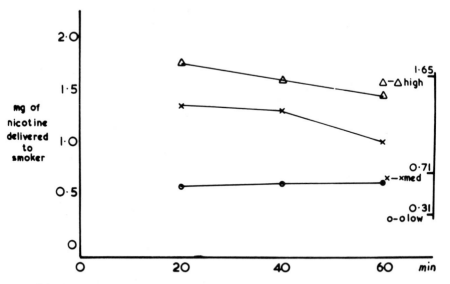

Fig. 3.3 The estimated nicotine intake to the mouth for the three cigarettes of each brand smoked during the vigilance session.

more than one would expect from the low nicotine cigarette and relatively less from the high nicotine brand. This pattern suggests that subjects are adjusting their intake to obtain an optimum dose of some constituent of the cigarette smoke. Adams

(1976, 1978) studied smoking habits using cigarettes with different nicotine levels and total particulate matter. He found that the type of cigarette affected the way that it was smoked; subjects adapted their habit in order to obtain what they need from the cigarette whether this need be for nicotine, tar or vapour phase. For ventilated cigarettes (i.e. low nicotine, low tar) there was clear evidence of compensation for about half of the magnitude of the reduction in smoke yield.

Compensation has also been demonstrated by Ashton and Watson (1970) for subjects smoking in a driving simulation task. They tested subjects in an easy driving task, a stressful driving task and at rest. In all situations they found that subjects took more frequent puffs at the low nicotine cigarettes (1.0 mg. nicotine in main-stream smoke) than the high nicotine cigarettes (2.1 mg. nicotine in main-stream smoke) and took into their mouths nearly the same amount of nicotine. The subjects abstracted more nicotine from the cigarettes during the more stressful driving test than the easier test, although the differences were not statistically significant. However, at rest the puffing rate was significantly higher than during the driving tests which suggests 'that the subjects were striving for a higher nicotine dose during the resting period' (p. 681), assuming of course that the cigarettes are being smoked for a dose of nicotine. These results suggest that not only does compensation occur, but that the smoking intensity varies during different activities.

As Armitage *et al,* (1968) have pointed out, subjects can vary the strength of a puff, the length of puff, the interpuff interval and the total number of puffs taken as well as the depth of inhalation in order to regulate the nicotine intake. This 'finger tip' control would enable the smoker to adjust the dose to his needs throughout a particular situation. In order to examine this possibility in our experiment we calculated the difference between the intake from the first cigarette of the session smoked at twenty minutes and the last cigarette taken at sixty minutes. We predicted in the Introduction that extraverts might smoke more at the end of a situation when they are bored and need nicotine to produce elctrocortical arousal. There was a tendency for this pattern to occur; the correlation coefficient rho is a +0.78 which is significant at $p < 0.01$ level for 1.65 mg. cigarette, but rho is only +0.46 ($p < 0.05$) for the 0.71 mg. cigarette. The direction of the correlations is consistent with the prediction. However, it should be noted that only two of the subjects are showing increments while the rest are showing decrements even though the majority of the group are extraverts. Once again the problem may be that the cigarette at twenty minutes is the first cigarette for those subjects for 12 hours and so the high initial intake on this cigarette would tend to reduce the size of the difference score.

In addition we examined the association between neuroticism and the smoking patterns over the session. There was a positive correlation between the decrement in intake across the session and neuroticism for both the 0.71 mg. cigarette (rho = 0.93; $p < 0.01$) and the 1.65 mg. cigarette (rho = 0.80; $p < 0.01$). Thus the more 'neurotic' subjects smoke harder at the beginning of the session than at the end.

We have hypothesised that the more neurotic subjects found the test situation stressful and so performed badly during the first twenty minutes. The results of Ashton and Watson (1970) are consistent with the idea that stress increases smoking intensity so our explanation for the smoking behaviour is that the more neurotic subjects are smoking more intensely because they are under stress i.e. subjects who are scoring highly on neuroticism have a need for some chemical from the cigarette in order to cope with the experimental test. In the next section we will consider the consequences of the smoking behaviour in terms of the performance of the subjects.

Effect of smoking on performance

The last aspect of the first study is the interaction between the smoking, performance and the individual. The effect of smoking on vigilance performance was calculated as a difference from baseline scores. Examination of the data for the whole session suggested that performance was better after the two cigarettes with the higher levels of nicotine (see Wesnes and Warburton, 1978). However, statistical analysis showed that only in the first twenty minutes was there any suggestion that performance was better for the medium and high cigarettes ($x_r^2 = 4.6$; $p = 0.10$ on a Friedman Analysis of Variance: Siegel, 1956). From a comparison of performance with the high and medium nicotine cigarette, vigilance performance in the first twenty minutes following the medium nicotine cigarette was significantly better at $p = 0.05$ level. We correlated the twenty minute difference scores for the medium nicotine cigarette with extraversion and neuroticism in order to discover the degree of association. We found that for neuroticism there was a 0.96 rho value which was significant at beyond the 0.01 level of significance. For extraversion the correlation coefficient, rho = 0.28 ($p > 0.10$). In other words smoking has produced greater improvement in the more neurotic subjects.

Results consistent with our findings were obtained by Kucek (1975) in an experiment where subjects were tested under conditions of information overload in which they were required to track a target and do mental arithmetic. A comparison of neurotic smokers assessed by the Maudsley Personality Inventory, allowed to smoke and neurotic subjects not smoking showed that smoking had a beneficial effect on the performance of neurotic subjects allowed to smoke. In another relevant study Myrsten et al, (1972) selected two groups of subjects on the basis of a questionnaire based on one by Frith (1971) about the situations in which they feel the need to smoke. One group smoked more in high arousal situations (to calm themselves) while the second group smoked when bored, i.e. low arousal. It was found that the high arousal smokers performed better in high arousal situations when they were allowed to smoke.

In the previous subsection it was shown that subjects who score highly on neuroticism take in more nicotine at the beginning of the session and the question arises whether their performance is related to the smoke intake. However, a correlation of intake on the first cigarette and performance over the subsequent twenty minutes resulted in a correlation coefficient rho = 0.32 ($p > 0.10$), which was not consistent with a simple relationship. Instead it suggests that each subject has a need for some constituent of cigarette smoke within the experimental situation, and that performance is the outcome of the interaction of the situation, the individual's constitution and smoking. In this study this need was related to the degree of neuroticism of the subject which suggests that it is the sedative properties of smoking which are important. In these studies we were only able to estimate the nicotine presented to the subject but it is conceivable that the sedative agent was the tar or vapour phase and there is no way of separating the influence of these variables.   The second experiment was designed to do this.

Effects of nicotine on performance

It is clearly essential to try to determine the important constituent of smoking which is involved in the sedative effects.   Nicotine is the most obvious candidate to test, and it is also the easiest to manipulate.   Thus the second study of vigilance performance tested nicotine tablets using a population of heavy smokers, light smokers and non-smokers with equal numbers of both sexes.   The personality characteristics and baseline performance of these subjects were considered earlier and we will first concentrate on the effects of nicotine on vigilance performance.   The subjects were given tablets at twenty, forty and sixty minutes so that the results would be directly comparable to the smoking study.   The dose levels were 0 mg., 1 mg. and 2 mg. and were the same for the three occasions during test sessions.   These doses were in the range of nicotine intake estimated from butt analysis in the previous study.   The tablets were held in the mouth for five minutes so that absorption was via the buccal mucosa.

The behavioural data from this study are discussed in more detail in Wesnes and Warburton (1978).   The main findings were that nicotine tablets improved the performance of both light and heavy smokers during the last forty minutes after the 1 mg. and 2 mg. dose, i.e. after the second tablet.   As no differences were observed in the effect of nicotine on light and heavy smokers, both groups are combined in the analysis of individual differences.

As we did in the previous study, we calculated a difference from baseline score in order to determine the vigilance decrement, or increment for the drug session and then a difference from placebo performance was calculated so that a positive score represents an improvement over placebo performance.   This difference from placebo score was then correlated with neuroticism and extraversion.   For neuroticism, shown in Figure 3.4, the degree of association on the Spearman Rank Correlation after correction for tied observations was 0.68 which was significant at the 0.01 level for the data for the whole group.   For males rho was 0.64 ($p < 0.01$) and for females rho was 0.44 ($p < 0.05$) so there are no grounds for concluding that there were any sex differences.   There was little evidence for any degree of association between extraversion and performance of all the subjects (rho = -0.124; $p > 0.10$).   As we pointed out before, the range of extraversion scores is narrow, which would reduce the likelihood of discovering an association between extraversion and performance.

This significant association with neuroticism is in agreement with the effects of smoking on performance and gives good evidence for the hypothesis that nicotine is the ingredient of cigarette smoke which is important in the effects of smoking on vigilance performance.   It follows from this idea that nicotine is having sedative effects which have a beneficial effect on the more neurotic subjects within the vigilance situation.   This finding was tested in another way by subdividing the smoker subjects into a 'high' neuroticism group and a 'low' neuroticism group about the mean neuroticism score for the group of 10.656.   The difference scores for the subjects in each group were compared by means of a Mann-Whitney U test for independent samples and it was found that there was a significantly ($p < 0.01$) greater effect of the nicotine on the high neurotic group (U = 48, n_1 = 17, n_2 = 15).

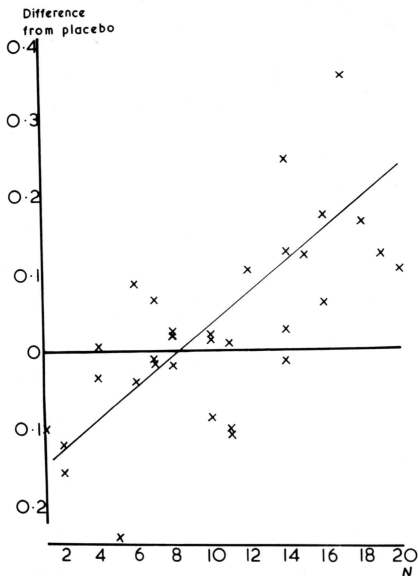

Fig. 3.4 Scattergram of the changes in performance after 2 mg. of nicotine and the neuroticism scores.

Smoking motives

In order to determine the smoking motives of our sample in everyday life, we gave the subjects a copy of the Smoking Motive Questionnaire (Russell *et al*, 1974). Russell *et al* compared the responses of a group of normal smokers with a sample of addicted heavy smokers attending smoking withdrawal clinics. He found that he could differentiate six types of smoking: stimulation, automatic, addictive, indulgent, sensorimotor and psychological. The first three of these factors make up a 'pharmacological addiction' dimension, which differentiated the heavy from the normal smokers. We compared the pharmacological addiction score for the heavy and light smokers in our study using a Mann-Whitney U test with correction for ties (Siegel, 1956). There was a clear difference between the two groups' scores on pharmacological addiction ($z = 3.12$; $p < 0.01$) with the heavy smokers scoring higher, which is what would have been predicted from the findings of Russell et al (1974). However, when we correlated these addiction scores with the nicotine-placebo difference scores the correlation coefficient rho, was 0.25 ($p > 0.10$) which gave no evidence for any degree of association with this variable. This was consistent with the finding that no differences in the effect of nicotine on performance were found in the comparison of heavy and light smokers (see Wesnes and Warburton, 1978).

It was also of interest to discover if there was any association between neuroticism and 'pharmacological addiction'; the correlation coefficient of -0.50 showed a significant ($p < 0.01$) negative degree of association for the data as a whole. In other words, the smoking subjects who scored high on neuroticism were less likely to be 'addicted' pharmacologically. If the stimulation component is considered alone (automatic smoking was more in our group in any case), the correlation of neuroticism with the stimulation factor was -0.43 ($p < 0.05$), which can be interpreted as meaning the subjects scoring high on neuroticism are less likely to smoke for stimulation. We might have predicted that extraversion would have had a significant correlation with the stimulation factor, but rho = 0.26 ($p > 0.10$) which gave no evidence for an association with this stimulation factor as defined by Russell et al, (1974).

The important finding is that subjects who had high scores on neuroticism were not stimulation smokers, and most smoke for some other reason. The obvious possibility is sedative smoking to reduce experimental stress. Russell et al, (1974) and others (e.g. Coan, 1973) were unable to find a sedative factor in their factorial analyses of smoking motives, but this fact has appeared in previous analyses (e.g. McKennell, 1970; Frith, 1971). If we examine the items on Russell et al's questionnaire for his general population sample, his clinic sample and our student population, the five items that occur in all three lists are smoking when worried (Item 6), when angry (Item 29), to help concentration (Item 16), after meals (Item 13), when resting (Item 21). The first two items provide measures of 'stress-induced' smoking and subjects gave great weight to these items. If we look at the percentage of subjects saying 'Yes' to these questions we find that 74% of the general, 93% of clinic and 88% of the student population in our study answered positively to smoking when worried. In psychological profiles of physicians who were non-smokers, light smokers (never more than twenty per day) or heavy smokers (sometimes more than twenty per day), Thomas (1973) found that cigarette smokers had significantly higher levels of anxiety and anger than non-smokers and that heavy smokers were not significantly more anxious than light smokers, but had significantly higher anger scores. Thomas concluded that 'heightened awareness of nervous tension, particularly feelings of anger and anxiety appears to lead to increased use of cigarettes......'

Consequently, we tested the hypothesis of high sedative smoking by subjects scoring high on neuroticism by subdividing our group into three classes on the basis of their replies to the two questions on smoking when worried and smoking when angry. The subdivisions were a high group (scores 5 and 6), intermediate group (scores 3 and 4) and a low group (scores 0, 1 and 2), so a high group would consist of subjects who checked 'Very much so' for both questions, or one question 'Very much so' and one question 'Quite a bit'. The neuroticism scores for these subjects in each group were compared by a Mann Whitney U test for independent samples and it was found that the high and low groups differed significantly (U = 19, n_1 = 8, n_2 = 10; p$<$0.05 on a one-tailed test). This is a marginal result based on small samples, but nevertheless it is consistent with our predictions that subjects scoring high on neuroticism would smoke when worried or angry i.e. 'under stress'. We also tried to test the relationship the other way round by partitioning the subject population into 'high' and 'low' neuroticism groups about the sample mean of 10.656 and testing the 'sedation smoking' scores, but no significant difference (p$>$0.05) was obtained on a one-tailed test (U = 98, n_1 = 13, n_2 = 19). A statistical explanation for the lack of significance is that sedative smoking was only measured on an ordinal scale from 0 - 6, which is too coarse for our purposes and gave too many tied ranks (see Siegel, 1956).

Cigarettes as self medication

The behavioural and smoking data can now be combined to form a coherent pattern. Subjects who had a high neuroticism score had poorer initial baselines for vigilance performance. When given a cigarette, there was some evidence that they took more smoke into their mouths than subjects who had low neuroticism scores. Their performance improved in the twenty minutes following the medium and high nicotine cigarette more than the more stable subjects. However, the absolute level of performance achieved did not differ across the subjects which showed that the effect of smoking was to bring the performance of the more neurotic subjects up to a level comparable with the more stable subjects. The nicotine tablet study showed that nicotine was one ingredient of cigarette smoke that produced this amelioration in the performance of the more neurotic subjects. Analysis of the Smoking Motive Questionnaire replies revealed that subjects who had high neuroticism scores were sedative smokers, i.e. they smoked in situations when they were worried or angry. We would like to argue that the amelioration of performance in the first twenty minutes of the session with these subjects was a consequence of the tranquillising effects of nicotine, which reduced situational anxiety in some way. In a survey at the Institute of Directors Medical Centre it was found that heavy smoking (more than twenty a day) was more common in patients judged by the examining doctor to be under excessive stress. One of the main reasons given by these patients for smoking was the tranquillising effect (Pincherle and Williamson, 1971).

Comparison of the nicotine intake across cigarettes suggests that the subjects were compensating in our situation by puffing relatively harder at the low nicotine cigarettes and relatively weaker at the high nicotine cigarettes compared with the medium nicotine cigarette. This finding dovetails well with the results of Ashton and Watson (1970) that subjects seek an optimum dose for a task and modify their smoking patterns to try to obtain this amount of nicotine. Evidence for self medication with drugs obtained from non-medical sources suggests that a person uses the classes of drugs which fulfil his own individual needs (Warburton, 1978a). Ashton and Watson's study and our study indicate that people will even select the dose to meet the immediate psychological need. We have extended the work of Ashton and Watson by showing that this need is determined by the characteristics of the individual as well as the requirements of the situation.

Thus the vigilance performance of the person in the situation is the outcome of a complex set of interactions. It is obviously determined by the characteristics of the situation, but also by the personality of the individual. This will determine the way in which the individual selects and interprets information within the situation, i.e. there is an interaction going on between individual factors and situational factors. It is one of the assumptions of this paper that individual differences have a constitutional basis and more specifically differences in the neurochemical pathways in the brain.

Another complex interaction occurs when a drug is given to a person. Drugs do not affect human performance directly, but they produce changes in behaviour as a consequence of their interaction with endogenous chemicals within the body. The end point of the interaction is when there are changes in neurochemical activity in the brain that alter the way in which the person interacts with his environment. Thus performance will not only reflect the nature of the drug but also the biochemical state of the person at that moment. In this paper we have presented evidence for an interaction between vigilance, neuroticism and nicotine and we will now discuss some possible neurochemical bases for the interaction between nicotine and neuroticism.

Some neurochemical speculations

One possible approach to suggesting a biochemical basis for the sedative action of nicotine is to reason by analogy. If nicotine is acting as a sedative drug then we would expect it to act in the same was as anxiolytic drugs like the more frequently prescribed antianxiety compounds, the benzodiazepines.

Anxiolytic hypothesis

In a review of the meagre evidence available, Warburton (1975b) concluded that stress steroids were released by an excitatory cholinergic pathway and were inhibited by an adrenergic pathway. The experience of 'anxiety' was a consequence of the feedback of stress steroids to release 5-hydroxytryptamine, and the person's interpretation of the situation. Benzodiazepines decrease the release of acetylcholine, noradrenalin and 5-hydroxytryptamine, but a tolerance develops to the adrenergic effects. Warburton proposed that the basis for the antianxiety action of the benzodiazepines is the decreased release of acetylcholine and 5-hydroxytryptamine. Other compounds that have been used as antianxiety agents like the tricyclic antidepressants probably act by inhibiting the stress steroid release in the hypothalamus by blocking the cholinergic pathways and increasing the activity in catecholamine neurones (Warburton, 1975b).   An ideal anxiolytic would increase catecholamine release and decrease the activity in acetylcholine and 5-hydroxytryptamine neurones. How does nicotine compare with this ideal anxiety drug ?

In the brain nicotine acts on cholinergic neurones but it increases the release of acetylcholines at the cortex (Armitage *et al,* 1968), but not only by a direct action on the cortical neurones (Armitage and Hall, 1968).   This is exactly the opposite of what we would have expected from a sedative drug because this action would increase stress steroid release.

The other possibility is that nicotine is producing its sedation by acting on the brain amines systems in the same way as anxiolytic drugs.   The effect of nicotine on the brain amines systems is not so simple.   It was found that nicotine did produce a statistically significant decrease in noradrenalin levels in the rat diencephalon, a decrease in the dopamine content of the rat striatum and an increase in 5-hydroxy-tryptamine in the rat striatum (Westfall *et al,* 1967).   These changes in the catechol-amine systems, noradrenalin and dopamine are consistent with increased release of these amines *in vivo,* whereas there is decreased release of 5-hydroxytryptamine. An *in vitro* study suggested that higher concentrations of nicotine increased the outflow of dopamine and noradrenalin from slices of rat hypothalamus and striatum (Westfall, 1974), but this has not been confirmed (Fuxe *et al,* 1977).   In the most recent study of catecholamine levels in the rat brain (Fuxe *et al,* 1977) nicotine showed a trend towards noradrenalin depletion in the whole brain and a significant depletion of noradrenalin and dopamine in the medial palisades zone of the basal hypothalamus.   An *in vivo* analysis showed that these effects could not be attributed to a direct action on amine release, uptake or storage mechanisms. Instead the authors concluded that nicotine acted on acetylcholine neurones which in some way increased the nerve impulse flow in the catecholamine systems.   As a consequence there was enhanced release of transmitter which could not be compen-sated for by increased synthesis.   In other words, any change in catecholamine release is secondary to an action on acetylcholine neurones.   There is no evidence on whether nicotine acts directly on 5-hydroxytryptamine neurones to inhibit release.

It can be seen that we would not expect nicotine to decrease the release of stress steroids because it does not decrease acetylcholine release or increase catecholamine release.   On the contrary we would expect an increase in stress steroid release, and this result has been obtained.   There was clear cut adrenal activation in the form of a rise in plasma adrenocorticotrophic hormone and plasma cortisol with 'normal' smoking, i.e. four per hour by habitual smokers (Winternitz and Quillen, 1977). The only possible mechanism for a direct sedative action on the nervous system would appear to be its blockade of serotonin release that would be induced by the feedback of stress steroids to the brain.

Attention hypothesis

The original hypotheses were phrased in terms of the action of nicotine on attentional pathways in the central nervous system, but the pattern of results favours the notion that nicotine is improving performance by reducing anxiety in the experimental situation. At first sight this sedative seems to be incompatible with the attention hypothesis, but there is one way of resolving this apparent paradox. Anxiety arises in situations of uncertainty when a person is subjected to an unpredictable pattern of stimuli, or is faced with uncertainty about which response to choose, or both. We have suggested that anxiety may arise in our situation due to the subject's uncertainty about his ability to respond appropriately. These preoccupations with failure act as distracting stimuli that will interfere with the main task; there is considerable evidence to show that a high incidence of day-dreaming and phantasising is correlated with poor vigilance performance (Warburton, in press).

An improvement of performance would be expected if these distracting preoccupations could be reduced. Warburton (1978b) has hypothesised that in increase in the activity of the cholinergic pathways ascending to the cortex will result in improved selection of information both from the internal and external world. The cortical desynchronisation produced by nicotine provides evidence that these pathways are being activated by this drug. It follows from this finding that nicotine should reduce the effect of distracting stimuli on performance and the enhanced performance of subjects tested on the Stroop test after nicotine (Wesnes and Warburton, 1978) supports this idea. It seems reasonable to conclude that nicotine will enable the distracting preoccupations with failure to be filtered out in a similar fashion and performance will improve. Subjects scoring highly on neuroticism will be more preoccupied with failure and so nicotine will restore their performance to the same level as more stable subjects by enhanced filtering of these distracting stimuli.

Acknowledgement

The research work in this paper was supported by a grant from The Tobacco Research Council.

References

Adams, P.I. (1976) Changes in personal smoking habits brought about by changes in cigarette smoke yield. *Proceedings of the Sixth International Tobacco Scientific Congress,* Tokyo, 102-108.

Adams, P.I. (1978) The influence of cigarette smoke yields on smoking habits *This volume.*

Armitage, A.K. & Hall, G.H. (1968) Further evidence relating to the mode of action of nicotine in the Central Nervous System. *Nature, London,* **214,** 977-978.

Armitage, A.K., Hall, G.H. & Morrison, C.F. (1968). Pharmacological basis for the tobacco smoking habit. *Nature, London,* **217,** 331-334.

Ashton, H. & Watson, D.W. (1970). Puffing frequency and nicotine intake in cigarette smokers. *British Medical Journal,* **3,** 679-681.

Bakan, P. (1959) Extraversion, introversion and improvement in an auditory vigilance task. *British Journal of Psychology,* **50,** 325-332.

Bakan, P. (1963). In *Vigilance: A Symposium,* ed. Buckner, D.A. & McGrath, J.J., pp. 88-100. New York: McGraw-Hill.

Bakan, P., Belton, J.A. & Roth, J.C. (1963). In *Vigilance: A Symposium,* ed. Buckner, D.A. & McGrath, J.J., pp. 22-28. New York: McGraw-Hill.

Beatty, J., Greenberg, A., Deibler, W.P. & O'Hanlon, J.F. (1974) Operant control of occiptal theta rhythm affects performance on a radar monitoring task. *Science,* **183**, 871-873.

Bendig, A.W. (1957) Extraversion, neuroticism and manifest anxiety. *Journal of Consulting Psychology,* **21**, 398-407.

Bendig, A.W. (1958. Identification of item factor patterns within the Manifest Anxiety Scale. *Journal of Consulting Psychology,* **22**, 158-169.

Berlyne, D.E. (1970) In *Attention: Contemporary Theory and Analysis,* ed. Mostovsky, D.J., pp. 25-50. New York: Appleton - Century - Crofts.

Broadbent, D.E. (1950) Applied Psychology Unit Report No. 130, Cambridge, England.

Broadbent, D.E. (1951) Applied Psychology Unit Report No. 160, Cambridge, England.

Brown, C.A. & Gunn, A.D.G. (1975) Tobacco smoking in a university community. *Public Health,* **89**, 199-205.

Cherry, N. & Kiernan, K. (1976) Personality scores and smoking behaviour. *British Journal of Preventive and Social Medicine,* **30**, 123-131.

Cherry, N. & Kiernan, K.E. (1978) A longitudinal study of smoking and personality. *This volume.*

Claridge, G.S. (1960) In *Experiments in Personality,* Vol. II. ed. Eysenck, H.J. pp. 369-383. London: Routledge and Kegan Paul.

Coan, R.W. (1973) Personality variables associated with cigarette smoking. *Journal of Personality and Social Psychology,* **26**, 86-104.

Colquhoun, W.P. & Corcoran, D.W.J. (1964) The effects of time of day and social isolation on the relationship between temperature and performance. *British Journal of Social and Clinical Psychology,* **3**, 226-231.

Corcoran, D.W.J. (1965) Personality and the inverted-U relation. *British Journal of Psychology,* **56**, 267-273.

Creighton, D.E. & Lewis, P.H. (1978) Effects of smoking pattern on smoke deliveries. *This volume.*

Davidson, W.Z., Andrews, J.A. & Ross, S. (1956) Effects of stress and anxiety on continuous high speed color naming. *Journal of Experimental Psychology,* **52**, 13-17.

Davies, D.R. & Hockey, G.R.J. (1966) The effect of noise and doubling the signal frequency on individual differences in visual vigilance performance. *British Journal of Psychology,* **57**, 381-389.

Dement, W. & Kleitman, N. (1957) Cyclic variations in EEG during sleep and their relation to eye movements, body motility and dreaming. *Electroencephalography and Clinical Neurophysiology,* **9**, 673-690.

Dunn, W.L. (1973) In *Smoking Behavior: Motives and Incentives,* ed. Dunn, W.L., pp. 93-112. Washington: V.H. Winston & Sons.

Dunnell, K. & Cartwright, A. (1972) *Medicine Takers, Prescribers and Hoarders.* London: Routledge & Kegan Paul.

Eysenck, H.J. (1957) *The Dynamics of Anxiety and Hysteria.* London: Routledge & Kegan Paul.

Eysenck, H.J. (1963a) Personality and cigarette smoking. *Life Sciences,* **3**, 777-792.

Eysenck, H.J. (1963b) *Experiments with Drugs.* Oxford: Pergamon Press.

Eysenck, H.J. (1965) *Smoking, Health and Personality.* London: Weidenfeld & Nicolson.

Eysenck, H.J. (1967) *The Biological Basis of Personality.* Springfield, 111: Charles C. Thomas.

Eysenck, H.J. & Eysenck, S.B.G. (1964) *Manual of the Eysenck Personality Inventory.* London: University of London Press.

Eysenck, H.J., Tarrant, M., Woolf, M. & England, L. (1960) Smoking and personality *British Medical Journal,* 2, 1456-1460.

Franks, C.M. (1956) Conditioning and personality: a study of normal and neurotic subjects. *Journal of Abnormal and Social Psychology,* 52, 143-150.

Frith, C.D. (1971) Smoking behaviour and its relation to the smoker's immediate experience. *British Journal of Social and Clinical Psychology,* 10, 73-78.

Fuxe, K., Agnati, L., Eneroth, P., Gustafsson, J.A., Hokfelt, T., Lofstrom, A., Skett, B. & Skett, P. (1977) The effect of nicotine on central catecholamine neurons and gonadotrophic secretion. I. Studies in the male rat. *Medical Biology,* 55, 148-157.

Gale, A. (1973) In *New Approaches in Psychological Measurement,* ed. Kline, P., pp. 211-225. London: Wiley.

Gale, A., Coles, M., Kline, P. & Penfold, V. (1971) Extraversion-introversion and the EEG: basal and response measures during habituation of the orienting response. *British Journal of Psychology,* 62, 533-542.

Gottlober, A.B. (1938) The relationship between brain potentials and personality. *Journal of Experimental Psychology,* 22, 67-74.

Grob, D., Harvey, A.M., Longworthy, O.R. & Lilienthal, J.L. (1947) Administration of diisopropylfluorosphosphate to man. The effect on the central nervous system with special reference to the elctrical activity of the brain. *Bulletin of the Johns Hopkins Hospital,* 81, 257-266.

Hendrickson, E. (1972) *An examination of individual differences in cortical evoked responses.* Doctoral Dissertation, University of London.

Kucek, P. (1975) Effect of smoking on performance under load. *Studia Psychologica,* 17, 204-212.

Kuhn, H. (1965) In *Tobacco, Alkaloids and Related Compounds,* ed. von Euler, U.S., pp. 102-109. Oxford: Pergamon Press.

Lacey, J.I. (1967) In *Psychological Stress: Issues in Research,* ed. Appley, M.H. & Trumbull, R. pp. 215-286. New York: Appleton-Century-Crofts.

Lawton, M.P. & Phillips, P.W. (1956) The relationship between excessive cigarette smoking and psychological tension. *American Journal of Medical Science,* 232, 397-402.

Lee, P.N. (1976) *Statistics of Smoking in the United Kingdom.* London: Tobacco Research Council.

McGrath, J.J. (1963) In *Vigilance: A Symposium,* ed. Buckner, D.N. & McGrath, J.J., pp. 3-18. New York: McGraw-Hill.

McKennell, A.C. (1970) Smoking motivation factors. *British Journal of Social and Clinical Psychology,* 9, 8-22.

Mackworth, N.H. (1950) Medical Research Council Special Report, Series No. 268. London: H.M. Stationary Office.

Matarazzo, J.D. & Saslow, G. (1960) Psychological and related characteristics of smokers and non-smokers. *Psychological Bulletin,* **57**, 493-513.

Meares, R., Grimwade, J., Bickley, M. & Wood, C. (1971) Smoking and neuroticism. *Lancet,* **2**, 770.

Moruzzi, G. & Magoun, H.W. (1949) Brain stem reticular formation and activation of the EEG. *Electroencephalography and Clinical Neurophysiology,* **1**, 455-473.

Myrsten, A.-L., Andersson, K., Frankenhaeuser, M. & Morth, A. (1972) Immediate effects of cigarette smoking as related to different smoking habits. *Reports of the Psychological Laboratories, University of Stockholm,* 378.

Ostfeld, A.M., Machne, X. & Unna, K.R. (1960) The effects of atropine on the electroencephalogram and behaviour in man. *Journal of Pharmacology,* **128**, 265-272.

Pincherle, G. & Williamson, J. (1971) Smoking and neuroticism. *Lancet,* **2**, 981.

Rae, G. (1975) Extraversion, neuroticism and cigarette smoking. *British Journal of Social and Clinical Psychology,* **14**, 429-430.

Russell, M.A.H., Peto, J. & Patel, U.A. (1974) The classification of smoking by factorial structure of motives. *Journal of the Royal Statistical Society,* A, **137**, 313-333.

Sarason, I.G. (1972) In *Stress and Anxiety,* vol. 2, ed. Sarason, I.G. & Spellberger, C., pp. 27-44. New York: Wiley.

Savage, K.D. (1964) Electrocerebral activity, extraversion and neuroticism. *British Journal of Psychiatry,* **110**, 98-100.

Sidman, M. (1960) *Tactics of Scientific Research.* New York: Basic Books.

Siegel, S. (1956) *Non-parametric Statistics for the Behavioral Sciences.* New York: McGraw Hill.

Taylor, J.A. (1953) A personality scale of manifest anxiety. *Journal of Abnormal and Social Psychology,* **48**, 285-290.

Thomas, C.B. (1973) In *Smoking Behavior: Motives and Incentives,* ed. Dunn, W.L., pp. 157-170. Washington: V.H. Winston & Sons.

Warburton, D.M. (1975a) *Brain, Drugs and Behaviour.* London & New York: Wiley.

Warburton, D.M. (1975b) Modern biochemical concepts of anxiety. *International Pharmacopsychiatry,* **9**, 189-205.

Warburton, D.M. (1978a) Internal pollution. *Journal of Biosocial Science,* (in press).

Warburton, D.M. (1978b) In *Chemical Influences on Behaviour,* ed. Brown, K. & Cooper, S.J. London: Academic Press (in press).

Waters, W.E. (1971) Smoking and neuroticism. *British Journal of Preventive and Social Medicine,* **25**, 162-164.

Wesnes, K. & Warburton, D.M. (1978) The effects of cigarette smoking and nicotine tablets upon human attention. *This volume.*

Westfall, T.C., Fleming, R.M., Fudger, M.F. & Clark, W.G. (1967) Effect of nicotine and related substances upon amine levels in the brain. *Annals of the New York Academy of Sciences,* **142**, 83-100.

Westfall, T.C. (1974) Effect of nicotine and other drugs on the release of ^{3}H-norepinephrine and ^{3}H-dopamine from rat brain slices. *Neuropharmacology,* **13**, 693-700.

White, R.P., Rinaldi, F. & Himwick, H.E. (1956) Central and peripheral nervous effects of atropine sulfate and mepiperphenidal bromade (Darstive) on human subjects. *Journal of Applied Physiology,* **8**, 635-742.

Williams, R.J. (1956) *Biochemical Individuality.* New York: Wiley.

Winternitz, W.W. & Quillen, D. (1977) Acute hormonal response to cigarette smoking. *Journal of Clinical Pharmacology,* **17**, 389-396.

4. Neuropsychology and tobacco

C IZARD

When our colleague Dr. Thornton asked me to come here to deliver a general paper entitled 'Neuropsychology and Tobacco', related to human beings (the area covered by part III of my monograph Neuropsychologie et Tabac) (Izard, 1976) I first thought it would be enough to have the text translated into English and then to read it with my special and inimitable pronunciation. I also thought - why not? - of delivering the lecture in French, which was more economical - and would have permitted me to keep myself in a divine loneliness quite suitable to my natural narcissism, and I could have looked upon you with some disdain - but it would not have been fair play. The first solution was equally impossible. It would have taken several hours and either you would have fallen into a sound relaxation or have left the room. Really, I don't think you would have offered me so terrible an affront.

Then, I'll give you an English text which is a summary of the third part of my book. A book which you are allowed to buy, of course! But it's a summary which is something more than an ordinary summing up. Indeed, I could not help adding and developing a few ideas which may appear somewhat amusing but which are - as in Alice in Wonderland - very earnest indeed.

I raise a corner of the veil and I tell you, for instance, that the time is come to cast a look at the neuropsychology of the unequalled champion in the fight against tobacco itself. I feel it makes your mouths water but, please, do wait a minute.

Quite correctly there have been many studies of the effects of nicotine in man and animal. A wide literature exists dealing with this - sometimes coherent and sometimes contradictory. The field of this research is far from being exhausted. Lots of unsolved questions remain and stimulate us, and that is why we are here together. It is known that the main alkaloid of tobacco has an effect on the central nervous system, especially on important structures such as the hypothalamus, the hippocampus and the reticular formation, through neurotransmitters. On the animal - and why should it be very different from man? - its action widely depends on the administered dose, on environment, motivation, experience and genetic constitution. But in man, things are not so simple because of the emergence of cognitive processes, of the power of symbols and imagination. It is also well known that nicotine may reinforce memory processes and delay extinction; it may make sexual behaviour easier in the male rat, depress or, on the contrary, make self-stimulation easier. But, before going on, I should like to draw your attention to the following points which are liable to encourage your optimism from two points of view and make your scientific curiosity more acute.

The first point is speculative. You know it is only since 1973 that we have been sure that specific receptors of morphinic substances exist in the brain and that the limbic system possesses many of them. You also know that this research on the identification and isolation of the morphinic receptor led to the discovery of enkephalins and endorphins which are small morphine-like drug peptides and the endogenous ligands of the receptor. But there is something more: recently, in Denmark, Squires and Braestrup (1977) discovered in the brain of the rat specific receptors for the remarkable anti-anxiety drugs such as diazepam and other benzodiazepines. As the authors write 'this suggests that there may be an unknown endogenous neurotransmitter which is the natural ligand for the benzodiazepine receptor'. It is on the level of this anxiety transmitter that this particular system could intervene. All those who are working in the field of neurochemistry and the ambivalent effects of 'Lady' nicotine in man ought to be interested in these important studies.

The second point leads us to a statement of fact.

The British Medical Journal of December 25th, 1976 brought us a gift for Christmas. Indeed, I learnt (as related by two eminent specialists), that tobacco consumption was negatively related to reticulo-endothelial system cancers and to Parkinson's disease. And I read this: 'Half the conditions in table III were positively related to smoking, some very strongly so, and one disease, Parkinsonism, was negatively related. To say that these conditions were related to smoking does not necessarily imply that smoking caused (or prevented) them (Doll and Peto, 1976). Well!

But let us leave nicotine for a time as it has a tendency to invade our scientists' conscience fields, to turn to that of smells. Indeed we can think that if nicotine is probably the most active molecule - neurochemically speaking - in tobacco smoke, it does not act alone in the pleasure taken by such and such a smoker. Paradoxically, this side of the problem does not seem to promote psychophysiological research, as we can see from the available publications, unless this research should be the object - and I'd not wonder at that - of some transcendental, then not communicable, meditation in the secret laboratories of the companies. Smells do not leave memory indifferent and reciprocally they are part of the swarm of the imponderables which govern human behaviour whose origin lies in the old brain. Smells bring emotions, sometimes very deep ones, because the sensations they induce may arouse in ourselves - often unaware - a strong affective imagery. 'If a girl whom in your youth you were fond of consistently wore a particular perfume, then if, fifty years later, you catch a whiff of that perfume from goodness knows where, your early love stands in front of you with disturbing clarity' (Moncrieff, 1977). I don't think the various and mixed perfumes of tobacco smoke are without action on behaviour and even on the prime motivation which leads to smoking since, in this last case, the subject does not yet know the various effects of nicotine. Olfaction and taste reinforce the vividness of the experience one has lived, *hic et nunc,* here and now. Olfaction and taste constantly interfere in our daily lives but the wide range of molecular perceptions is probably due to olfaction.

It was related, after fragmentary and rudimentary research, that the heavy smoker could experience some olfactive deficiency as to vanilla, pyridine, citral or phenol for instance. However, other workers report that there is no difference between smokers and nonsmokers.   On the whole the results reported by different authors do not agree too well and they are sometimes contradictory. It is true that olfaction appeals to delicate physiological and neuropsychological mechanisms which are difficult to explore. The fact has sometimes been stressed that the subjects submitted to olfactometric experiments must avoid olfactive weariness; they must not be under the influence of medicine which may cause hypo or, on the contrary, hypernosmia, and must endeavour not to smoke.

Experienced perfumers think that cigarettes have little effect on olfactive acuteness and even, from that point of view, it may be favourable. As to taste, some workers have studied the gustatory reactivity of smokers, to various molecules such as phenyl-thiocarbamide, saccharin, citric acid, sodium chloride or quinine for instance. Generally speaking it does not seem that large differences exist between smokers and nonsmokers as to salt, acid and sweet tasting compounds. But, conversely, the threshold of perception for quinine (i.e. the bitter sensation) would be higher for smokers.

It was suggested that nicotine would cause a fatigue of the mechanisms of the recognition of bitter taste. But no definitive proof has been given yet. Therefore it is wiser not to give too hasty a generalisation. Gustative sensitivity and behaviour - such as mnesic olfactive sensitivity - are more or less related to certain personality features, congenital or acquired ones. We know, for instance, that some subjects are not very sensitive to the bitter taste of phenylthiocarbamide and that this lack of perception is related to a recessive homozygote gene. There would be, of course, many other things to say on qualitative discriminations of smells by smokers and on the bioelectrical or neurochemical aspects but we must go on.... and I can only ask you to turn to specialised literature.

A lot of research has been done dealing with the study of the smoker's and non-smoker's personalities. But when we approach this problem we find ourselves in front of the fundamental question : what is personality? These questions are of high value because the methodology, and conscious or unconscious direction of the experimental process will depend on them. When we speak of personality we com-prehend a dynamic process which has a beginning, which develops and fixes, whose origin lies in a genetic and constitutional basis. Personality genesis implies a complex integration of numerous elements, related to education, to social and cultural surroundings, to a number of frustrations and rewards, of failures and success, of various emotional shocks, the acceptance or refusal of some ethical or religious options which are expressed through a certain language and behaviour. It is charac-terised by a unity and a continuity, a resistance and adaptation to the environment, and identity through which the individual feels himself as a whole through his psychism and physiological activities; we know that any lasting modification of these various characteristics may bring troubles which are the pathology of person-ality.

In front of this existential complexity, we must be reserved as to the real efficacy of our investigations. But what can be drawn from the studies made on smokers and nonsmokers? Many approaches have been made with a view to defining the smoker's personality. Most of them, I mean those which dealt with big populations, were carried on in Scandinavian and Anglo-Saxon countries so that their results, more or less in agreement but sometimes contradictory are not so useful when countries with different social and cultural conditions are concerned. And, moreover, even inside a well determined culture it is always difficult and rash to generalise from observations made on populations and samples more or less representative, or even self selected, or, still, as some dared to do it, from observations made only in hospitals or in psychiatric clinics. I have no time to develop this idea here. Let us say that, as a rule, if it is admitted that smokers are different from nonsmokers on some characteristics, it is, in no way, possible to define one variable which would be present either in one group or in the other.

The values obtained with Taylor's anxiety scale or Cornell's Medical Index may show that smokers are different from nonsmokers but the average of these differences is not important. If, on the whole, the surveys show that, on average, the smoker is more anxious than the nonsmoker, we must admit that, in numerous cases, just the contrary occurs. Then, it is difficult to state that a specific smoker's personality does exist. On the other hand, many have stated that the millions of smokers from such or such country are not likely to belong to the same well defined type of personality. This remark, of course, does not - *a priori* - exclude a certain differentiation on the level of similar factors. Besides, everyone knows Eysenck's valuable work about this emotional instability factor which he thinks to be underlying all neurotic personalities and which he calls 'neuroticism', a factor which regulates introversion and extraversion in the healthy as well as in the sick man. If it is admitted that the autonomic nervous system is related functionally to the manifestation of neuroticism, it seems that neurotic personality could be characterised by an unstable and easily excitable autonomic nervous system, largely due to hereditary factors. As to introversion and extraversion, Eysenck, taking into account the Pavlovian concepts of excitation and inhibition and considering the more recent data on cortical electrogenesis, the arousal and various functions of the reticular system, thinks that extraverted people have a cortical activity lower than introverted people. Roughly speaking and using the vocabulary of electrogenesis, the extravert would show a predominance of the alpha rhythm. Then, it could be possible that the different behaviour of the extravert and introvert should correspond to the expression of cortical and reticular functions which are partly innate but which can be influenced by drugs.

After his research, Eysenck was led to postulate that the extravert subject would be likely to find from the cigarette a certain level of stimulation which he lacks. Nicotine would permit him to increase his cortical activation level and so to be, or to feel, more efficient, able to stand the painful trials of daily life more easily. The introvert would profit by the sedative action of the alkaloid. However, it is worth noting that there is some doubt as to the role of neuroticism here.

Surveys made in France and in other countries would show that many smokers think themselves anxious and nervous and take tobacco as an anxiolytic which permits them to fight against a vulnerability of character by helping them to control some manifestations of anxiety and depression.

As a rule, all the authors who are working on this line concluded that the extravert would look for the stimulating effect of cigarette, whereas the introvert and anxious subjects would use it as a tranquilliser. We can hardly see how it could be possible to determine the features of 'the smoker's personality'. So much that the same subject may be led - without being maniaco-depressive - according to circumstances and his mood of the moment, to feel the effects of cigarette differently. We are turning round and round and are saying things already known but we cannot do otherwise, being enclosed in the psychometric field.

We'll now look toward another trend insisting upon the fact that smoking moderately is one thing and smoking with a compulsive behaviour is another. In the latter case, we find ourselves obliged to consider the problem of oral frustration. Whatever our personal attitude may be, as well as the reservation that one can have toward psychoanalytic ideology and dogmatism, we cannot reject the fact that its concepts have entered and impregnated the normal and pathologic field of psychology. Whether or not we consider its declarations as more or less false, whether we follow such or such thought: Freud, Adler, Young, Klein or Horney; we can hardly ignore the possibilities of investigations and interpretations that depth psychology offers us. We know that the general needs of an individual are related to an intrapsychologic whole more or less elaborated from the child/mother relationship and we understand that the child may, symbolically or not, look for compensations or gratifications. We also know that frustration - oral frustration more especially - may be the source of behaviours in which anxiety, depression and even aggressivity are predominant. As an adept of Adlerian thought, I'll say that the child - if we consider his organic deficiencies and his mother's attitude - compensates in his way and makes his personal way of living among the community and social reality; the lack of maternal affection, or his mother's hardness or coolness are experienced negatively by the child. Such a child will be inclined to become neurotic and a heavy smoker who will present - when compared to the average smoker and to the nonsmoker - an amplification of concomitant stigmata of frustration, that is: rebellion, impetuosity, the looking for dangerous situations, disdain toward authority and the feeling of great difficulty in living.

At the thought level of the value of a model, the orality and impulsivity concepts are likely to explain, at least partly, the behaviour of the heavy smoker, which does not exclude motivation based upon the research of a higher level of cortical arousal or relaxation. We must not, of course, conceal the reality of neurophysiology and pharmacology of nicotine, because of psychoanalytic investigations.

It was impossible to define the personality of the normal smoker according to criteria, more or less specific, of such or such School in spite of a greal deal of research, the methodological implications of which have a touch of naivety which could make us only smile if the conclusions drawn by some workers were not so confusing. However, it is to be noted that the concepts of orality, anxiety, extraversion, are liable to explain the heavy smoker's behaviour. From various observations I should be inclined to support the following thesis: the heavy smoker seems to correspond to a particular typology in which the various personality features taken arbitrarily apart are particularly pronounced; besides, it is from observations on heavy smokers that it was possible to find out these characteristics, the amplification of which opens onto the neurotic field. But, putting all the smokers in such a deviating sub-group has no sense.

In some way, motivation and personality are parts of the same problem. Here again, it is noted that most research dealing with the smoker's motivations has been carried on as *a posteriori*, either from psychological and physiological models centered on nicotine pharmacological action, or from psychological models. But, of course, a synergy does exist between psychical manifestations and the reinforcement effects likely to be exerted by the alkaloid. It is difficult to understand or analyse why one starts smoking, why one goes on or stops smoking. The answers vary according to the idea one can have *a priori*, the motivation itself, or even the personality features which are applied to the smoker versus the nonsmoker. After some very elaborate studies on factors which are quite remarkable by their objective character, it seems that smokers could be associated with the following ones: relaxation need, stimulation need, habit, need of manipulation, pleasure, social need.

But we have spoken of the oral aspect which does not appear clearly in these studies. Considering the compulsive smoker again we cannot ignore the presence of neurotic factors, even masochistic ones. In this case, the cigarette could be seen as a pacifying oral means, an exterior and repetitive sign, a comforting sign helping to overcome anxiety. A great deal has been written about the first tobacco smoke intake being unpleasant, the symbol of the passage from adolescence to adult age, of affirmation, power and virility among a group sharing the same rites. In fact, when we consider the problem of the smoker's motivation we see at once there is a whole composed of many factors imbricated all together. Motivations are associated to the whole of the individual; that is why, in turn, all the terms of compulsion, pleasure, curiosity, entertainment, social relationship, frustration, conflict, emotion, power, self-estimation and fear are taken apart.

Tobacco smoking is a real social phenomenon proper to our time and expresses the strong needs of the individual in the face of life's problems. Besides the great existential crises - the death of a loved person, disease or serious surgical operation or loss of a job - it is known that our society and our culture facilitate the generalisation of what we call, by euphemism, slight 'nervous troubles', as a consequence of the acute reactions before the event we are experiencing. If we used the word stress, we should say it is the result of psychological, social and biological factors. And it is exactly in this psychological and neurophysiological background that the use of tobacco takes place. The situations in which stress is predominant could help starting the smoking habit as well as its continuation. We have learnt that nicotine could be active by giving out noradrenalin from the hypothalamus with the consequence of inhibiting the production of corticosteroids by the adrenal cortex. On the other hand, we don't know much about the possible effect of nicotine on histidine decarboxylase and histamine at the level of the diencephalon main structures.

Tobacco smoking could also be related to a reinforcement process in which nicotine would play a positive part, and experiments on monkey and man seem to indicate that nicotine causes a rapid and notable reduction of the effects of a stressing and unpleasant stimulation by reducing usual reflexes and reinforces the reactions tending to suppress stress. In other research on the masseter muscle contraction in man, it was found that nicotine administration caused a reduction of both the frequency and intensity of contractions. It seems now quite certain that the absorption of small amounts of nicotine, that is to say, at least, reasonable tobacco smoking, is likely to induce a differential reduction in behaviours associated with aggressivity and irritability when the subject finds himself in an environment which he feels as hostile. After a recent study it seems that stress could be a precipitating factor of psychiatric illness (Schless *et al,* 1977). I dare to dream of a preventive prescription:

ten to twenty cigarettes a day of your favourite blend, but avoid the obsessional idea of tar and nicotine rates

don't smoke your cigarettes

get new stock every day or twice a day when it is raining or if you feel blue...

Tobacco smoking is not - however - a stereotyped act. There are large differences between individuals. Each smoker is modifying - consciously or unconsciously - his behaviour and knows how to find the dose of nicotine which suits him according to his personal experience, his present state, the environmental factors, and, of course, the type of cigarettes he is smoking, the cigar or the pipe he is smoking, the strength, the pH and flavour of them and so on. That's why it seems to me it is not a realistic view to attribute the whole of smokers' behaviours to the sole action of nicotine, though this is unquestionable. We know how to standardise our smoking machines, and those who are working in this line know that all is not so easy. But it seems to me it is quite a Utopian idea to try to standardise smokers, from research carried on in laboratories. Of course I don't say such research is not necessary; I only state that we must be aware of the psychological and physiological constraints it implies and we must not generalise.

Many works have been done these last years about the effects of nicotine and smoke on brain electrogenesis in man whether smoker or nonsmoker, and in smokers deprived of tobacco. Most of them take into account, in the experiment, vigilance tasks more or less complicated and resting times; the analysis of the data gets more and more sophisticated. Besides, and quite rightly, some of these studies differentiate the heavy smoker from the average smoker or the light smoker, though the criterion on which such differentiation is based may appear more or less arbitrary. It is known that smoke does reactivate the EEG of the smoker momentarily deprived of tobacco; the desynchronisation which goes with the reduction of alpha rythm being associated with a vigilance increase. Some works have a tendency to show - if not to demonstrate - that some differences exist at the level of the EEG between nonsmokers and smokers. Moreover, there would be a relation between the modification of the pattern and tobacco consumption whether a nonsmoker, an average smoker or a heavy smoker are concerned. In so far as it is possible to determine the nature of the modifications, smokers may have on an average an alpha rhythm with a higher frequency and an increase of beta rhythm amplitude; but heavy smokers could form a group apart, especially as regards the abundance of the three rhythms, alpha, beta and theta. Then it is possible - if not probable - we should be faced with the expression of genetic or constitutional factors proper to this group of smokers, in this last case. Whether these modifications be the expression of innate characters or acquired ones they are supporting the thesis I have spoken of about studies on personality, and according to which the 'compulsive' smoker would belong to a specific group very near the neurotic field.

French workers have recently tried to determine the influence of cigarette contents of nicotine on cortical activation after a time of deprivation which causes a synchron-isation of the EEG. The conditions of experiments were elaborate and included, with the measures of Hjorth Descriptors (activity, mobility, complexity), the frequency of the critical flicker fusion and of the decisional, or cognitive tasks. These works confirm that the 'frequency of critical flicker fusion' is systematically increased by cigarettes and more especially as the content of alkaloid is greater. But there was a 'placebo effect' (e.g. lettuce-made cigarettes), Besides, though mobility and complexity are almost unvarying with lettuce-cigarettes, they are significantly stronger with tobacco cigarettes and these effects are all the clearer as the nicotine content is higher. In this study - as well as in others carried on elsewhere - the evidence desynchron-isation brought about by tobacco after a time of deprivation seems to be related to nicotine. But as I have already said, I don't think that in daily life, out of experi-mental constraints, things are as easy! One the other hand, the study of the average visual evoked potentials is concordant with those carried on with the EEG. Besides, the research dealing with the 'contingent negative variation' shows that the cigarette effect depends on the behaviour of the smoker himself and on the amount of nicotine he chooses to take. Indeed, the increase or decrease of the CNV average value are respectively correlated to the central nervous system stimulation or depression; these last being more or less related to the degree of introversion and extraversion of individuals.

In another view, it was shown that tobacco is likely to have a favourable and immediate action of the habituation speed to a repetitive noise and it is known that such acceleration is generally associated to a sedative effect. Once more we are coming back to Nesbitt's paradox.

The smoker absorbs only a part of the nicotine present in smoke. The alkaloid passes into blood rapidly, at very low concentrations. It is immediately metabolised mostly to cotinine and then eliminated. On the other hand, the amount of adrenalin excreted is increased in smokers, some of which react by a transitory hyper-glycaemia, perhaps because of a compensatory mechanism for a bioenergetial deficiency. I cannot, once more, develop the idea widely but in the average smoker, cigarettes, in most cases, seem to help memory storage processes.

When sexuality is concerned, all is still to be said, but some experiments carried out on rats, with all that is known about psychophysiological responses to sexual stimulation, make us think that tobacco could have a facilitating influence, ejaculatory performances being not - you will agree with me - the only criterion to be considered when man is concerned and neither is it for women of course! However, we know that at least once in history tobacco did facilitate sexual relations. It is well known that tobacco helped a lot to increase the US population, and perhaps some of the Americans who are among us today in this room, owe their lives to tobacco. If some of you have forgotten the history of the beginnings of the American Adventure I remind them of this passage by A. Nevis and Commager (America, the History of a Free People 1942). 'By 1619 Virginia had no more than two thousand people. That year was notable for three events. One was the arrival of a ship from England with ninety 'young maidens' who were to be given as wives to those settlers who would pay a hundred and twenty pounds of tobacco for their transportation. This cargo was so joyously welcomed that others like it were soon sent over....'   As you can see, if Americans sent tobacco to get women, the English exchanged women against tobacco!

Tobacco can regulate the average smoker's temper; and here I must insist upon the necessity of agreeing on the semantic content of words such as mood, affect, emotion, feeling..... and so on .....; the various authors using these words in more or less different meanings. Tobacco can facilitate mental efficiency, increase or decrease vigilance and behavioural arousal according to the individual's needs, to the existential situation in which he finds himself. Besides, it never provokes personality troubles and psychical disorders such as those which are seen in real drug addicts.

I should like to come back to the beginning of my lecture. I think it would be very interesting to start a neuropsychological study - not of the smoker or the exsmoker who both are respecting the other's freedom, but of people who are displaying a great deal of reaction of aggressive or obsessional nature when they are with people who are smoking. The fight against tobacco is apparently based on ethical grounds and takes as its own the following statements whether unproved or false: tobacco kills people; for the sake of morals, the smoker must be protected in spite of himself, whatever he may think; advertising is urging people to smoking; advertising which is urging people to self-destruction must be suppressed; the smoker is a danger to the nonsmoker; the smoker is a burden to the community; everything must be done for the number of smokers to decrease; mothers and children must be protected against tobacco; people must be compelled to submit themselves by means of kindliness, science or power. In the course of time - not very long ago - ethnic groups or minorities have disappeared, victims of violence, who pretended not to conform to the established usage, not to yield to a normative pressure. But what seems to me more serious is that some persons may find an alibi so as to give free course to their violence - which may be expressed in different ways - in the incongruous declarations immoderately propagated by some undue compaigns. I'll not speak now of the psychoanalytical mechanisms which lie under such psychopathic behaviours. But I'll say we are far from true altruism which leads to the understanding of others and tolerance, which is born from humour and unconstraint.

At last, I apologise for not giving the names of all my friends, whether distant or near: I should have been obliged to give a list of 250 quotations. As you can see I don't lack friends. I prefer to present this work as a collective one which is far from being over. Perhaps have you have got an impression of finding yourselves in a sort of mist which is blurring the outlines and make us doubt of the reality of things, quite as in some of Turner's paintings. But don't be afraid: we'll find again the hard reality of experimentation and scientific language.

References

Doll, R. & Peto, R. (1976) Mortality in relation to smoking: 20 years' observations on male British doctors. *British Medical Journal*, **2**, 1525-1536.
Izard, C. (1976) *Neuropsychologie et Tabac*. Paris: Masson

Moncrieff, R.W. (1977) Emotional response to odours. *Soap, Perfumery and Cosmetics,* **50,** 24-25.

Schless, A.P., Teichman, A., Mendels, J. & Di Giacomo, J.N. (1977) The role of stress as a precipitating factor of psychiatric illness. *British Journal of Psychiatry,* **130,** 19-22.

Squires, R.F. & Braestrup, C. (1977) Benzodiazepine receptors in rat brain. *Nature, London,* **266,** 732.

5. The use of event-related slow potentials of the brain as a means to analyse the effects of cigarette smoking and nicotine in humans

HEATHER ASHTON, V R MARSH, J E MILLMAN, M D RAWLINS, ROSEMARY TELFORD AND J W THOMPSON

Introduction

It is generally accepted that nicotine has actions on the human brain, but direct evidence for this supposition is scanty. Although smokers often comment that subjectively they feel either 'relaxed' or 'stimulated' after a cigarette, depressant and stimulant effects on brain activity are difficult to demonstrate objectively. Electroencephalographic changes after smoking have in general shown only stimulant effects and these have not been fully quantified or related to nicotine dosage. By contrast, in animals Armitage, Hall and Sellers (1969) have clearly shown that nicotine and cigarette smoke can exert both stimulant and depressant effects on the brain, both on electrocortical activity and on the release of acetylcholine from the cerebral cortex, and that these effects are dose-related.

It has been clear for some time that to measure effects of nicotine and other centrally acting drugs on the brain in man, an objective measure, which is sensitive, reproducible and quantifiable, is needed. For this reason, we investigated the effect of drugs on the electroencephalographic phenomenon known as the contingent negative variation (CNV), first described by Walter *et al,* (1964). The CNV is the archetype of event-related slow potentials of the brain. It is recorded between electrodes on the vertex and mastoid or ear lobe and consists of a small negative potential which slowly builds up between a warning signal and an imperative signal requiring the subject to carry out some response, usually a motor response such as pressing a button. The CNV thus occurs in an expectancy situation and is sometimes referred to as an expectancy wave.

Although the immediate source of the slow potential probably resides in the cortex, there is evidence that the origin of the CNV is in the arousal systems of the brain, including the ascending reticular activating system (Rebert, 1972) and probably the limbic system (Routtenberg, 1968). The magnitude of the CNV is thought to reflect the degree of activity in these arousal systems and so is related to the degree of alertness of the subject. For this reason it seemed likely that drugs which altered the degree of alertness in either a positive or negative direction might alter the magnitude of the CNV in a corresponding way. Therefore we tested the effect of some centrally active drugs and of cigarette smoking on the CNV.

Method

The method of recording the CNV has previously been described in detail (Ashton *et al,* 1974), but slight modifications have been introduced in later experiments. Briefly, the subject sits in a chair or may lie on a couch. The CNV is recorded from surface electrodes on the vertex and linked ear lobes or mastoids, and the subject is earthed via an electrode on the forehead. An additional electrode is placed at the nasion to pick up voltages generated by eye movements and blinks. A proportion of the nasion signal can then be subtracted from the vertex signal in order to compensate for any artefacts due to eye movements.

The voltages are amplified by a high gain AC amplifier with a long time constant (9 s). The amplifier signals are fed into a PDP8/E computer, programmed to average ten time-locked individual CNVs. The averaged CNVs are displayed on an oscilloscope and traced out by an X-Y recorder fed from the computer. The whole assembly is driven by a timing circuit which is itself triggered by a punched paper tape.

Generators for the warning and imperative signals are triggered by the timing circuit. The warning signal is either a flash of light (0.49J; 100 ms) or a tone (4,000 Hz, 20 ms) and the imperative signal is another tone (1,500 Hz, 400 ms). The interval between the two signals is 1.25 s and the time between pairs of signals is varied randomly between 4 and 10 s. The subject is presented with a number of series of ten paired signals and instructed to press a button as soon as he hears the imperative signal.

Results

Effects of central stimulant and depressant drugs on the CNV

If CNV magnitude does reflect alertness, then central stimulant drugs should increase and central depressant drugs should decrease CNV magnitude. To test this hypothesis, the effects of caffeine, nitrazepam, pemoline and diazepam on the CNV were measured. The effects of caffeine and nitrazepam are shown in Fig. 5.1. As described previously (Ashton *et al,* 1974), caffeine caused a significant increase and nitrazepam a significant decrease in CNV magnitude. These changes occurred after small oral doses (caffeine citrate 300 mg, nitrazepam 2.5 mg) which produced virtually no subjective effects.

Another central stimulant drug, pemoline (20 mg orally) caused a significant increase in CNV magnitude in seven subjects while diazepam in two oral doses, 5 mg and 7.5 mg, caused a signficant decrease in CNV magnitude (Ashton *et al,* 1976, 1978). We concluded that the CNV is a sensitive and reliable indicator of drugs with central stimulant and depressant effects.

Effects of cigarette smoking on the CNV

We predicted that cigarette smoking might have a dual effect on the CNV, with stimulant effects of nicotine on the brain increasing CNV magnitude and depressant effects decreasing it. This prediction was tested in 22 smokers, smoking standard cigarettes in their normal manner. The results showed that smoking did have a significant effect on CNV magnitude which was increased in some subjects and decreased

C*

in others (Ashton *et al*, 1973, 1974).   Fig. 5.2 shows CNV recordings from individual subjects showing a typical increase and a typical decrease in CNV magnitude after smoking, while Fig. 5.3 shows the mean percentage changes in CNV magnitude in the 22 subjects.

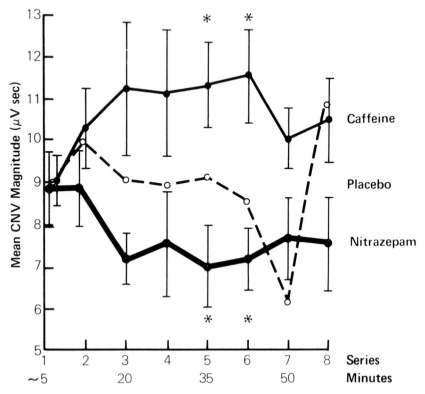

Fig. 5.1 Mean changes in CNV magnitude ($\pm$ S.E. in bars) after 2.5 mg nitrazepam (12 subjects), 300 mg caffeine citrate (13 subjects) and placebo (three subjects). Significant changes from CNV magnitude in Series 1 occurred during Series 5 and 6 in both nitrazepam and caffeine subjects, as denoted by * (nitrazepam: Series 5, t = 1.9167, p < 0.05; Series 6, t = 2.2554, p < 0.05; caffeine: Series 5, t = 1.981, p < 0.05; Series 6, t = 1.9511, p < 0.05; one-tailed "t" test). Significant differences also occurred between caffeine and nitrazepam subjects in Series 3 and 4 (p < 0.05) and Series 5 and 6 (p < 0.01).

Repeat experiments in 11 of the 22 subjects showed CNV changes in the same direction after smoking as had previously been observed.   Sham smoking (puffing on an unlit cigarette) had no effect on the CNV and there was no relation between CNV change and changes in heart rate, blood pressure, fingertip temperature or blood carboxyhaemoglobin level after smoking.   We concluded that the effects of cigarette smoking on the CNV were due to a central action which was most likely to be due to the nicotine in the cigarette smoke.

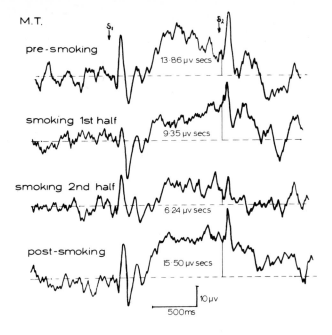

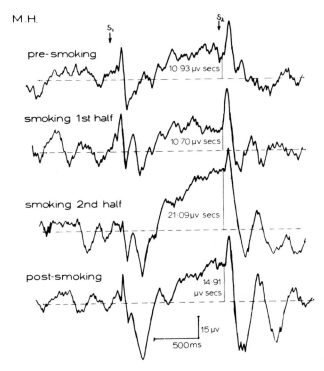

Fig. 5.2 CNVs obtained from two subjects showing changes in magnitude in different directions. Subject M.T. shows a decrease and subject M.H. shows an increase after smoking. S_1 and S_2 = light and tone signals.

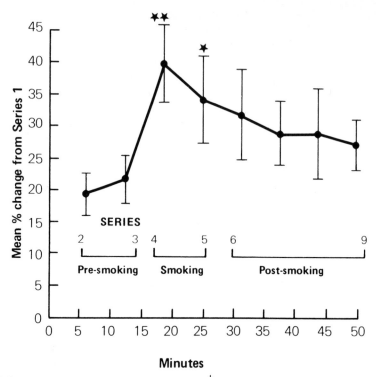

Fig. 5.3 Mean change in magnitude of CNV ($\pm$S.E. between bars) associated with smoking in 22 subjects. The points represent the mean % change in CNV size between the first pre-smoking series (Series 1) and each subsequent series. When compared with Series 1, the % change in CNV size was significantly greater in Series 4 (** p 0.001) and Series 5 (* p 0.02) than in either of the presmoking series (Series 2 and 3). Mean changes in CNV magnitude are based on changes in either direction, positive or negative.

Relationship between personality, nicotine,intake and CNV magnitude. In 16 of the 22 subjects the degree of extraversion/introversion was rated by means of the Eysenck Personality Inventory and the rate of nicotine intake was estimated by analysis of the cigarette butts. Correlation of these data with changes in CNV magnitude showed that the eight more extraverted subjects took a smaller dose of nicotine per minute and showed a mean increase in CNV magnitude after smoking, while the eight more introverted subjects took a larger dose of nicotine per minute and showed a mean decrease in CNV magnitude. These findings are consistent with the work of Armitage *et al,* (1969) who showed that in animals small doses of nicotine produced stimulant effects and larger doses could produce depressant effects. It appears that this dose-dependent action in man interacts with personality factors so that under certain conditions extraverts and introverts tend to select different doses of nicotine when smoking so as to obtain stimulant and depressant effects respectively.

Effects of pure nicotine administered intravenously on the CNV

Since cigarette smoking produced both stimulant and depressant effects on the brain, in terms of changes in the magnitude of the CNV, it became necessary to find out whether these effects could be accounted for by the nicotine in the cigarette smoke.

We were already aware of the work by Armitage and his colleagues (1969) who had shown that in animals intravenous nicotine can imitate the effects of cigarette smoking provided that the drug is given in the form of intermittent 'shots' but not if it is administered as a continuous infusion. A number of volunteers were given intermittent intravenous injections of nicotine and physiological saline as a control. The method used to prepare the nicotine for injection was that described by Armitage and his colleagues (1975) in which the solution of nicotine bitartrate was neutralised with sodium bicorbonate in order to prevent pain on injection. Under these conditions, subjects were unable to distinguish between an infusion of nicotine bitartrate and one of physiological saline.

The dose of nicotine in each 'shot' and the total amount of drug delivered to each subject was similar to that which would be obtained by a smoker who inhaled a cigarette of a brand belonging to the middle tar range i.e. 1-2 mg nicotine and 17-22 mg tar per cigarette (Health Departments of Great Britain, 1975).

Methods.   The method of recording the CNV was the same as that used for the experiments with cigarette smoking with the exception that each subject lay on a couch with the head propped up sufficiently to see the flashing light which was arranged to be on a level with his eyes. The button was held in the preferred hand and the infusion of neutralised nicotine bitartrate or physiological saline was made into an antecubital vein of the opposite arm via an indwelling 'butterfly' needle. The 'butterfly' needle was slowly flushed with physiological saline throughout the experiment apart from each occasion when intermittent 'shots' of nicotine or physiological saline were given when the rate of infusion was increased from twenty seconds before to twenty seconds after each 'shot' in order to ensure that it was well flushed through the infusion system. In some experiments the 'shots' were delivered automatically from a modified Harvard Infusion Apparatus and in others they were delivered from a manually operated syringe.

Effects of a single dose of nicotine.   In order to determine whether or not nicotine could produce similar changes in the CNV to those produced by smoking, subjects who had taken part in the smoking experiments were tested with a single dose of intravenous nicotine (given as 'shots'). In each instance it was found that the change in the magnitude of the CNV was in the same direction as occurred after smoking.

Each subject received several control infusions of physiological saline before and after two infusions of nicotine which were also separated by not less than one infusion of saline. The total dose of nicotine for each infusion was calculated to be similar to that which the subject obtained from a standard cigarette of known nicotine content.

Fig. 5.4. shows the results from a subject (T.L.) in whom nicotine produced an increase in CNV magnitude. After two saline controls, five 'shots' of 100 μg nicotine were given I.V. each minute over a period of five minutes (total = 500 μg) and increased the size of the CNV to 160% when compared with the mean saline control. After the second five 'shots' of 100 μg nicotine the size of the CNV was increased again although on this occasion to 124% compared with the mean saline control. During the subsequent post-nicotine saline injections there was a steady fall in magnitude of the CNV to values either the same as or slightly less than control values. These results are typical of those obtained in four experiments carried out on three volunteers.

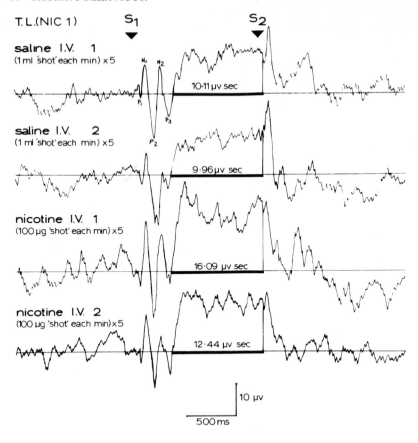

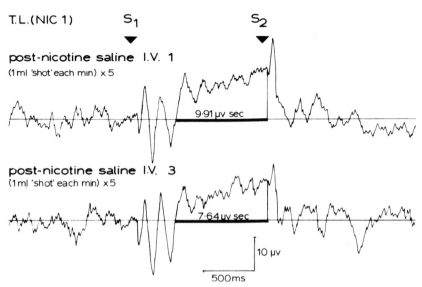

Fig. 5.4 Increase in magnitude of CNV in subject T.L. after two doses of I.V. nicotine 500 μg (given as five 'shots' of 100 μg over five minutes). Physiological saline control (five 'shots' of 1 ml over five minutes) given before and after nicotine. S_1 = flash, S_2 = tone, calibration 500 ms and 10 μV; CNV measured as area under curve in μVs.

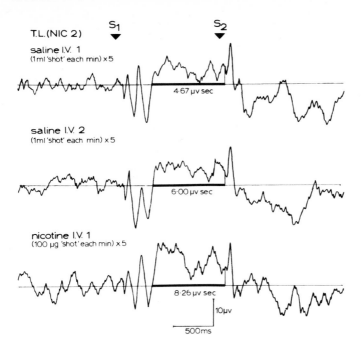

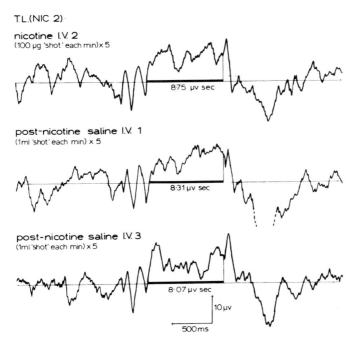

Fig. 5.5 Repeat experiment in same subject (T.L.) as in Fig. 5.4 showing increase in magnitude of CNV after two doses of I.V. nicotine 500 μg (given as five 'shots' of 100 μg over five minutes). Physiological saline control (five 'shots' of 1 ml over five minutes) given before and after nicotine. Symbols and calibration as in Fig. 5.4.

The experiment shown in Fig. 5.4 was repeated in the same subject (T.L.) after an interval of several months with similar results.

Fig. 5.5 shows that in this repeat experiment the control CNV's were smaller than in the first experiment (i.e. compared with Fig. 5.4) probably because on the second occasion the subject had become familiar with the experimental procedure with the result that he was less aroused.   After two saline controls, five 'shots' of 100μg nicotine I.V. (total 500μg) increased the size of the CNV to 156% as compared with the mean saline control value.   After the second five 'shots' of 100μg nicotine the magnitude of the CNV was a little larger (165%) than after the first dose of nicotine.   After each of the post-nicotine saline injections the size of the CNV's began to fall slowly although they did not reach control values by the end of the experiment.

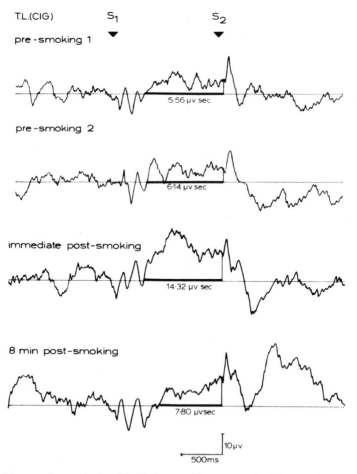

Fig. 5.6 Increase in magnitude of CNV after smoking one standard cigarette in same subject (T.L.) as in experiments of Figs. 5.4 and 5.5. After two control CNV's note increase in size of immediate post-smoking CNV; eight minutes later CNV is still larger than control levels. S_1 = flash, S_2 = tone; calibration 500 ms and 10 μV.

In another experiment the same subject (T.L.) smoked a cigarette and this produced similar effects on the CNV as those produced by intravenous nicotine. Fig. 5.6 shows that after two control CNV's, the subject smoked a standard cigarette (nicotine content 2.1 mg). Immediately after finishing the cigarette the size of the CNV increased to 245% whereas eight minutes after the end of the cigarette the size of the CNV had fallen to only 133% of the control value. This result, which was typical for all subjects, illustrates that the effect of smoking a single cigarette and receiving comparable dose of nicotine intravenously (in the form of intermittent 'shots') produces similar changes in the CNV both in magnitude and direction.

Fig. 5.7 shows the results from a subject in whom nicotine caused a decrease in the size of the CNV. After three reproducible responses to saline, five 'shots' of 150 μg nicotine (total 750 μg) the size of the CNV was reduced to 45% of its control value. After a second series of five 'shots' of 150 μg nicotine the CNV was reduced to 60% of the control value, rather less than after the first dose of nicotine. After each of the four post-nicotine salines the magnitude of the CNV steadily increased until finally it was slightly larger (14%) than the mean control value. This result is typical of those which were obtained in a total of four experiments carried out on three volunteers.

Dose-response relationship of nicotine and the CNV. The results of the experiments with single doses of nicotine showed that in some subjects nicotine produced an increase in CNV magnitude whilst in other subjects it produced a decrease. The next step was to determine whether or not the response of each subject depended upon the dose of nicotine or whether it depended upon the individual and was largely or completely independent of dose. This was examined by carrying out another set of experiments in order to determine the dose-response relationships between nicotine and the CNV.

Six volunteers received seven different doses of nicotine bitartrate although not all of the subjects received every dose in the series. As with the experiments using a single dose of nicotine, each total dose was divided into five equal intravenous 'shots' given once a minute over a period of five minutes. The total doses given in random order were 12.5, 25, 50, 100, 200, 400 and 800 μg nicotine and these were presented as five equal 'shots' of 2.5, 5, 10, 20, 40, 80 and 160 μg respectively, at minute intervals. Armitage, Hall and Morrison (1968) calculated that the average cigarette smoker obtains 1-2 μg nicotine per kg per puff so that a 70 kg man obtains 70-140 μg per puff, i.e. an average of about 100 μg per puff. Thus, the equivalent 'puff' doses of nicotine given to our subjects extended over a range from 2.5% to 160% of the average dose based on the predictions of Armitage *et al,* (1968).

Figs. 5.8 and 5.9 show the dose-response relationships in two subjects which were characteristic for the whole series. The striking feature is the unusual form of the dose-response curve such that with lower doses the magnitude of the CNV increases as the dose of nicotine is increased but thereafter further increases of dose result in a progressive reduction in the size of the CNV. The biphasic pattern is characteristic for all subjects although the precise shape of the dose-response curve differed for each subject.

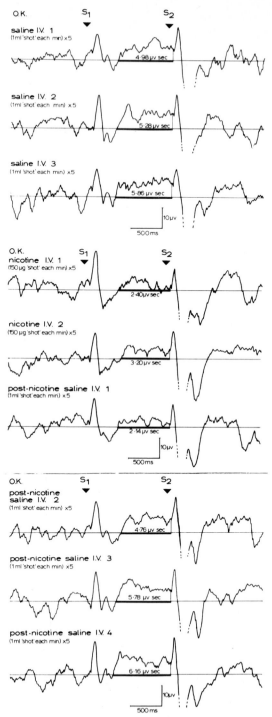

Fig. 5.7 Decrease in magnitude of CNV in subject O.K. after two doses of I.V. nicotine 750 μg (given as five 'shots' of 150 μg over five minutes). Physiological saline control (five 'shots' of 1 ml over five minutes) given before and after nicotine. S_1 = flash, S_2 = tone, calibration 500 ms and 10 μV.

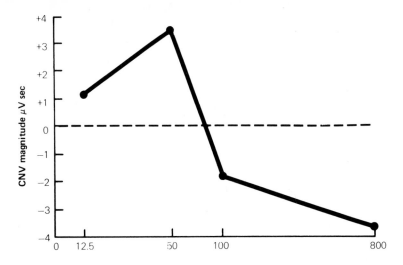

Fig. 5.8 Dose-response curve of subject A.R.H. showing effect of intravenous nicotine (each dose given as five 'shots'), expressed as increase or decrease (in μVs) from immediately preceding saline injection (0).

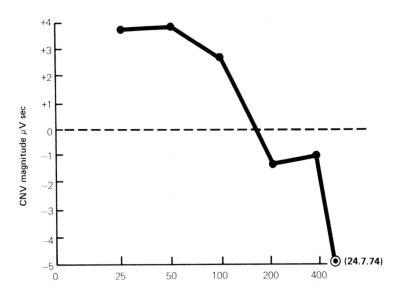

Fig. 5.9 Dose-response curve of subject I.S. showing effect of intravenous nicotine (each dose given as five 'shots'), expressed as increase or decrease (in μVs) from immediately preceding saline injection (0). Note highest dose given in separate experiment.

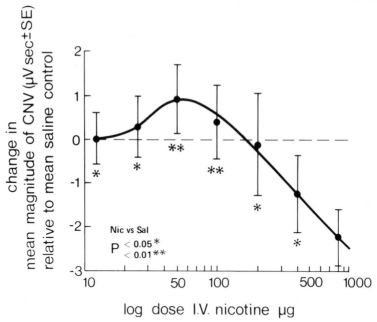

Fig. 5.10 Mean dose-response curve in six subjects showing effect of intravenous nicotine (each dose given as five 'shots') expressed as change in mean magnitude of CNV relative to mean saline control.   Note biphasic shape of curve so that smaller doses produce an increase in CNV magnitude (stimulant effect) and larger doses produce a decrease in CNV magnitude (depressant effect) relative to saline control. Abscissa: log dose I.V. nicotine μg.
Ordinate: change in mean magnitude relative to mean saline control (μVs $\pm$ 1 S.E.) Correlated t test for significance of difference between mean CNV with nicotine and mean CNV with saline for each dose * p$<$0.05 and ** p$<$0.01.

Fig. 5.10 illustrates the biphasic dose-response curve which represents the mean results obtained from the six experiments. The change in magnitude of the CNV in response to each dose of nicotine was significantly different from that of the corresponding saline (p$<$0.05–0.01) with the exception of the largest dose (800μg) which was given to only a small number of the subjects.

From the results of the experiments with intravenous nicotine we have drawn the following conclusions. (1) Cigarette smoking and nicotine produce effects on the CNV which are closely similar. (2) Nicotine causes biphasic effects on the CNV which are dose-related.   It is already known that cigarette smokers can adjust their intake of nicotine by altering their puffing rate (Ashton and Watson, 1970). If it is assumed that the biphasic effect of nicotine on the CNV reflects its ability to produce stimulant and depressant effects on the brain, it is reasonable to postulate that cigarette smokers adjust their intake of nicotine (mainly by puffing rate) so as to place themselves at an appropriate point on their individual dose-response curve to achieve the desired effect i.e. a stimulant or depressant effect.   It seems most likely that the part of the curve which would be automatically chosen by the average smoker is that which extends from the highest point across the baseline to the lowest (depressant) part of the curve.   By adjusting the intake of nicotine appropriately, a smoker should be able to adjust the degree of alertness to suit a particular occasion.

If the situation demanded maximum attention the smoker would adjust the intake of nicotine so as to maintain his or her brain at the highest point of the dose-response curve. Conversely, when the task had been accomplished and it was desired to produce a relaxed state the smoker would then need to increase the intake of nicotine so as to convert the stimulant effect to a depressant effect.

It is well known that at a simple synapse, such as the superior cervical ganglion of the cat, nicotine produces a biphasic response (Langley and Dickinson, 1889; Paton and Perry, 1963). The stimulant effect is due to an initial depolarisation of the ganglion cells whereas the depressant or paralytic effect is due to a sustained depolarisation which is probably followed by some reversible membrane changes. It seems likely that nicotine produces analagous changes in certain nervous elements in the brain which result in a stimulant or depressant effect depending on the dose. An alternative explanation is that nicotine may act on the brain by stimulating two opposing systems one of them excitatory and the other inhibitory, the effect manifest representing the resultant of its action on these two antagonistic systems. Such a possibility is not unlikely and would be in accord with the two-arousal hypothesis suggested by Routtenberg (1968) in which the reticular activating system and the limbic system may represent the controlling elements.

Acknowledgements

The authors wish to thanks Mrs. Valerie Wright for her efficient help with data processing and secretarial work. This work has been generously supported by the Tobacco Research Council. The figures appear by kind permission of the Journal of Clinical Pharmacology.

References

Armitage, A.K., Hall, G.H. & Morrison, C. (1968) Pharmacological basis for the tobacco smoking habit. *Nature, London,* **217**, 331-334.

Armitage, A.K., Hall, G.H. & Sellers, C.M. (1969) Effects of nicotine on electrocortical activity and acetylcholine release from cat cerebral cortex. *British Journal of Pharmacology,* **35**, 156-160.

Armitage, A.K., Dollery, C.T., George, C.F., Houseman, T.E., Lewis, P.J. & Turner, D.M. (1975) Absorption and metabolism of nicotine from cigarettes. *British Medical Journal,* **4**, 313-316.

Ashton, H. & Watson, D.W. (1970) Puffing frequency and nicotine intake in cigarette smokers. *British Medical Journal,* **3**, 679-681.

Ashton, H., Millman, J.E., Telford, R. & Thompson, J.W. (1973) Stimulant and depressant effects of cigarette smoking on brain activity in man. *British Journal of Pharmacology,* **48**, 715-717.

Ashton, H., Millman, J.E., Telford, R. & Thompson, J.W. (1974) The effects of caffeine, nitrazepam and cigarette smoking on the contingent negative variation in man. *Electroencephalography and Clinical Neurophysiology,* **37**, 59-71.

Ashton, H., Millman, J.E., Telford, R. & Thompson, J.W. (1976) A comparison of some physiological and psychological effects of propranolol and diazepam in normal subjects. *British Journal of Clinical Pharmacology,* **3**, 551-559.

Ashton, H., Millman, J.E., Telford, R. & Thompson, J.W. (1978) A comparison of some physiological and psychological effects of Motival (fluphenazine and nortriptyline) and diazepam in normal subjects. *British Journal of Clinical Pharmacology* (in press).

Health Departments of Great Britain (1975) *Tar and Nicotine Yields of Cigarettes.*

Langley, J.N. & Dickinson, W.L. (1889) On the local paralysis of peripheral ganglia, and on the connexion of different classes of nerve fibres with them. *Proceedings of the Royal Society, B,* **46**, 423-431.

Paton, W.D.M. & Perry, W.L.M. (1953) The relationship between depolarisation and block in the cat's superior cervical ganglion. *Journal of Physiology,* **119**, 43-47.

Rebert, C.S. (1972) Cortical and subcortical slow potentials in the monkey's brain during a preparatory interval. *Electroencephalography and Clinical Neurophysiology,* **33**, 389-402.

Routtenberg, A. (1968) The two-arousal hypothesis: reticular formation and limbic system. *Psychology Review,* **75**, 51-80.

Walter, W.G., Cooper, R., Aldridge, V.J., McCallum, W.C. & Winter, A.L. (1964) Contingent negative variation: An electric sign of sensorimotor association and expectancy in the human brain. *Nature, London,* **203**, 380-384.

6. The effect of cigarette smoking on the contingent negative variation (CNV) and eye movement

C D BINNIE AND A KAY COMER

The contingent negative variation (CNV) was first described by Walter *et al,* (1964). It is usually recorded between the vertex and mastoid electrodes and is a small negative potential which occurs between two signals when the first is a warning and the second requires a decision or action by the subject. It has been shown to be related to motivation, attention and level of arousal (e.g. Tecce, 1972; Knott and Irwin, 1973). Ashton *et al,* (1973, 1974) have found that cigarette smoking can affect the magnitude of the CNV in man. It was therefore decided to conduct a preliminary investigation into the effects of smoking on the CNV, as part of a larger study on the electroencephalogram (EEG). Particular care must be taken when recording the CNV to avoid contamination due to eye movement. A number of types of eye movement potential can be recorded at the vertex and these may resemble the shape of the CNV. Some types of eye movement are known to be affected by drugs (e.g. Stern, Bremer and McClive, 1974), but the effect of smoking on involuntary changes in eye fixation has not been investigated. We therefore recorded both CNV and eye movement before and after cigarette smoking. Since the way in which a cigarette is smoked may play a part in determining the physiological effect produced, we also recorded details of smoking behaviour.

Methods

The CNV was recorded between vertex and left mastoid sites using chlorided silver stick-on electrodes. Recordings were made with a bandwidth of 0.125 - 30 Hz. The CNV was evoked by paired auditory signals (S_1 and S_2), 1000 Hz. tone pulses, 60 dB above threshold, 1.2 seconds apart. The interval between stimulus pairs was random, between three and eight seconds. The subject responded to S_2 by pressing a hand-held button. Eye movement was minimised by asking subjects to fixate on the pupil of their own eye in a mirror (as suggested by Papakostopoulos, Winter and Newton, 1973). The electrooculogram and 12 channels of EEG (including C_z - A_1) were recorded on paper and on magnetic tape for subsequent off-line analysis. Smoking behaviour was recorded using the smoking analyser and data logger (Creighton, Noble and Whewell, 1978).

Subjects were 18 male and 18 female cigarette smokers who were members of B.A.T. staff at the Group Research and Development Centre, Southampton. Their ages ranged from 19 to 55 years and they represented a wide range of occupations. Subjects were chosen for this study so that there were equal numbers of people who consistently took high, medium and low average total smoke volume when smoking a standard cigarette on previous occasions. The CNV and eye movement were recorded before and after smoking one king-size filter tipped cigarette (1.7 mg nicotine, 27 mg TPM by machine smoking).

All subjects had previously completed the Eysenck Personality Inventory (E.P.I., Eysenck and Eysenck, 1964). A mood adjective check list (Nowlis, 1965) was administered before and after the experiment. Scores were obtained for the factors of aggression, anxiety, surgency, pleasantness, concentration, fatigue, vigour and sadness.

Experimental procedure

CNV recordings were made at the end of an experiment during which a number of other EEG measurements were made. Before subjects arrived for the experiment they abstained from smoking and drinking tea, coffee and alcohol for at least thirty minutes. Electrode application and completion of questionnaires took about 25 minutes. Background EEG and evoked responses were then recorded for 45 minutes (no smoking). CNVs were recorded after this, in blocks of twenty stimulus pairs. Blocks started at five minute intervals, allowing subjects a short rest between them. Three blocks of CNVs were recorded before smoking and five afterwards. The subjects, who had been deprived from smoking for almost two hours, smoked their cigarettes through a small holder (see Creighton *et al*, 1978) and no instructions were given about the way in which they should smoke. All subjects were familiar with the equipment to record smoking behaviour. Recordings were made in a large, well-ventilated room with the subject seated in an upright chair. The recording equipment was in the same room as the subject but it was partially obscured by screens. Conversation between experimenters and subjects during the test was not allowed, but all instructions were given verbally and queries about procedure were answered.

Analysis of results

It had been hoped that asking subjects to fixate on their eyes in a mirror would minimise eye movements. Most subjects, however, found this surprisingly difficult, especially if they were anxious or becoming drowsy. It was therefore necessary to correct the CNV measurements for the effects of eye movements. Epochs containing the most extreme examples of artifact in the CNV were rejected. The remaining CNVs were corrected by computer using what is, effectively, a software adaptation of the potentiometer correction method (McCallum and Walter, 1968). The computer then calculated the area of the averaged CNVs for each block. Eye blinks were counted from the paper record for each block. Eye movement during the CNV was determined by planimetry from an average for each block obtained from a small computer and written out on paper. All results were analysed in terms of CNV change for each subject. Preliminary results for this experiment, before computer analysis of the CNV, have already been reported (Comer *et al*, 1975).

Results

Eighteen subjects showed an increase in CNV magnitude after smoking (mean 104.7% increase) and 18 subjects showed a decrease (mean 29.6% decrease). Both these changes were statistically significantly different from zero ($p \leqslant 0.05$) and the mean increase was significantly greater than the mean decrease ($p \leqslant 0.05$).

The mean pre-smoking CNV and eye movement magnitudes and number of eye-blinks were compared with the post-smoke mean values using the Welch modified t-test (Brownlee, 1965) which makes no assumptions about the variance of the two samples to be compared.

Since this was a preliminary study to determine whether to investigate the CNV/ smoking relationship further, it was decided that any changes significant at the 90% confidence level or above would be included in comparisons of smoking behaviour.

Of 35 subjects, three showed a decrease and seven and increase in CNV magnitude ($p \leqslant 0.1$), all other subjects showing no significant change. For eye movement during the CNV, eight subjects showed a significant decrease and two an increase. Five subjects showed a significant increase in eye blinks during post-smoking blocks and four a decrease.

In order to investigate any relationship between CNV and eye movement changes, smoking behaviour and personality, subjects were divided into groups according to the direction and significance of physiological change. The means for each group were compared using Student's t-test for the measurements shown in Table 6.1. Of all the comparisons made, only those shown in Table 6.2 were significant ($p \leqslant 0.05$).

Table 6.1 List of measurements which may be related to physiological changes during the CNV experiment.

Puff Number	Average Inter-puff Interval
Average Puff Volume	Total Inter-puff Interval
Total Puff Volume	Total Time Cigarette was Alight
Average Puff Duration	Butt Length
Total Puff Duration	Butt Nicotine
Rate of Nicotine Intake	

(Estimated Nicotine Delivery $\div$ Total Time Alight)
Rate of Smoke Intake
(Total Volume $\div$ Total Time Alight)
Percentage Time Spent Puffing
(Total Puff Duration $\div$ Total Time Alight)
Number of Cigarettes Smoked Per Day
E Score (Extraversion-Introversion Scale of E.P.I.)
N Score (Neuroticism-Stability Scale of E.P.I.)

Table 6.2 Smoking behaviour and changes in CNV and eye movement.

Significant Change in CNV vs. No Significant Change:
   Greater total puff volume and faster rate of nicotine intake for significant change
   Greater average puff volume for males with significant change

Significant Decrease in CNV vs. Nonsignificant Decrease:
   Larger average puff volume for significant decrease.

Significant Increase in CNV vs. Nonsignificant Increase:
   Faster rate of nicotine intake for significant increase.

Significant CNV Increase vs. Significant CNV Decrease:
   Shorter average interpuff interval for increase.

Any CNV Increase vs. Any CNV Decrease:
   Subjects with increase smoked less cigarettes per day
   Female subjects with increase had shorter total time alight and shorter total
      inter-puff internal.

Significant Change in Number of Eyeblinks vs. Nonsignificant Change:
   Average inter-puff interval shorter for significant eyblink change.

Significant Change in Eye Movement during CNVs vs. Nonsignificant Change:
   Less cigarettes smoked per day by subjects with significant change.

Significant Increase in Eye Movement vs. Significant Decrease:
   Total inter-puff interval shorter, total time alight shorter, rate of nicotine
      intake faster and percentage time puffing higher for increase in eye
      movement.

   Some of the subgroups are too small for firm conclusions to be drawn about possible relationships. It can be said in summary, however, that there was a tendency for subjects showing a significant CNV change to have smoked more intensely than those showing no significant change and that a CNV increase was associated with greater smoking intensity than a CNV decrease. There was no apparent relationship between smoking behaviour and personality for these subjects. The only scores on the mood adjective check list which changed significantly were those for concentration and vigour, both of them showing a decrease.

Discussion

The rather blurred relationship between our measurements of smoking behaviour and physiological effect may have a number of explanations. It is probable that at least part of the effect of smoking on the CNV is due to nicotine. The amount of nicotine entering the blood-stream of a smoker and going to his brain will depend both on the way in which the cigarette is smoked and on the depth and duration of smoke inhalation (Rawbone *et al*, 1978).   In the absence of blood nicotine or inhalation measurements, we are only able to take account of smoking behaviour, and this may give insufficient information for a meaningful relationship between smoking and physiological change to emerge.   Other interpretive difficulties can also arise from the possible effect of the initial state of arousal of the subject, both on base-line CNV and on any action of smoking.   The relationship of CNV magnitude to arousal level appears to be an inverted-U curve (Tecce, 1972; Tecce and Hamilton, 1973).   Using this model it is possible that a subject in a sub-optimum state of arousal would show a CNV increase from a given dose of nicotine while another person in a high state of electroencephalographic arousal would show a CNV decrease with the same nicotine dose.   Thus the effect of nicotine and smoking on the CNV need not necessarily be dose related and could be solely unidirectional in terms of arousal.

Ashton and her colleagues (Ashton *et al*, 1973, 1974) have found that smoking may cause increases or decreases in CNV magnitude and that the direction of change is related to personality and rate of nicotine intake. We have also found CNV changes in both directions, but these do not appear to be related to smoking behaviour in the same way. There are, however, a number of important methodological differences between our study and that of Ashton. Our results tend to suggest that a significant CNV change is associated with intense smoking, regardless of direction of change. Most of our subjects showed no significant CNV change, despite smoking more intensely than they had done outside the experiment (Comer and Creighton, 1978), and they may therefore have been near their optimum arousal level for CNV task performance. It can be suggested, however, that more subjects were below their optimum level than were above it, since more of the significant changes involved CNV increase and the overall mean increase in CNV magnitude was greater than the mean decrease.

While the results from the mood adjective check list do not give information relating directly to mood at the time of smoking, they do tend to indicate that many subjects found the experiment tiring and/or boring.   Verbal reports confirmed this although it was known that some subjects were anxious during the experiment and perceived themselves to be under stress.

Ashton and her colleagues have suggested that the effects of smoking and of intravenous nicotine on the CNV are very similar (Ashton *et al*, 1978).   There are, however, several important differences between the two methods of nicotine administration.   In one case the smoker is given a specific dose and in the other he has exact control over his nicotine intake.   There may also be psychological factors involved in smoking which affect the CNV and brain activity independently of nicotine dose.

In order to determine the possible effect of initial state of the subject and of psychological factors, further work must be done, and ideally this would include measurement of CNV changes after smoking and intravenous injection of nicotine in subjects whose arousal levels were manipulated in some way. Any such experiments should include some measurement of dose of nicotine retained in the body during smoking.

The changes in eye movement after smoking are of interest since this has not previously been studied. Eye movement during the CNV were minimised by asking subjects to fixate on the pupil of their own eye in a mirror. This was found to be surprisingly difficult by many subjects and was considered by them to be a task in itself. In general, eye movements are most prominent in anxious or drowsy subjects. The effects of smoking which were seen are unlikely to have been caused by side-stream and exhaled smoke from the cigarette since the experiment was conducted in a large, well-ventilated room. We were, therefore, measuring the effects of smoking on involuntary changes in eye fixation. It seems possible that the subjects who experienced a decrease in eye movement after smoking had used smoking to increase their ability to concentrate on the task by facilitating eye fixation. This could occur as a particular action of smoking or as a result of changes in arousal level. The former possibility seems most likely since subjects who showed marked eye movement changes did not show significant changes in CNV magnitude. Smoking may, therefore, aid task performance by decreasing eye movement and this could be particularly important during vigilance tasks. It is unlikely, however, that there is any practical significance in the observed changes in number of eye blinks.

It can be suggested that people may smoke in a way which enables them to optimise performance in a given situation. This may be achieved both by changes in brain activity and in eye-fixation ability.

Acknowledgements

We would like to thank Mrs. C.E. Darby, Miss L. Burnett, Miss C.A. Smith and Mrs. J.R.M. Lavier for skilled technical assistance.

References

Ashton, H., Millman, J.E., Telford, R. & Thompson, J.W. (1973) Stimulant and depressant effects of cigarette smoking on brain activity in man. *British Journal of Pharmacology,* **48,** 715-717.

Ashton, H., Millman, J.E., Telford, R. & Thompson, J.W. (1974) The effects of caffeine, nitrazepam and cigarette smoking on the contingent negative variation in man. *Electroencephalography and Clinical Neurophysiology,* **37,** 59-71.

Ashton, H., Marsh, R.V., Millman, J.E., Rawlins, M.D., Telford, R. & Thompson, J.W. (1978) The use of event-related slow potentials of the brain as a means to analyse the effects of cigarette smoking and nicotine in humans. *This volume.*

Brownlee, K.A. (1965) *Statistical Theory and Methodology in Science and Engineering,* 2nd edn., p. 299. New York: John Wiley & Sons, Inc.

Comer, A.K., Binnie, C.D., Burnett, L., Darby, C.E. & Thornton, R.E. (1975) The effect of cigarette smoking on the contingent negative variation (CNV) and eye movement. (Abstract) *Electroencephalography and Clinical Neurophysiology,* **39,** 222.

Comer, A.K. & Creighton, D.E. (1978) The effect of experimental conditions on smoking behaviour. *This volume.*

Creighton, D.E., Noble, M.J. & Whewell, R.T. (1978) Instruments to measure, record and duplicate human smoking patterns. *This volume.*

Eysenck, H.J. & Eysenck, S.B.G. (1964) *Eysenck Personality Inventory.* University of London Press.

Knott, J.R. & Irwin, D.A. (1973) Anxiety, stress and the contingent negative variation. *Archives of General Psychiatry, 29,* 538-541.

McCallum, W.C. & Walter, W.G. (1968) The effects of attention and distraction on the contingent negative variation in normal and neurotic subjects. *Electroencephalography and Clinical Neurophysiology, 25,* 319-329.

Nowlis, V. (1965) Research with the mood adjective check list. In *Affect, Cognition and Personality,* ed. Tomkins, S.S. & Izard, C.E. pp. 352-389. Tavistock Publications.

Papakostopoulos, D., Winter, A. & Newton, P. (1973) A new technique for the control of eye potential artifacts in multichannel CNV recordings. *Electroencephalography and Clinical Neurophysiology, 34,* 651-653.

Rawbone, R.G., Murphy, K., Tate, M.E. & Kane, S.J. (1978) The analysis of smoking parameters, inhalation and absorption of tobacco smoke in studies of human smoking behaviour. *This volume.*

Stern, J.A., Bremer, D.A. & McClive, J. (1974) Analysis of eye movements and blinks during reading: effects of valium. *Psychopharmacologia, 40,* 171-175.

Tecce, J.J. (1972) Contingent negative variation (C.N.V.) and psychological processes in man. *Psychological Bulletin, 77,* 73-108.

Tecce, J.J. & Hamilton, B.T. (1973) C.N.V. reduction by sustained cognitive activity (distraction). *Electroencephalography and Clinical Neurophysiology,* **Suppl. 33,** 229-237.

Walter, W.G., Cooper, R., Aldridge, V.J., McCallum, W.C. & Winter, A.L. (1964) Contingent negative variation: An electric sign of sensorimotor association and expectancy in the human brain. *Nature, London,* **203,** 380-384.

7. The effect of experimential conditions on smoking behaviour

A KAY COMER AND D E CREIGHTON

Introduction

Although a considerable amount of work has been reported on the way in which smoking behaviour may vary with changes in cigarette design, few workers have investigated the effects of different conditions on the smoking of one cigarette type. Ashton and Watson (1970) found that cigarettes were smoked more intensely by subjects under relaxed conditions when compared with smoking during a simulated driving task. Similarly, Fuller and Forrest (1973) have observed a greater rate of smoking in a low-arousal compared with a high-arousal situation. Glad and Adesso (1976) were unable to detect any differences in the amount of smoking in their high- or low-arousal social situations. They found that smokers were sensitive to the presence or absence of other smokers in a group. Their subjects increased the number of cigarettes smoked, puffs taken, flicks on the cigarette and minutes spent smoking, when everyone around them smoked.

In spite of these suggested differences in behaviour there seems to have been a general tendency to assume that the way in which a person smoked during an experiment will give information which is in some way relevant to more 'normal' or 'natural' situations. In order to investigate this we have compared the smoking of one cigarette type under various experimental and social conditions.

Subjects and methods

All subjects were members of B.A.T. staff at the Group Research and Development Centre, Southampton.

In the laboratory, smoking behaviour was recorded using the smoking analyser and data logger described in this volume (Creighton, Noble and Whewell, 1978). This gave information on puff number, volume, duration and pressure, and the interval between puffs. Butt length was also measured.

Surreptitious monitoring of smoking was accomplished using small tape recorders and hand-held controls concealed in the handbags of trained female observers. The Sony T.C.55 cassette recorder was used with a control which generated a 400Hz tone to record the interval between puffs. When a puff was observed a 4KHz tone was produced by pressing a small button on the control. There was also a microphone in the control so that details such as subject's name, location, time, type of cigarette and butt length could be recorded verbally immediately after observation. Butt length was estimated visually and puff number, duration and interval between puffs were obtained by decoding the tone pattern on the cassette tape.

Experimental procedure and environment

Experiment 1

This was conducted in a purpose-built smoking laboratory which is a sound-attenuated and pleasantly decorated room. Subjects were seated in a comfortable chair and listened to music of their choice. All subjects smoked the same type of cigarette (king size filter tipped, 27 mg TPM, 1.7 mg nicotine by machine), on four different occasions. Smokers were alone in the smoking room during experiments but could be observed through a one-way mirror.

Experiment 2

Only subjects who smoked consistently in Experiment 1 in terms of number of puffs and total smoke volume were eligible for Experiment 2. Equal numbers of subjects were chosen from groups with high, medium and low average total smoke volumes.

During Experiment 2 (which is described elsewhere in this volume - Binnie and Comer, 1978) electroencephalographic (EEG) recordings were made. Subjects had not smoked for about two hours when asked to do so in this experiment.

The procedure was conducted in a large room in which EEG equipment, the smoking analyser and data logger and experimenters were partially obscured by screens. Subjects were seated in an upright chair and there was little background noise during smoking. Each subject smoked one cigarette of the type used in Experiment 1.

Data available for 16 male and 16 female subjects who took part in both Experiment 1 and Experiment 2.

Experiment 3

This experiment took place in the same laboratory as Experiment 1, but one year later.

Subjects smoked the same cigarette type as for the previous experiments. On four occasions this was under 'normal' conditions (as in Experiment 1) and on a further four occasions subjects abstained from smoking for at least one hour before smoking in the laboratory. The order of conditions was randomised and no subject completed more than one test in a day. There were 14 male and ten female subjects who took part in Experiments 1, 2 and 3.

Experiment 4

Subjects from the previous experiments were observed surreptitiously while they smoked in a coffee lounge at work, during lunch times. This is an uncontrolled social environment and subjects were unaware of the observations being made.

If possible each subject was observed smoking on four separate occasions. This was achieved for 15 male and six female subjects. For a further 32 males and 13 females who took part in Experiment 1 it was only possible to observe one, two or three cigarettes of the same type being smoked in the lounge.

Results

Table 7.1 shows a comparison of measurements of smoking behaviour for Experiments 1 and 2. Both males and females have smoked more intensely during Experiment 2 (EEG) and have changed a number of different aspects of their smoking behaviour. Male smokers have tended to show a greater change in smoking than have females.

Differences between the two conditions were analysed statistically using a sign test, since a t-test was considered to make too many assumptions about the underlying distributions in the populations from which the observations were taken. A summary of the results of this analysis appears in Table 7.2. This shows that many of the changes seen are statistically significant.

Table 7.3 shows a comparison of smoking behaviour under normal laboratory conditions and after a period of smoking deprivation (Experiment 3). There are no differences between the conditions which can be detected by the sign test at the 95% confidence level or above. Since it may be expected that any effects of smoking deprivation would be most marked over the first part of the cigarette this has also been analysed separately.

Table 7.4 shows a comparison for the first four puffs taken on the cigarettes. Only the total of the intervals between puffs for male smokers has changed significantly ($p < 0.05$). These results suggest, therefore, that a short period of smoking deprivation is unlikely to account for the changes in smoking behaviour which are seen when Experiments 1 and 2 are compared.

Table 7.5 shows a comparison of normal laboratory smoking during Experiment 3 with that recorded one year previously in Experiment 1. The sign test reveals that only the butt length has changed significantly but this change is numerically very small and is unlikely to be of practical significance. This indicates that smoking behaviour has remained stable over a one-year period.

Table 7.6 shows a comparison between smoking in the laboratory (Experiment 1) and in the coffee lounge (Experiment 4). Subjects smoked a similar cigarette in the lounge to that used in the laboratory and four sets of measurements were obtained for each location. The sign test was again used and it can be seen that the average puff number is significantly lower in the social situation and there is a tendency for the average interval between puffs to be longer.

Table 7.7 shows a similar pattern of results for subjects who were observed smoking one, two or three cigarettes in the lounge. These results could not be analysed statistically by the sign test but there is an indication that changes are in the same direction as those shown in Table 7.6.

Table 7.1 Comparison of Experiment 1 (EEG) and Experiment 2 (Laboratory). Figures are group means. Each subject smoked four cigarettes in Experiment 1 and one cigarette in Experiment 2.

Subjects	Test	Total Volume of Smoke (ml)	Total Puff Duration (sec)	Total Inter-puff Interval (sec)	Total Puff Pressure (cm W.G.)	Average Puff Number	Average Puff Volume (ml)	Average Puff Duration (sec)	Average Inter-puff Interval (sec)	Average Puff Pressure (cm W.G.)	Average Draw Resistance (cm W.G.)	Total Time Alight (sec)	Average Butt Length (mm)
Male (16)	EEG	525.8	33.0	320.9	517.3	14.2	39.3	2.35	26.4	38.0	16.2	354	30.6
	Laboratory	385.8	26.6	390.8	406.1	11.6	34.1	2.30	39.3	35.8	15.6	411	30.0
	% Difference	+36	+24	−18	+27	+22	+15	+2	−33	+6	+4	−14	+2
Female (16)	EEG	481.4	28.4	354.5	444.3	14.3	35.1	2.04	28.3	34.0	17.1	379	30.6
	Laboratory	391.8	24.4	416.5	407.1	12.4	32.6	2.01	40.0	32.0	16.3	442	28.4
	% Difference	+23	+16	−15	+9	+15	+8	+1	−29	+6	+5	−14	+8
All Subjects (32)	EEG	503.6	30.7	337.7	480.8	14.3	37.2	2.20	27.4	36.0	16.7	366.5	30.6
	Laboratory	388.8	25.5	403.7	406.6	12.0	33.4	2.16	39.7	33.9	16.0	426.5	29.2
	% Difference	+29.5	+20	−16	+18	+19	+11.5	+2	−31	+6	+4.5	−14	+5

D

Table 7.2   Summary of statistical analysis comparing Experiment 1 (EEG) and Experiment 2 (Laboratory)

	Males		Females	
	Direction of Change	Significance	Direction of Change	Significance
Total Volume of Smoke	EEG Greater	***	EEG Greater	**
Total Puff Duration	EEG Longer	***	EEG Longer	*
Total Inter-Puff Interval	Laboratory Longer	***	Laboratory Longer	***
Total Puff Pressure	EEG Higher	***	EEG Higher	***
Butt Length	–	N.S.	EEG Higher	**
Puff Number	EEG Higher	***	EEG Higher	**
Average Puff Volume	EEG Greater	*	–	N.S.
Average Puff Duration	–	N.S.	–	N.S.
Average Inter-puff Interval	Laboratory Longer	***	Laboratory Longer	***
Average Draw Resistance	–	N.S.	–	N.S.
Average Total Time Alight	Laboratory Longer	***	Laboratory Longer	***

N.S. = Not significant   *** $p \leq 0.01$ ** $p \leq 0.05$ * $\bar{p} \leq 0.1$

Table 7.3 Comparison of 'normal' and 'deprived' smoking (Experiment 3). Figures are group means. Each subject smoked four cigarettes in each condition

Subjects	Test	Total Volume of Smoke (ml)	Total Puff Duration (sec)	Total Inter-puff Interval (sec)	Total Puff Pressure (cm WG)	Average Puff Number	Average Puff Volume (ml)	Average Puff Duration (sec)	Average Inter-puff Interval (sec)	Average Draw Resist-ance (cm WG)	Total Time Alight (sec)	Average Butt Length (mm)
Male (14)	Deprived	441.5	28.1	371.4	380.6	12.1	36.6	2.33	33.5	13.5	399.5	29.2
	Normal	399.6	25.2	391.4	357.2	11.1	35.8	2.26	38.6	14.2	416.5	29.8
	% Difference	+10.4	+11.5*	−5.1	+6.6	+9.0	+2.2	+3.1	−13.2	−4.9	−4.1	−2.0*
Female (10)	Deprived	414.4	24.8	416.1	364.4	12.4	33.5	2.00	36.6	14.7	440.9	27.5
	Normal	412.3	24.7	424.5	360.4	12.5	32.9	1.97	36.9	14.6	449.3	27.7
	% Difference	+0.5	+0.4	−2.0	+1.1	−0.8	+1.8	+1.52	−0.8	−0.7	−1.9	−0.7
All Subjects (24)	Deprived	430.2	26.7	390.0	373.9	12.2	35.3	2.19	34.8	14.0	416.7	28.5
	Normal	404.9	25.0	405.2	358.6	11.7	34.6	2.13	37.8	14.4	430.2	28.9
	% Difference	+6.3	+6.8	−3.8	+4.3	+4.3	+2.0	+2.8	−7.9	−2.8	−3.1	−1.4

* $p \leqslant 0.1$

Table 7.4 Comparison of 'normal' and 'deprived' smoking (Experiment 3) (first four puffs)

Subjects	Test	Total Volume of Smoke (ml)	Total Puff Duration (sec)	Total Inter-puff Interval (sec)	Total Puff Pressure (cm WG)	Average Puff Number	Average Draw Resistance (cm WG)	Time Alight for 4 puffs
Male (14)	Deprived	185.8	11.5	74.3	166.8	4	14.5	85.8
	Normal	174.2	10.9	98.5	160.4	4	14.7	109.4
	% Difference	+6.7	+5.6*	−24.6**	+4	0	−1.4	−21.6*
Female (10)	Deprived	162.4	10.1	78.1	147.2	4	14.6	88.2
	Normal	163.6	10.2	82.7	147.6	4	14.5	92.9
	% Difference	−0.7	−0.8	−5.6	−0.3	0	+0.7	−5.1
All Subjects (24)	Deprived	176.1	10.9	75.9	158.6	4	14.5	86.8
	Normal	169.8	10.6	91.9	155.0	4	14.6	102.5
	% Difference	+3.7	+3.0	−17.4*	+2.3	0	−0.7	−15.3

*   P ≤ 0.1
** P ≤ 0.05

Table 7.5 Comparison of Experiment 3 (normal smoking) with Experiment 1 (laboratory smoking) one year previously. Figures are group means. Each subject smoked four cigarettes in each experiment.

Subjects	Test	Total Volume of Smoke (ml)	Total Puff Duration (sec)	Total Inter-puff Interval (sec)	Total Puff Pressure (cm WG)	Average Puff Number	Average Puff Volume (ml)	Average Puff Duration (sec)	Average Inter-puff Interval (sec)	Average Draw Resistance (cm WG)	Total Time Alight (sec)	Average Butt Length (mm)
Male (14)	Normal	399.6	25.2	391.4	357.2	11.1	35.9	2.26	38.6	14.2	416.5	29.8
	Laboratory	391.7	26.7	387.7	403.0	11.5	34.0	2.31	36.8	15.1	414.3	30.4
	% Difference	+2.0	−5.6	+0.9	−11.4	−3.5	+5.6	−2.2	+4.9	−6.0	+0.5	−2.0**
Female (10)	Normal	412.3	24.7	424.5	360.4	12.5	32.9	1.97	36.8	14.6	449.3	27.7
	Laboratory	386.8	22.6	434.4	366.7	12.2	31.7	1.85	38.7	16.2	457.2	28.1
	% Difference	+6.6	+9.4	−2.3	−1.7	+2.5	+3.8	+6.5	−4.9	−9.9	−1.7	−1.4
All Subjects (24)	Normal	404.9	25.0	405.2	358.6	11.7	34.6	2.13	36.4	14.4	430.2	28.8
	Laboratory	389.6	25.0	407.1	387.9	11.8	33.0	2.11	36.3	15.5	432.2	29.4
	% Difference	+3.9	0	−0.5	−7.6	−0.9	+4.9	+1.0	+0.3	−7.1	−0.5	−2.0**

** P ≤ 0.05

Table 7.6 Comparison of Experiment 1 (Laboratory) and Experiment 4 (Surreptitious). Figures are group means. Each subject smoked four cigarettes in each experiment.

Subjects	Test	Average Puff Duration (sec)	Average Inter-puff Interval (sec)	Average Puff Number	Average Butt Length (mm)
Male (15)	Laboratory	2.10	41.9	11.5	27.8
	Surreptitious	2.04	51.6	9.3	27.9
	% Difference	−3	+23	−19	0.4
Female (6)	Laboratory	1.69	38.0	12.5	30.0
	Surreptitious	1.61	55.7	8.7	29.0
	% Difference	−5	+47	−30	3
All (21)	Laboratory	1.98	40.8	11.8	28.4
	Surreptitious	1.92	52.7	9.1	28.2
	% Difference	−3 NS	+29 *	−23 **	0.7 NS

NS   =   Not significant
* $P \leqslant 0.1$
** $P \leqslant 0.05$

Table 7.7 Comparison of Experiment 1 (Laboratory) and Experiment 4 (Surreptitious) Figures are group means. Each subject smoked four cigarettes in Experiment 1 and one, two or three cigarettes in Experiment 4.

Subjects	Test	Average Puff Duration (sec)	Average Inter-puff Interval (sec)	Average Puff Number	Average Butt Length (mm)
Male (32)	Laboratory	2.20	41.0	12.1	28.0
	Surreptitious	1.95	47.6	9.7	28.4
	% Difference	−13	+16	−20	+1.5
Female (13)	Laboratory	1.75	37.1	12.6	31.5
	Surreptitious	1.65	50.6	8.1	30.5
	% Difference	−6	+36	−36	−3
All (45)	Laboratory	2.07	39.8	12.2	29.0
	Surreptitious	1.87	48.4	9.2	29.0
	% Difference	−10	+22	−25	0

Discussion

When smoking in a relaxed laboratory environment was compared with smoking during an EEG experiment a number of aspects of smoking behaviour were found to have changed. All subjects tended to smoke more intensely during the EEG experiment, especially the males. Two main factors could have contributed to the observed changes in smoking pattern. Firstly, subjects had been deprived from smoking for about two hours when they were asked to smoke during the EEG experiment. A further experiment showed, however, that a short period of smoking deprivation had almost no effect on smoking behaviour under laboratory conditions. It therefore seems unlikely that the changes seen were due to deprivation. The second factor was the difference in environment in which the subjects smoked. It is probable that this was a major influence on their smoking behaviour. There is evidence (see Binnie and Comer, 1978) that some of the subjects became tired and bored with the lengthy experimental procedure once the initial novelty had worn off. Other subjects may have considered themselves to be under stress during the EEG experiment. They were able to see unfamiliar equipment and some of them were worried that their brain activity might be abnormal or that an EEG recording could reveal their thoughts, despite reassurance to the contrary. Subjects were asked to smoke in the middle of a part of the experiment during which they were required to complete a simple task (pressing a button after the second of a pair of auditory stimuli and fixating on the pupil of their own eye in a mirror). Subjects in the EEG experiment could, therefore, have been smoking to obtain stimulation, to relieve stress or to improve their task performance. Unfortunately, we are unable to distinguish between these possibilities for each subject but can conclude that the overall effect of the experimental conditions on our sample of 32 subjects was to give an observed intensification of smoking. We must, however, remember that we did not measure difference in smoke/nicotine intake which may have occurred due to variations in depth of inhalation under the different conditions.

We have shown that, although smoking behaviour may vary according to experimental conditions, it remains remarkably stable over time if the same type of cigarette is smoked under the same laboratory conditions. A comparison of average smoking parameters for four cigarettes during each of two experiments, one year apart, showed very similar patterns for a number of aspects of smoking behaviour.

Knowing that smoking patterns could be altered by experimental procedures it was of particular interest to compare laboratory and social smoking. The differences seen could be due to several factors. In the laboratory, subjects smoke through a small cigarette holder (see Creighton et al, 1978) and know that they are being observed, although they are alone while they smoke. In the coffee lounge where social smoking was observed there were no restrictions on smoking; subjects were unaware of observation and were free to indulge in social interactions. It should also be noted that laboratory smoking data are based on averages for two cigarettes smoked in the morning and two in the afternoon, whereas all social smoking observations took place at lunchtime. It is thought that the differences in smoking behaviour which were detected were not due to the presence or absence of the cigarette holder, since this is most likely to affect butt length, which did not alter significantly. It is also unlikely that time of day had an effect, since we have never found any significant differences between smoking in the morning and in the afternoon. Differences were probably due mainly to the surrounding environment and social interaction. In the laboratory subjects have nothing to do but smoke and listen to music, whereas in the coffee lounge they may be far less aware of the fact that they are smoking, especially while they are engaged in conversation. They therefore tend to take fewer puffs, less often, in the social environment. They may also be seeking a different effect from the cigarette in the two different situations.

In summary it can be said that people really do smoke the same type of cigarette in different ways under different conditions, as has always been suspected. Intensity of smoking was increased during an EEG experiment and decreased in a social situation, when compared to smoking in a solitary, relaxed laboratory environment. In this laboratory, smoking behaviour was stable with time and unaffected by a short period of smoking deprivation. It seems reasonable to suggest that people tailor their smoking behaviour to obtain a desired physiological (and possibly psychological) effect and that their requirements will differ according to the situation in which they find themselves. Our results indicate that care must always be taken if results of laboratory smoking, during an experiment, are extrapolated to a wider context, and that it is always necessary to consider the ways in which the experimental procedure may itself alter smoking behaviour.

Acknowledgement

We would like to thank Mr. M.J. Derrick, Mrs. U.C. Hopkins, Mrs. J.R.M. Lavier and Miss C.A. Smith for skilled technical assistance.

References

Ashton, H. & Watson, D.W. (1970) Puffing frequency and nicotine intake in cigarette smokers. *British Medical Journal,* **3,** 679-681.

Binnie, C.D. & Comer, A.K. (1978) The effect of cigarette smoking on the contingent negative variation (C.N.V.) and eye movement. *This volume.*

Creighton, D.E., Noble, M.J. & Whewell, R.T. (1978) Instruments to measure, record and duplicate human smoking patterns. *This volume.*

Fuller, R.G.C. & Forrest, D.W. (1973) Behavioural aspects of cigarette smoking in relation to arousal level. *Psychological Reports,* **33,** 115-121.

Glad, W. & Adesso, V.J. (1976) The relative importance of socially induced tension and behavioural contagion for smoking behaviour. *Journal of Abnormal Psychology,* **85,** 119-121.

8. An 'enhancement' model of smoking maintenance?

G L MANGAN AND J GOLDING

Introduction

The research reported in this paper is concerned with factors maintaining smoking behaviour, although these factors obviously play a role in recruitment of the smoking population, and in the difficulties experienced by smokers in giving up.

Currently, the most widely accepted theories of smoking maintenance are the addiction and arousal modulation theories.

Physiological Addication Theories

Physiological addiction theories (Schachter *et al*, 1977, e.g.) postulate that certain CNS receptors, probably located in the median forebrain bundle, become addicted to nicotine, i.e. they signal punishment when the nicotine level at these sites falls below a critical level. From this point of view, we might regard the desire to smoke as a consequence of nicotine 'hunger' in the classical drive sense, the purpose of smoking being to maintain nicotine homeostasis, just as regular heroin injections maintain opiate homeostasis at the CNS opiate receptors.

There are two main lines of evidence supporting an addiction model:

'withdrawal effects' following cessation of smoking;

variations in smoking rate following experimental manipulation of nicotine levels in the smoker.

Despite the fact that behavioural effects such as increases in irritability, in eating, mannerisms, laziness, depression are commonly reported, especially in heavy smokers (Ryan, 1973; Schachter *et al*, 1977), as well as psychophysiological effects, usually in the direction of decreased arousal - lowered frequencies of dominant EEG (Ulett and Itil, 1969; Knott and Venables, 1977), decreased evoked potential envelopes (Hall *et al*, 1973) and reductions in pulse rate and diastolic blood pressure (Knapp, Bliss and Wells, 1963) - there is no evidence of withdrawal effects in any way comparable with those reported by subjects going 'cold turkey' in heroin addiction, or by alcoholics 'drying out'. On this basis, it is also difficult to account for the fact that some smokers can abstain for a day or more with little consciously experienced craving.

Even if significant withdrawal effects were to be demonstrated, however, it is a moot point whether this would constitute direct support for an addiction hypothesis insofar as the total population of smokers is concerned. While such effects may be a 'rebound' phenomenon, suggesting that nicotine tolerance has occurred, particularly in long-term, heavy smokers, it is equally plausible that these effects may signal a return by some subjects to a more 'normal' constitutional level of functioning, a possibility strongly suggested by Brown's (1973) data, comparing EEG characteristics of groups of heavy and light smokers, ex-smokers and non-smokers. Indeed, Brown's (1973) findings may be cited as indirect evidence for an arousal modulation theory of smoking maintainence.

More convincing empirical support comes from studies in which nicotine levels in the smoker are artificially manipulated, and the effects on smoking rate assessed. These may be roughly divided into those studies concerned with *internal,* and those concerned with *external* manipulation of nicotine delivery.

Internal

Direct pharmacological control of nicotine supply to postulated mid-brain receptors has been obtained by intravenous or oral administration of nicotine or lobeline (Lucchesi, Schuster and Emley, 1967), of nicotine receptor antagonists such as mecamylamine, which readily pass the blood-brain barrier (Stolerman *et al,* 1973) or through varying nicotine excretion rates by manipulating urinary pH (Schachter *et al,* 1977). These studies claim to demonstrate that the smoker will adjust his smoking rate in the appropriate direction. Observed changes, however, have been relatively small.

A number of factors, however - two in particular - could have depreciated treatment effects.

In the case of oral ingestion of nicotine or lobeline, since there is considerable degradation by the liver of nicotine before the active molecule can reach the brain, nicotine dosage levels to mimic smoking may have been radically underestimated by experimenters.

With regard to cigarette smoking, nicotine may have to arrive at the CNS receptors in a concentrated bolus form, which suggests the method of pulsed microinjections into the carotid to mimic the *in vivo* effects of cigarette smoking. While Russell (1976) reports minimal effects on smoking of discrete, rapid, intravenous nicotine injections, at a rate designed to mimic *in vivo* 'boli', this may be in part a function of bolus dispersion due to venous mixing.

External

Attempts to vary smoking rate by manipulating the maximum possible nicotine delivery of a cigarette have produced conflicting results. While Frith (1971) and Schachter (1975) report significant variations in number of cigarettes smoked under these conditions, the present authors and Goldfarb, Jarvik and Glick (1970) report no relationship.   There is, however, some relevant evidence concerning smoking style. It has been reported that the number of puffs increases as the nicotine delivery of the cigarette is reduced (Frith, 1971; Ashton and Watson, 1970). It may be that other aspects of smoking style, such as puff strength, for example, are also critical in determining the amount of nicotine extracted from a cigarette.

Another factor, which has general relevance in studies involving manipulation of nicotine delivery, is that smoking quickly acquires secondary reinforcing properties - nicotine is a potent drug, the latency between the conditional stimulus (CS), (lighting up, lip contact, taste, inhalation) and the unconditional stimulus (US) (arrival of nicotine at the appropriate CNS receptors) is short - approximately ten seconds - and the smoker has experienced many thousands of CS-US pairings. Secondary reinforcement undoubtedly operates as a confounding variable when we attempt to measure the effects of manipulation of smoking rates.

Arousal Modulation Theories

Arousal modulation theories suggest that the smoker uses nicotine to maintain a steady state, approximating an 'optimal arousal state' (Berlyne, 1971). Nicotine clearly has both a stimulant and depressant effect on animal brains (Armitage, Hall and Sellers, 1969) depending on dosage (Paton and Perry, 1953; Armitage *et al*, 1969). However, while data from human EEG studies generally support the stimulant effect of nicotine (Phillips, 1971), there is as yet only indirect evidence that nicotine can have a tranquillising effect on the CNS (Brown, 1973).

Nicotine addiction theorists regard these postulated beneficial effects - relaxation or stimulation - as a subjective rationalisation for the feeling of relief produced by the arrival of nicotine at depleted CNS sites. Thus, in learning theory terms, nicotine can be regarded as producing reward more or less directly (arousal modulation), or by avoiding punishment (addiction). Since omission of punishment is regarded by some theorists (e.g. Gray, 1971) as equivalent to reward, the only way to resolve the relative contribution of beneficial arousal effects, compared with avoidance of aversive withdrawal effects, on smoking maintenance, is to compare the effects of smoking on naive smokers, ex-smokers and current smokers. Critical studies on this issue, however, are lacking.

In addition to maintenance of optimal arousal level, however, nicotine facilitates performance in a number of tasks - vigilance (Frankenhaeuser *et al*, 1971), acquisition and retention, in both animal (Garg, 1969 e.g.) and human subjects (Anderson, 1975, for example). The precise mechanisms involved are unknown. It may be that the effect can be accounted for simply in terms of increased arousal, leading to narrowing of the attentional focus (Wachtel, 1967), with consequent improvement in performance. However, this would hardly account for improved retention, as distinct from acquisition. Whatever the case, it seems obvious that arousal modulation (psychological 'comfort') theory of smoking maintenance needs to be broadened to accommodate such enhancement effects on behaviours which have important adaptive significance.

General Research Plan

Five experiments are reported in the present paper. The first concerns the effects of external manipulation of nicotine delivery on smoking rate, where possible confounding variables of taste and inferred strength of cigarette are partialled out. Experiments 2 and 3 examine the effects of smoking on arousal and response suppression, measured in the electrocortical and autonomic systems, under 'neutral' conditions, and under conditions of stress and mild sensory isolation. Experiments 4 and 5 report data on the effects of smoking on vigilance and learning.

Subjects in all these experiments were selected from a pool of forty volunteer habitual smokers (smoking between five and thirty cigarettes a day) in the age range 18-25 years, recruited from undergraduate classes, technical and clerical staff of the department of experimental psychology, and by advertisement from the general public. Subjects in experiments 2 through 5 received a standard payment, and were familiarised with the laboratory environment a few days prior to the experiments. All cigarettes used (apart from experiment 1) were proprietary 1.3 mg nicotine filter tipped cigarettes. Subjects were asked to smoke only 1.3 mg cigarettes for at least three days, to refrain from alcohol or other drugs for one day, and from cigarettes, tea and coffee for at least two hours prior to the experimental sessions.

All psychophysiological responses were recorded on a six channel Devices Model M19 physiograph. All recording and programming equipment was located externally to the test room, which was sound dampened, and maintained at a constant temperature of $21^{\circ}C$.

Experiment 1: Effects of external manipulation of nicotine delivery on smoking rate

Design

The present study was undertaken to test predictions from the smoking maintenance models described. The design called for subjects (Ss) to *ad lib* smoke anonymised cigarettes, which did not differ in taste or draw resistance but did differ in nicotine content.

Procedure

Ss were invited to participate in a market research exercise involving judgement of the taste of three brands of commercially available cigarettes. They were asked to neither give, nor accept cigarettes from others during the test run.

Each night S rated the taste of the day's cigarette and his general mood on a seven point scale. The mood scale was anchored by the descriptive terms 'depressed, irritable' at value 1, and 'buoyant, elated' at value 7.

S was informed that since taste is affected by the number of cigarettes consumed, it was important to record cigarette consumption, so that each day he was to return any unused cigarettes from the previous day's supply. As an incentive, he was told that the number returned each day would be recorded, and that at the end of the experiment he would be credited with the number returned, but of his preferred brand. From post-experimental enquiry, no S appeared to be aware of the real nature of the experiment, nor did any suggest that smoking rate was suppressed to build up a surplus of preferred cigarettes. Subsequently, when Ss were informed about the real purpose of the experiment, many commented that they detected little difference between the brands, which in most cases appeared to be similar to those they normally smoked.

The four brands used yielded 0.9 (A), 1.1 and 1.3 (B) and 1.7 (C) mg/nicotine per cigarette. In a pre-test, 12 Ss had been unable to discriminate between these four brands in terms of taste, 'strength' or draw resistance. All brands were filter tipped, and measured 53, 50, 49 and 50 mm respectively. All cigarettes were anonymised by covering exactly 10 mm immediately above the filter with a strip of gummed paper.

In Series 1, Ss were 10 males and 11 females. For the male group, the 0.9, 1.1 and 1.7 mg/nicotine brands were used, and for female Ss, the 0.9, 1.3 and 1.7 mg/nicotine brands. For each S, brands were counterbalanced over the six day run, using an abccba sequence, with all possible abc combinations. Mean nicotine/tar consumption per day for each S was calculated by multiplying the number of cigarettes smoked by nicotine/tar delivery (mg) for that brand, and by a factor of either 0.811, 0.80, 0.796 or 0.80 respectively, to compensate for the amount of shortening due to the anonymising procedure.

In Series 2, the same procedure was adopted, except that Ss smoked only brands A and C, each brand for four consecutive days. Brands were counterbalanced. Ss were five males and four females.

Results

Series 1

Mean number of cigarettes smoked by male and female Ss, and daily average consumption of nicotine/tar over the six day period, by brand, are shown in Table 8.1.

The t tests of differences between means of the three brands for male and female groups, and for total sample, were non-significant. Irrespective of the amount of nicotine/tar ingested, Ss maintained a stable consumption rate over the six day period, which did not differ very greatly from estimated normal consumption.

Figures for the four heaviest and the four lightest smokers were independently analysed. Results replicated those for the total sample - both light and heavy smokers maintained a stable rate of consumption, which was unrelated to brand of cigarette.

Mood ratings for the six days are presented in Table 8.2.

Table 8.1 Mean numbers of cigarettes smoked per day, by brand, and average nicotine/tar consumption, in mgs, for male and female Ss over the six day run.

| | Brand | | | Estimated Daily Consumption |
	A (0.9mg)	B (1.3mg)	C (1.7mg)	
Males	20.1	21.7	20.6	19.0
Females	18.7	17.8	19.1	18.2

	Estimated mgs nicotine/tar ingested			
Males	14.7/235.2	19.1/312.4	28.0/395.5	24.7/361
Females	13.7/212.9	18.4/256.3	25.9/366.7	23.6/345.8

Table 8.2 Mood ratings for days on which different brands were smoked for male and female Ss.

| | Brand | | |
	A	B	C
Male	3.95	3.74	4.00
Females	4.95	4.82	4.73

Clearly, there are large between-sex mood differences, but these are of no immediate concern. Within-sex, there are no significant differences in rated mood, as a function of brand smoked, when tested by t test.

Series 2
Results, which are presented in Table 8.3, are very similar to those reported in Series 1.

Table 8.3 Mean consumption of low (A) and high (C) nicotine/tar yield cigarettes over the eight day period.

			Brand				
	A Day				C Day		
1	2	3	4	5	6	7	8
20.0	22.25	22.75	22.0	19.75	21.75	22.5	22.5
Mean:	21.75 (15.9/264.7)			Mean:	21.6 (29.4/414.6)		

Estimated mean consumption for sample, 20.0 (26.0/390)

	C Day				A Day		
1	2	3	4	5	6	7	8
22.3	22.6	24.8	24.4	24.8	25.2	23.4	21.2
Mean:	23.6 (32.1/453)			Mean:	23.6 (17.2/287.3)		

Esimated mean consumption for sample, 23.0 (39.1/448.4)

In both sequences, amount consumed on the fifth day - the first day following the change to the stronger or weaker cigarette - did not differ significantly from mean rates recorded for the preceeding days when tested by t test.

Conclusions

It is not suggested that the present study is a critical test of the addiction hypothesis. Despite the fact that this group of Ss normally ingest approximately 24 mg nicotine per day, it is possible that the 14 mg ingested while they were smoking the low nicotine yield cigarettes was sufficient to maintain nicotine homeostasis. It is also possible, of course, that Ss were managing to compensate for the differences in nicotine delivery between brands by means of smoking style - variations in puff rate, strength, duration and depth of inhalation. In this case, however, one might ask why these Ss habitually smoke middle nicotine/tar yield cigarettes, which are not discriminably different, in an addictive sense, from safer low nicotine/tar yield cigarettes.

The absence of within-sex differences in rated mood when Ss were smoking low nicotine yield cigarettes would also suggest tentatively that nicotine is not a critical factor in mood control. Again, of course, we might comment that mood control may require nicotine ingestion equivalent to, or less than that offered by the lowest nicotine yield cigarette.

These reservations notwithstanding, the obvious implication of the present results is that the addictive element in smoking cigarettes appears much less pronounced than a simple addictive model would suggest, certainly not strong enough to endorse the rather simple-minded hypothesis that when subjects smoke cigarettes offering a substantially lower nicotine yield than those to which they are accustomed, they increase their consumption to maintain nicotine homeostasis.

Experiment 2: Effects of smoking on measures of arousal, response suppression and excitation/inhibition balance

The fact that nicotine increases cortical arousal is well attested from both animal (Armitage et al , 1969; Cheshire, Kellett and Willey, 1973) and human studies (Murphree, Pfeiffer and Price, 1967; Philips, 1971; Brown, 1973; Knott and Venables, 1977), arousal being measured by EEG desynchronisation, attenuation or frequency shift of alpha activity.   A similar inference might also be derived from studies reporting decreased arousal as one consequence of giving up smoking (Knapp et al, 1963; Ulett and Itil, 1969; Hall et al, 1973; Knott and Venables, 1977). We note, however, that in all the animal, and in most of the human studies, nicotine supply is maintained by intravenous or oral administration, and, as previously mentioned, this procedure could produce somewhat different results from those obtained from smoking cigarettes.

The depressant effect of nicotine on human EEG, however, is less well established. The only relevant studies, to the author's knowledge, are reports by Ashton et al, (1974) of reduction in contingent negative variation (CNV) - although precisely what the CNV is measuring is open to some question - and by Friedman, Harvath and Meares,(1974) of a significant acceleration of habituation rate, measured by the alpha-block component of orienting response to auditory stimuli, following smoking.   Although Murphree et al, (1967) generally conclude that smoking has a stimulant rather than depressant effect on human EEG, some of their Ss demonstrated a depressant effect. They suggest that the effects of drugs on the CNS are dependent to some degree on the state of S before dosage, an observation which has also been made in a number of animal studies (cf. Domino, 1973, e.g.).

Clearly, there is some uncertainty about whether, and under what conditions, stimulant or depressant effects can be expected from smoking. Dosage, and the state of S before dosage, may be important factors. The latter condition, however, has seldom been manipulated in smoking research. Another difficulty in interpreting available research findings is that the response measure, particularly with human Ss, has been electro-cortical. And although theories of general arousal still enjoy a wide acceptance, the weight of psychophysiological evidence suggests that the various arousal subsystems - electro-cortical, autonomic and somatic - may not be totally synergistic.

Design

The present study aimed to investigate the effects of smoking on phasic responding, response suppression, and excitation/inhibition balance under 'neutral' conditions, using measures of autonomic arousal. Electrodermal reactivity was selected as response measure, since approximately 90 - 95% of Ss show electrodermal reactivity to stimulus onset (Venables, 1977), percentages being considerably lower in other response modes.

Three measures were employed - skin conductance response (SCR), measured as initial amplitude of orienting response to neutral tones, which is considered to reflect phasic arousability (Mangan, 1974), orienting response (OR) habituation rate, which indexes speed of development of internal or extinctive inhibition (Nebylitsyn, 1972), and rate of spontaneous fluctuations (SF) or SCR in resting Ss, which is regarded as a measure of excitation/inhibition balance, or the relative stability of excitatory and inhibitory processes (Koepke & Pribram, 1966).

The Spiral After-Effect (SAE) was also included as a dependent variable. SAE refers to the movement after-effect following fixation of a previously rotated Archimedes Spiral, which is thought to be due to adaptation of the neurones responsive to movement in the appropriate visual field. Removal of the adapting stimulus produces a movement after-effect, due to the release of units signalling movement in the opposite direction from lateral inhibition of the previously adapted units (Gregory, 1972).

SAE decline following massed trials has been considered a measure of reactive inhibition (Eysenck, 1967) and SAE recovery as a measure of dissipation of inhibition following a rest pause. Stimulant and depressant drugs appear to affect SAE in the expected direction - stimulant drugs such as d-amphetamine and caffeine increasing the duration of the SAE, and depressant drugs such as amytal or mepro-bromate decreasing duration (Eysenck and Easterbrook, 1960). On this basis, we might expect cigarettes to shorten or lengthen SAE duration, depending on whether nicotine is acting as a stimulant or depressant.

Procedure

Electrodermal responding

Twelve Ss were tested, using a counterbalanced design, in two sessions, one week apart. In the treatment session, S smoked one cigarette in the ten minute interval immediately prior to tone presentation. In the control session, S relaxed for ten minutes.

SCR was recorded using a preamplifier sensitivity of 1 mm of pen deflection equal to 500 ohms. Ag-AgC1 cup electrodes, in contact with standard electrolyte jelly, were fixed by adhesive discs above the whorls of the finger tips to the first and third fingers of S's left hand. The electrode area was 0.7 cm^2, and an impressed current of $8 \mu A$ DC produced a current density of $11.4 \mu A \text{ cm}^2$.

Amplitude criterion for evoked SCRs was change in log conductance equivalent to a pen deflection of 1 mm at the lowest resistance expressed by any S in the sample (20 K Ohms). The criterion was 0.011 log μmhos. SCRs greater than 0.011 log μmhos occurring within the period 1 to 5 sec from stimulus onset, using as baseline values tonic skin conductance level (SCL) in the 5 sec period preceding the stimulus, were judged to be changes evoked by the stimulus.

Procedure and equipment for measuring auditory SCRs, habituation rate and spontaneous fluctuation rate have been described fully elsewhere (Siddle and Mangan, 1971). The stimuli in the two series, 2 sec tones of frequencies 1000 and 360Hz, intensity 60 dB (re .0002 dyne/cm^2) were randomly ordered at intervals of 18, 20 and 22 sec. These were delivered to S through a set of stereophonic earphones from a Sony tape recorder.

SCR was recorded as the mean of the first two trials. Primary habituation was judged to have occurred when S recorded three consecutive response failures. SF rate was calculated by comparing the number of above-criterion responses in the first and last two minutes of the ten minute control or treatment sessions preceding tone presentation. Under the treatment condition, S smoked a cigarette in the intervening six minutes.

SAE

Twelve Ss were tested in two sessions, one week apart, using a counterbalanced design. On both occasions S received five massed SAE trials, followed by a ten minute period in which S either smoked one cigarette (treatment) or relaxed (control). A further five massed SAE trials followed.

The spiral, reproduced from Robbins *et al*, (1959) was rotated in a clockwise direction at 100 rpm for 30 sec under standard illumination. Following a demonstration of the effect, S, who was seated 2 m from the spiral, was instructed to concentrate on the centre of the spiral, to report onset of apparent movement, and the point at which the after-effect (contraction) appeared to stop. This procedure was followed for the two blocks of five trials in each session, the blocks being separated by a ten minute interval. Within each block of trials the inter-trial interval (ITI) was 20 sec.

Three SAE values were calculated under each condition.

Decline within first and second blocks of trials, measured as ratio of duration of effect on trials 1 and 2 to duration of effect on trials 4 and 5 (6 + 7: 9 + 10).

SAE recovery, measured as ratio of SAE duration on trials 6 and 7 (post-rest) to duration on trials 4 and 5.

Results

SCR data

Initial amplitude of OR (mean of first two trials) was significantly smaller under treatment than under control conditions. Means were 5.13K ohms and 8.58K ohms respectively, the differences being significant (t = 2.58, p $<$0.05). Thus, under these conditions, phasic arousal appears to be significantly depressed.

Mean number of trials to OR habituation in the control and treatment conditions were 8.8 and 3.2 respectively. Differences between conditions are significantly different (t = 3.68, p$<$0.01). In line with studies of habituation of electro-cortical responses following smoking (Friedman *et al*, 1974, e.g.), in the present case habituation of the electrodermal component of OR is significantly accelerated under treatment condition.

Rates of spontaneous fluctuation in SCR in the initial and final two minute epochs of the ten minute period preceding tone presentation in both control and treatment sessions were calculated.

In the control condition there is no significant change from first to second epoch. Under treatment, however, there is a highly significant reduction in SF rate in the second, compared with the first epoch (t = 4.17, p$<$0.01), and in the second treatment epoch compared with the second control epoch (t = 4.65, p$<$0.01) when tested by t test.

SAE data

SAE duration over the two blocks of five trials under control and treatment conditions are shown in Figure 8.1.

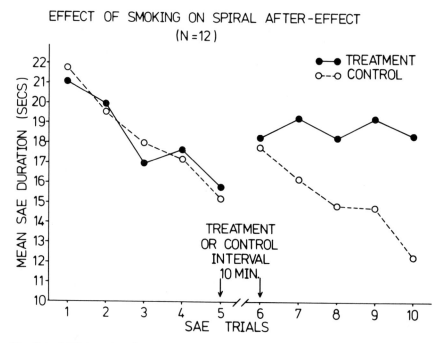

Fig. 8.1 SAE duration for treatment and control groups.

From the graph, the expected decline in SAE duration is evident over the first block of five trials under both conditions. Values between conditions are not significantly different when tested by t test. Following treatment, or control rest pause during the ten minutes between blocks, there is clearly substantial recovery, although treatment and control Ss are not significantly different on trial 6. However, during trials 7 - 10, the treatment group maintains SAE, whereas the control group shows a significant decline. Differences in SAE decline between treatment and control data are highly significant when tested by t test (p$<$0.01).

Conclusions

Results from the two sets of data, superficially at least, appear to be somewhat contradictory. Smoking a 1.3 mg nicotine cigarette immediately prior to tone presentation appears to significantly depress SCR to initial stimuli, to accelerate habituation rate, which can be regarded as a measure of rate of development of internal or extinctive inhibition, and to smooth out transient fluctuations in arousal, as measured by spontaneous fluctuation rate.

The results of smoking versus control, therefore, seem to be to swing the excitation/inhibition balance of the electrodermal system in the direction of inhibition, a result which is consistent with Friedman et al's (1974) finding that habituation rate to non-aversive tone stimuli, measured by EEG desynchronisation, is hastened by cigarette smoking. These latter data also add some substance to our claim that the effect is not simply due to nicotine acting peripherally on the electrodermal system by cutaneous vasoconstriction, an effect which is well established (Sarin, 1974).

On the other hand, smoking appears to prevent the buildup of inhibition when measured by SAE decline (trials 6 - 10), rather than increasing the dissipation of inhibition, as measured by 'recovery' from trial 5 to trial 6. On the basis of the electrodermal data, we might have expected a greater recovery effect when comparing treatment with control.

The reasons for this are not at all obvious. We might comment, however, that in the habituation series, S was instructed not to attend to the stimuli, while in the SAE experiment he was required to report the beginning and termination of the after-effect. Possibly the different task demands account for the different effects reported.

Experiment 3: Psychophysiological effects of smoking under conditions of stress and mild sensory isolation

Arguing from arousal modulation theory, and in view of the reported findings from animal studies that the effects of nicotine are biphasic, i.e. can be stimulant or depressant, depending on dosage (Armitage et al, 1969), it was hypothesised that under conditions of stress and mild sensory isolation, S will attempt to manipulate his level of arousal to maintain an optimal state through self-titration with nicotine.

As to the actual method of self-titration, a number of possibilities suggest themselves. The most obvious is that S attempts to bring himself to the stimulant (low nicotine) or depressant (high nicotine) portions of the biphasic dose-response curve by manipulating one or more of the smoking style variables - frequency, strength and duration of puffing. Data relevant to this issue were also examined in this study.

Design

Twenty-four Ss were randomly allocated to one of three groups (N = 8 in each case).

'Real smoking' group, where each S smoked a cigarette during the indicated period;

'Activity control' group, where S sham-smoked an unlit cigarette (puffed and inhaled as in normal smoking), while smoke from a lit cigarette in the ash-tray floated around;

'Situation control' group, where S did nothing, but was told that he was one of a control group, and that the two light flashes were presented to equate conditions between groups.

There were two conditions within the experiment. In the sensory isolation (SI) condition, S lay on a soft bed with head supported by a low pillow, and with eyes open. After twenty minutes relaxation, the last five minutes of which were taken as the baseline period, S smoked a cigarette for five minutes (or sham-smoked, or did nothing), onset and termination of this period being indicated by light flashes. S then relaxed for a further seven minutes.

In the stress (ST) condition, bursts of white noise were relayed through earphones at randomly determined points throughout the 15 minute experimental period. S smoked (or sham-smoked, or did nothing) during the middle five minute period, the beginning and end of which were indicated as in the SI condition, by light flashes.

The total duration of white noise during the 15 minute experimental period was 61 sec, distributed randomly in 23 episodes, of duration 1, 2, 3 or 4 sec. Tone onset and duration were controlled by a tape programmer and solid-state logic, and displayed on a polygraph marker channel from associated relay equipment. White noise was at an intensity 106 dB (re.0002 dyne/cm^2) as rated by a Dawe sound level meter located at the earphones.

The order of the two conditions was randomised between Ss to avoid serial order effects. During the twenty minute interval between conditions S relaxed and talked with the experimenter.

Data analysis

Electrodermal (SC) and electroencephalographic (EEG) responses were recorded throughout the sessions. Concerning SCR, methodology has been described in Experiment 2. The only additional response taken was SCL in the SI condition. This was read at every 10 sec event mark throughout the 17 minute period, except where such points coincided with S's actual smoking. Mean SCL values for successive 30 sec periods were derived from these readings. Units of measurement, as before, were logμmhos.

EEG was recorded using SLE miniature electrodes placed in the midline frontal and left occipital areas (F_z and 0_1, Jasper, 1958) referenced to the opposite mastoid (A_2). The recording channel was filtered for 8 - 13 Hz activity, calibrated to yield a pen deflection of 1.5 cm for an average peak alpha burst. Care was taken to ensure that any large 8 - 13 Hz output was not the result of any 13 - 14 Hz spindle activity. The calibration was performed during the eyes open baseline period preceding the relevant experimental condition.

An arbitrary criterion of 0.75 cm was employed so that alpha activity had to be at least 50% of the average peak amplitude to be counted. Bursts of 8 - 13 Hz alpha waves during one sec intervals constituted an alpha unit. The total record for each condition was utilised. The five minutes preceding the two experimental periods were employed to establish baseline values. Percentage alpha deviation from baseline values were plotted in one minute blocks.

Puff frequencies were recorded for both smoking and sham-smoking groups throughout the session.

Results

Psychophysiological variables

Results are presented in Figures 8.2, 8.3 and 8.4.

Analyses of variance were computed on EEG, SCR and SCL data. Results were as follows.

EEG: Main effects and order effects were non-significant. The following interactions were significant: condition x activity (5% level, $F = 3.55$, df 2, 18), condition x period (1% level, F 13.15, df 2, 76), and condition x period x activity (5% level F 2.63, df 4, 76). From inspection of means and from the appropriate t tests calculated, it is clear that the main effect occurs during the smoking period, as a function of condition, period and activity.

SCR: The main effects for activity ($F = 4.78$, df 2, 21) and for period ($F = 32.42$, df 2, 42) are significant at the 5% and 1% levels respectively. The period x activity interaction is also significant (5% level, $F = 3.13$, df 4, 42). These results suggest that the main source of variation is between sham and real smoking, versus situation control activity, during the smoking period, and, to a lesser extent, during the pre-smoking period.

SCL: The main effect for period is marginally significant at the 5% level ($F = 2.91$, df 2, 40) and the period by activity interaction significant at the 5% level ($F = 3.39$, df 4, 42). From inspection of means and from the t tests calculated, these results suggest that the main source of variation is real smoking during both the smoking and post-smoking periods.

Overall, the most striking feature of the psychophysiological data is the reversal of the EEG effect for real and sham-smoking according to condition. It is obvious that percentage alpha is increased during stress, and decreased during sensory isolation by smoking. The activity control produces similar but smaller effects to real smoking. In the situation control, the only significant change is that between the second and third five minute periods. This is presumably the effect of the second signal to S (cf. procedural details), which may produce relief at the knowledge that the session will finish in another five minutes or so.

The fact that the activity control group produce roughly 50% of the real smoking effect suggests that some of the effects of the latter are due simply to activity - to having an object to manipulate, for example. Many Ss stated that the reason they found smoking in a stress situation relaxing was that it diverted their attention. It is also likely that the smell of smoke, puffing, and the sight of the cigarette itself is a conditional stimulus (CS) producing a conditioned response (CR) (change in arousal level), which is part of the activity control effect.

As regards the role of nicotine, undoubtedly this accounts for some of the difference between sham and real smoking. Under the SI condition the alpha-blocking effect from real smoking lasts well into the seven minute post smoking period. This is probably the time required for nicotine clearance. This, however, is not the case

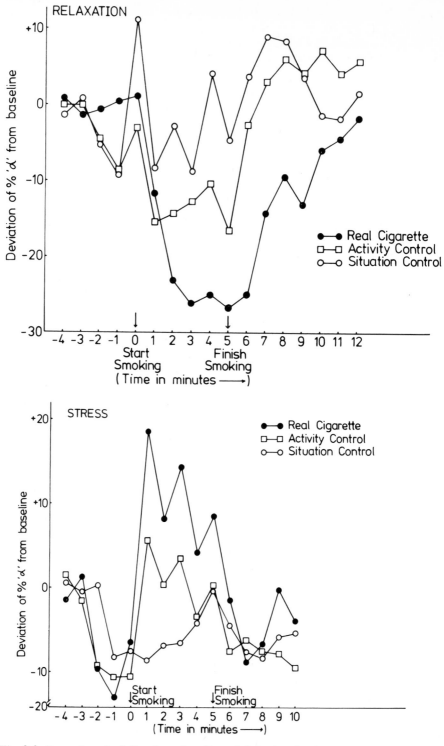

Fig. 8.2 Percentage deviation from baseline of alpha for the three groups under conditions of stress and sensory isolation.

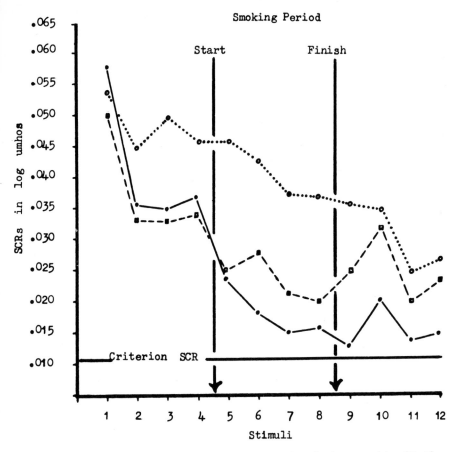

Fig. 8.3 SCRs to aversive stimuli for real smoking (●—●), sham smoking (□··□) and situation control (O-O) groups.

in the ST condition, which may reflect the shorter clearance time for nicotine during stress, because of heart rate acceleration due to white noise, for example.

Smoking style variables
Puff frequency data are shown in Table 8.4. Although real and sham smokers puffed

Table 8.4 Puff frequencies under stress and sensory isolation conditions.

	Stress	Sensory Isolation	p
Real	10.3	8.9	NS
Sham	11.1	9.9	NS

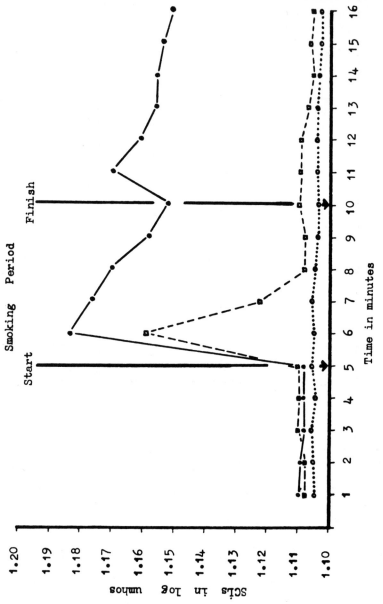

Fig. 8.4 SCLs for real smoking (●——●) sham smoking (□··□) and situation control (O·O) groups throughout the 16 minute sensory isolation period.

more frequently under stress than under sensory isolation, the differences between conditions are not significant.

In a subsequent experiment, which is not reported in this paper, but which replicated the present design, similar puff frequency data were reported; in this case the critical smoking style variable is puff strength, measured by pressure drop in a plumbed cigarette holder. Relevant data are shown in Table 8.5.

Table 8.5 Differences in smoking style variables between real and sham smoking Ss under conditions of stress and sensory isolation.

Real smoking		Stress	Sensory Isolation	p
Puff frequency	N	15.75	13.75	NS
Puff strength	mm/merc.	1.062	0.772	0.001
Puff duration	sec	2.19	2.07	NS
Butt weight	gms	0.61	0.55	0.05
Sham smoking				
Puff frequency	N	18.71	14.71	NS
Puff strength	mm/merc.	1.166	0.843	0.01
Puff duration	sec	2.19	2.30	NS

Note also that sham smokers have a significantly higher puff rate under both stress (F = 7.44, df 6, 11, p<0.01) and sensory isolation (F = 4.56, df. 11, 6, p<0.05), suggesting an overshoot when the sham smoking - predictably - fails to produce the desired effect. Sham smokers also puff more strongly than real smokers under both stress and sensory isolation conditions, but in neither case are the differences significant.

The question of how these postulated nicotine effects are mediated remains unanswered. Nicotine is well documented as a CNS stimulant, having an effect mainly on the ascending reticular activating system (ARAS). Thus the alpha-blocking caused by smoking in the SI condition is to be expected. In the stress condition it is possible that nicotine is producing the relaxation effect by blockading the neuro-muscular junction or ganglions, an effect which has been reported by Goodman and Gilman (1971) and Domino and von Baumgarten (1969), thus relieving some of the muscular tensions. This in turn would reduce the feedback of neurones monitoring muscular tensions into the ARAS, the balance between the central and peripheral effects of nicotine leading to the direction of observed change in alpha.

Experiment 4: The effects of smoking on vigilance performance

Some evidence has been reported that smoking improves performance on a prolonged vigilance task (Heimstra, Bancroft and Dekock, 1967; Frankenhaeuser et al, 1971). The reasons for this, however, are unclear, in view of the fact that other data reported point to effects which render untenable the obvious interpretation - that increased arousal increases alertness.

The results of Experiment 2, and those reported by Friedman *et al,* (1974) demonstrate that smoking reduces SF rate and accelerates habituation, i.e. rate of inhibitory growth. These psychophysiological measures have been shown to be consistently and significantly correlated (Koepke and Pribram, 1966; Bohlin, 1976 e.g.), high SF rate being associated with slow habituation rate. It has also been reported, however, that fast habituation rate in the modality of the target stimuli predicts poor vigilance behaviour (Siddle, 1972), due to generalised inhibition which interferes with detection of such stimuli. On this basis, we might predict that smoking, since it facilitates inhibitory growth, should produce poorer vigilance behaviour.

No explanation for this conflict of evidence is immediately obvious. The experimental tasks, of course, are quite different - in typical habituation studies, S is instructed to ignore the (non-signal) stimuli, while in vigilance experiments, S is required to attend to all stimuli, and to respond appropriately to those differing from background stimuli in some designated fashion. We might suggest that enhanced vigilance performance following smoking could be due to increased arousal improving detectibility, or to a more stable excitatory/inhibitory balance (i.e. fewer spontaneous fluctuations) reducing the frequency of false positives.

The latter alternative is suggested in animal data reported by Nelsen and Goldstein (1973). They report that nicotine significantly reduces errors of commission (corresponding to our false positives), while having no effect on correct responding (detection rate) in an 'attention' task.

The present experiment was planned to examine these possibilities.

Design

Twelve Ss were used. Each was tested in two sessions, one week apart, using a counterbalanced design. In one of the sessions, S smoked a cigarette in a ten minute period prior to the vigilance task (treatment), in the other he relaxed during the ten minute period (control). 600 events - 360 Hz or 1000 Hz tones (frequency was counterbalanced within Ss and between sessions) of 60 dB intensity - were presented at a rate of one every three sec. Thirty target stimuli, signal tones of the same frequency, but of 65dB intensity, were randomly positioned throughout the series. S's task was to press the button provided in response to every target stimulus.

S was given two practice periods. In the first of these, twenty pairs of 60 and 65 dB tones were presented in a paired comparisons sequence to give S experience of the intensity differences involved. In the second practice period, sixty background and five interspersed target stimuli were presented, and S given knowledge of his performance.

Results

Relevant data are presented in Figures 8.5 and 8.6. Treatment appears to have little effect on errors of omission - detection rate - compared to control, when measured by t test (t = 1.03, NS). However, smoking significantly decreases the number of errors of commission - false positives (t = 6.35 p<0.001).

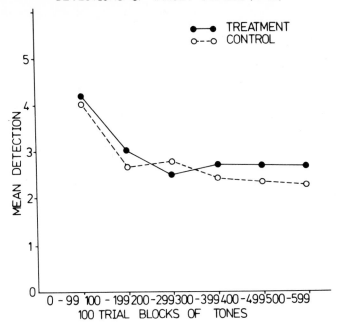

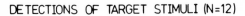

Fig. 8.5 Detection rate of target stimuli for treatment and control groups.

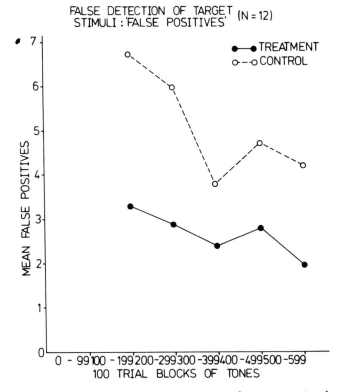

Fig. 8.6 False detection (false positive) frequency for treatment and control groups.

d^1 values were calculated using Swets (1964) tables. This value takes into account both correct detections and false positives. d^1 values for treatment and control conditions are significantly different when tested by t test (t = 4.80, p 0.001).

These results indicate conclusively that under the experimental conditions, smoking improves vigilance performance by decreasing S's false positive rate rather than by improving his detection rate.

Experiment 5: The effects of smoking on acquisition and retention in verbal learning tasks

A good deal of evidence from rat studies indicates that nicotine may facilitate acquisition and retention in various learning tasks - maze learning (Garg, 1969), shock avoidance (Domino, 1973; Evangelista, Gattoni and Izquierdo, 1970), operant behaviour such as bar pressing to obtain water (Morrison, 1967; 1968) and visual discrimination (Bovet-Nitti, 1969) for example. The effect seems to be biphasic i.e. facilitatory or inhibitory, depending on dosage, although the relevant data are difficult to evaluate, primarily because different investigators have employed different routes and rates of nicotine injection.

A number of findings, however, seem relatively clearcut and unambiguous. Small doses of nicotine facilitate, and larger doses inhibit acquisition of active avoidance (pole jump response) in the rat (Domino, 1973). Large doses also seem to depress established avoidance behaviour (Domino, 1973). Finally, improved consolidation measured, for example by greater retention of shuttle box learning following post-trial injections of nicotine, seems well established (Evangelista *et al,* 1970).

With human Ss, there is some evidence that smoking impairs verbal rote learning, but improves subsequent recall (Andersson, 1975), suggesting an effect on consolidation. There is also evidence that smoking interferes with incidental learning in an immediate serial recall task (Andersson and Hockey, 1977).

In the present experiment, we examined the effects of smoking on acquisition and consolidation in two verbal learning tasks, paired associate learning and serial learning.

Design
Paired-associate learning
The stimuli were sets of twenty monosyllabic words selected randomly from Waugh's (1961) list, approximately matched for frequency of usage in printed English. Both high and low interference lists were constructed. For the low interference condition, the associations within pairs, and between members of different pairs, were low, for example

shoe   bean
hike   pick

while in five of the ten pairs in the high interference list, the associations between members of different pairs were high, for example

miss   white
black   take

Twelve Ss were tested in four sessions, one week apart, using a counterbalanced design.   In one session, high interference, and in the second, low interference lists were learned to a criterion of two successive error-free trials.   In the remaining two sessions, the procedure was repeated, but each S had a cigarette during the ten minute interval before the session.

The pairs of words were presented on a memory drum, one word every three seconds, using a serial anticipation method.   After S had reached the criterion level of response, he was given a book and asked to read for thirty minutes, at which point he was retested.

Results
Data for both high and low interference lists, under treatment and control conditions, are presented in Figures 8.7 and 8.8.

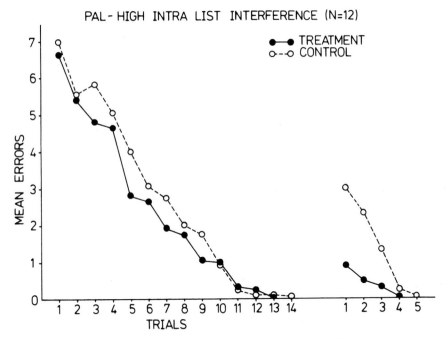

Fig. 8.7 Error frequency for treatment and control groups on high interference lists.

There are no significant differences in acquisition rate between treatment and control conditions, for either high or low interference lists, when number of trials to criterion are compared, using t test.   Not unexpectedly, control Ss learned the low interference lists significantly faster than the high interference lists ($t = 4.09$, $p < 0.001$), although differences in learning rate under treatment condition are not significant.

When retention is measured after the thirty minute rest period, highly significant differences emerge between conditions.   There are significantly fewer errors under

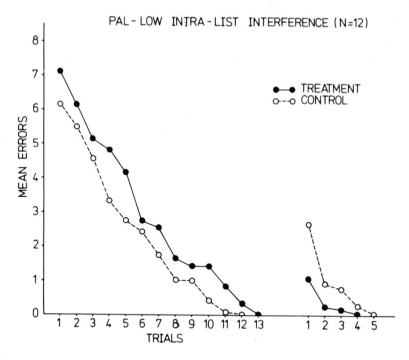

Fig. 8.8 Error frequency for treatment and control groups in low interference lists.

treatment than under control conditions for both low (t = 2.72, p <0.01) and high (t = 7.45, p <0.001) interference lists.

It seems clear, therefore, that smoking significantly improves consolidation, more particularly in the case of high interference lists. From the graphs, initial learning of low interference lists is impaired - though not significantly - by smoking, a finding similar to that reported by Andersson (1975). However, smoking improves the initial learning - though again not significantly - of high interference lists. It might be that smoking focusses attention on the immediate task demand, thus reducing the interference caused by high association values between stimulus members of different pairs. This inhibition of 'irrelevant' features of the stimulus array is congruent with the finding that smoking reduces recall of irrelevant information (Andersson and Hockey, 1977).

Serial learning

Eight Ss were tested in two sessions, one week apart, using a counterbalanced design. Stimuli were two sets, each of 12 lists (four practice, eight experimental) of twenty words, randomly selected from Waugh's (1961) list. In each session, the words were presented to S in a memory drum, one word every three sec, and S recorded his responses immediately following each trial. The inter-trial interval was 30 sec.

In one session, S smoked a cigarette immediately prior to the task.
Recall was measured as number of words correctly identified from each list.
Correct responses were allocated to primacy, intermediate and recency categories,
using as cut-off point a 4/8/8 split.
Frequencies in the primacy category were doubled for comparison purposes.
Results are shown in Figure 8.9.

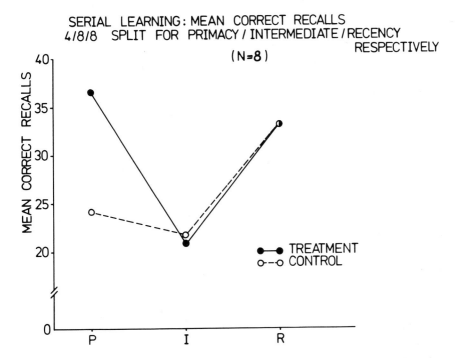

Fig. 8.9 Effects of smoking in primacy, intermediate and recency in serial learning.

The only difference between control and treatment data is the significant increase
in mean number of correct recalls in the primacy category (t = 6.07, p<0.001).
Clearly the facilitatory effect of smoking is shown on long rather than short term
memory.

Summary and discussion

The general thrust of the results reported in this paper is to demonstrate that smoking
has beneficial effects in both the short and long term. Clearly, smoking confers some
advantage in coping with extremes of arousal, thus contributing to psychological
'comfort', and enhances various types of performance over a longer time scale.
From the overall results, a number of conclusions about mechanisms mediating
these beneficial effects seem justified.
1. Experiments 1 and 3 are taken as strong evidence for the secondary reinforcing
nature of the smoking behaviour itself. Thus we would assert that while some

compensation for varying nicotine yield in Experiment 1 could occur by changes in smoking style, the major reason for the lack of control exerted by varying nicotine yield on smoking rates is the strong secondary reinforcing nature of smoking behaviour. Such secondary reinforcement, we believe, accounts for the observation that in Experiment 3 'Activity Control' accounts for roughly half the difference observed between 'Real' smoking and 'Situation Control' Ss. This is spite of the fact that sham smoking is only a very poor approximation to a true placebo, which would evoke the full conditioned response.

2. Some of the improvements observed in the performance measures of experiments 4 and 5 appear to issue from psychophysiological effects initially observed in experiment 2. Thus smoking could be improving vigilance behaviour by inhibiting momentary imbalances in autonomic arousal. During the vigilance task skin conductance measures were taken, and it was observed that false positives occurred most often immediately following a spontaneous fluctuation (Figure 8.10).

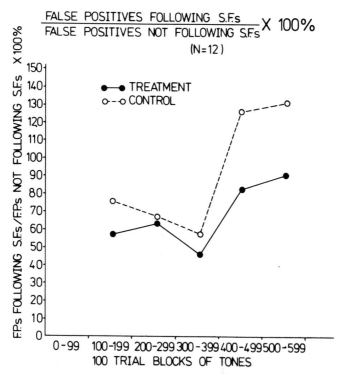

Fig. 8.10 False positives following SFs under treatment and control conditions.

A momentary increase in arousal prior to a stimulus may result in a 60dB tone appearing to be more intense. Since S is alert to a slight increase in the intensity of the tone stimulus - a target - he might well make a false positive response at this juncture.

Since we know from experiment 2 that spontaneous fluctuations are significantly reduced by smoking, it seems reasonable to infer that in the vigilance experiment, smoking was reducing the number of false positives by increasing the stability of the autonomic arousal system. At first sight this relationship has a paradoxical quality, since it is generally known that fast habituation rates and low spontaneous fluctuations predict poor vigilance performance. However, efficiency of vigilance, d^1, involved a trade-off between detections and false positives. In this experiment, reduction in false positives wins out, possibly due to the low number of target stimuli, and the difficulty in discriminating between target and non-target stimuli (65 dB versus 60 dB).

3. The smoking style data from experiment 3 indicate that S titrates himself with nicotine to produce the desired arousal or dearousal effect largely by varying strength of puff, rather than puff frequency or puff duration.

4. It seems clear that smoking, while having little effect on acquisition in verbal learning tasks, significantly improves consolidation, more so with high than with low interference lists. The neural mechanisms involved can only be surmised; this is hardly surprising, however, in view of the current general state of ignorance about the consolidation process.

It is, of course, theoretically possible that what we are regarding as enhancement effects from smoking are really decremented performance from the non-smoking, i.e. control Ss, due to nicotine withdrawal. To the extent that this is true, the data reported would generally support an addiction theory of smoking maintenance. While we would suggest that withdrawal effects are hardly likely to be experienced within two hours, we acknowledge that the only way to resolve this dilemma is to establish and compare psychophysiological and performance base rates from longitudinal studies of smokers at different stages in the course of their smoking habit - for example, at stages of naive, light and heavy smoking, and possibly after giving up.

On balance, however, we feel that the data reported support an arousal modulation rather than an addiction model of smoking maintenance, although, as previously suggested, a more robust model to incorporate performance enhancement as well as psychological comfort factors seems necessary to accommodate the penumbra of variables underlying smoking maintenance.

Acknowledgement

The research reported in this paper was completed during the tenure by the senior author of an SSRC Fellowship in the Psychology of Smoking.

References

Andersson, K. (1975) Effects of cigarette smoking on learning and retention. *Psychopharmacologia,* **41**, 1-5.

Andersson, K. & Hockey, G.R. (1977) Effects of cigarette smoking in incidental memory. *Psychopharmacologia,* **52**, 223-226.

Armitage, A.K., Hall, G.H. & Sellers, C.M. (1969) Effects of nicotine on electrocortical activity and acetylcholine release from the cat cerebral cortex. *British Journal of Pharmacology and Chemotherapy,* **35**, 152-160.

E

Ashton, H. & Watson, D.W. (1970) Puffing frequency and nicotine intake in cigarette smokers. *British Medican Journal,* **3**, 679-681.

Ashton, H., Millman, J.E., Telford, R. & Thompson, J.W. (1974) The effect of caffeine, nitrazepam and cigarette smoking on the contingent negative variation in man. *Electroencephalography and Clinical Neurophysiology,* **37**, 59-71.

Berlyne, D.E. (1971) *Aesthetics and Psychobiology.* New York: Appleton.

Bohlin, G. (1976) Delayed habituation of the electrodermal orienting response as a function of increased level of arousal. *Psychophysiology,* **13**, 169.

Bovet-Nitti, F. (1969) Facilitation of simultaneous visual discrimination by nicotine in four inbred strains of mice. *Psychopharmacologia,* **14**, 193-199.

Brown, B.B. (1973) Additional characteristic EEG differences between smokers and non-smokers. In *Smoking Behaviour: Motives and Incentives,* ed. Dunn, W.L. pp. 67-8. Washington: V.H. Winston & Sons.

Cheshire, P.J., Kellett, D.N. & Willey, G.L. (1973) Effects of nicotine and arousal on the monkey EEG. *Experientia,* **29**, 71-73.

Domino, E.F. (1973) Neuropsychopharmacology of nicotine and tobacco smoking. In *Smoking Behaviour: Motives and Incentives,* ed. Dunn, W.L., pp. 5-31. Washington: V.H. Winston & Sons.

Domino, E.F. & von Baumgarten, A.M. (1969) Tobacco cigarette smoking and the patellar reflex depression. *Clinical Pharmacology and Therapeutics,* **10**, 72-79.

Evangelista, A.M., Gattoni, R.C. & Izquierdo, I. (1970) Effect of amphetamine, nicotine and hexamethonium on performance of a conditioned response during acquisition and retention trials. *Pharmacology,* **3**, 91-96.

Eysenck, H.J. (1967) *The Biological Basis of Personality,* Springfield, Ill.: C. Thomas.

Eysenck, H.J. & Easterbrook, J.A. (1960) The effects of stimulant and depressant drugs on visual after-effect of a rotating spiral. *Journal of Mental Science,* **106**, 842-844.

Frankenhaeuser, M., Myrsten, A-L., Post, B. & Johansson, G. (1971) Behavioural and physiological effects of cigarette smoking in a monotonous situation. *Psychopharmacologia,* **22**, 1-7.

Friedman, J., Horvath, T. & Meares, R. (1974) Tobacco smoking and a 'stimulus barrier'. *Nature, London,* **248**, 455-456.

Frith, C.D. (1971) The effect of nicotine content of cigarettes on human smoking behaviour. *Psychopharmacologia,* **19**, 188-192.

Garg, M. (1969) The effect of nicotine on two different types of learning. *Psychopharmacologia,* **15**, 408-414.

Goldfarb, T.L., Jarvik, M.E. & Glick, S.D. (1970) Cigarette nicotine content as a determinant of human smoking behaviour. *Psychopharmacologia,* **17**, 89-93.

Goodman, L.S. & Gilman, A (1971) *Pharmacological Basis of Therapeutics.* 4th Ed., Macmillan.

Gray, J.A. (1971) *The Psychology of Fear and Stress.* Weidenfeld & Nicolson.

Gregory, R.L. (1972) *Eye and Brain: The Psychology of Seeing.* Weidenfeld & Nicolson.

Hall, R.A., Rappaport, M., Hopkins, H.K. & Griffin, R. (1973) Tobacco and evoked potential. *Science, N.Y.,* **180**, 212-214.

Heimstra, N.W., Bancroft, N.R. & DeKock, A.R. (1967) Effects of smoking upon sustained performance in a simulated driving task. *Annals of the New York Academy of Sciences*, **142**, 295-307.

Jasper, H.H. (1958) The ten-twenty electrode system of the International Federation. *Electroencephalography and Clinical Neurophysiology*, **10**, 371-375.

Knapp, P.H., Bliss, C.M. & Wells, H. (1963) Addictive aspects of heavy cigarette smoking. *American Journal of Psychiatry*, **119**, 966-972.

Knott, V.J. & Venables, P.H. (1977) EEG alpha correlates of non-smokers, smokers, smoking and smoking deprivation. *Psychophysiology*, **14**, 150-156.

Koepke, J.E. & Pribram, K.H. (1966) Habituation of GSR as a function of stimulus duration and spontaneous activity. *Journal of Comparative and Physiological Psychology*, **61**, 442-448.

Lucchesi, B.R., Schuster, C.R. & Emley, G.S. (1967) The role of nicotine as a determinant of cigarette smoking frequency in man with observations of certain cardiovascular effects associated with the tobacco alkaloid. *Clinical Pharmacology and Therapeutics*, **8**, 789-796.

Mangan, G.L. (1974) Personality and conditioning; some personality, cognitive and psychophysiological parameters of classical appetitive (sexual) GSR conditioning. *Pavlovian Journal*, **9**, 125-135.

Morrison, C.F. (1967) Effects of nicotine on operant behaviour in rats. *International Journal of Neuropharmacology*, **6**, 229-240.

Morrison, C.F. (1968) The modification by physostigmine of some effects of nicotine on bar-pressing behaviour in rat. *British Journal of Pharmacology and Chemotherapy*, **32**, 28-33.

Murphree, H.B., Pfeiffer, C.C. & Price, L.M. (1967) EEG changes in man following smoking. *Annals of the New York Academy of Sciences*, **142**, 245-260.

Nebylitsyn, V.D. (1972) *Fundamental Properties of the Human Nervous System.* English translation. ed. Mangan, G.L. New York: Plenum Press.

Nelsen, J.M. & Goldstein, L. (1973) Chronic nicotine treatment in rats: acquisition and performance of an attention task. *Research Communication in Chemical Pathology and Pharmacology*, **5**, 681-693.

Paton, W.D.M. & Perry, W.L.M. (1953) The relationship between depolarisation and block in the cat's superior cervical ganglion. *Journal of Physiology, London*, **119**, 43-53.

Philips, C. (1971) The EEG changes associated with smoking. *Psychophysiology*, **8**, 64-74.

Robbins, E.S., Weinstein, S., Borg, S., Rifkin, A., Wechsler, D. & Osley, B. (1959) The effect of electroconvulsive treatment upon perception of the spiral aftereffect; a presumed measure of cerebral dysfunction. *Journal of Nervous and Mental Diseases*, **128**, 239-242.

Russell, M.A.H. (1976) Tobacco smoking and nicotine dependence. In *Research Advances in Alcohol and Drug Problems.* Volume 3, ed. Gibbins, R.J. *et al.* pp. 1-47. New York: Wiley & Sons.

Ryan, F.J. (1973) Cold turkey in Greenfield, Iowa: a follow-up study. In *Smoking Behaviour: Motives and Incentives.* ed. Dunn, W.L. pp. 231-241. Washington: V.H. Winston & Sons.

Sarin, C.L. (1974) Effects of smoking on digital blood-flow velocity. *Journal of the American Medical Association,* **229,** 1327-1328.

Schachter, S. (1975) Eat bicarbonate and smoke less. *New Scientist,* **65,** 931, 54.

Schachter, S., Silverstein, B., Kozlowski, L.T., Perlick, D., Herman, C.P. & Leibling, B. (1977) Studies of the interaction of psychological and pharmacological determinants of smoking. *Journal of Experimental Psychology: General,* **106,** 5-40.

Siddle, D.A.T. (1972) Vigilance decrement and speed of habituation of the GSR component of the orienting response. *British Journal of Psychology,* **63,** 2, 191-194.

Siddle, D.A.T. & Mangan, G.L. (1971) Arousability and individual differences in resistance to distraction. *Journal of Experimental Research in Personality,* **5,** 295-303.

Stolerman, I.P., Goldfarb, T., Fink, R. & Jarvik, M.E. (1973) Influencing cigarette smoking with nicotine antagonists. *Psychopharmacologia,* **28,** 247-259.

Swets, J.A. (ed) (1964) *Signal Detection and Recognition by Human Observers.* New York: Wiley & Sons.

Ulett, J.A. & Itil, T.M. (1969) Quantitative EEG in smoking and smoking deprivation. *Science,* **164,** 969-970.

Venables, P.H. (1977) The electrodermal psychophysiology of schizophrenics and children at risk for schizophrenia: controversies and developments. *Schizophrenia Bulletin,* **3,** 28-48.

Wachtel, P.L. (1967) Conceptions of broad and narrow attention. *Psychological Bulletin,* **68,** 417-429.

Waugh, N. (1961) Free versus serial recall. *Journal of Experimental Psychology,* **62,** 496-502.

9. Smoking, EEG and input regulation in smokers and non-smokers

VERNER J KNOTT

In the 1967 symposium on 'Effects of Nicotine and Smoking on the Central Nervous System' sponsored by the New York Academy of Sciences, Dr. McKeen Cattell made the opening remark that though much was controversial regarding the effects of smoking, there could be no disagreement that the answer to the question 'Why do we smoke?' must involve the central nervous system (CNS), and it was only through the study of effects, either direct or reflex, of the constituents of smoke on central functions that we were likely to come up with the correct answer. As the scalp-recorded electroencephalogram (EEG) is the most direct measure currently available for assessment of the human CNS, a number of investigations have examined EEG activity in an attempt to objectively interpret the relationship between smoking and cortical activity. The outcomes of these empirical investigations have by no means been uniform in nature. They have yielded variable and contradictory results such that if one were to interpret them within cortical 'arousal' theory (Lindsley, 1970) they would indicate smokers to have been either more or less aroused than non-smokers and for smoking to have either increased or decreased arousal.

Though future EEG investigations would certainly produce greater uniformity of results with more effecient control over pharmacological and non-pharmacological variables, it is within reason to suggest that alternative, more sophisticated experimental designs may be an important ingredient which will enhance clarity of results in smoking - EEG research. Dunn (1973) has reviewed the experimental designs commonly employed in smoking research and he has discussed them in terms of their potential to yield information relevant to the critical factors underlying smoking motivation. Two of the designs discussed have been used throughout the smoking - EEG literature. One design involves a comparative analysis of smokers and non-smokers while the second design involves an analysis of the effects of smoking or smoking deprivation. In employing the first design, the experimenter is essentially asking - do smokers show different EEG characteristics from non-smokers? In employing the second design one is asking - does smoking or smoking deprivation affect the EEG?

To date, very few studies in smoking research in general, and not one study involved with EEG has attempted to incorporate both questions within one experimental design to ask - do smokers show different EEG characteristics from non-smokers and what are the effects of smoking or smoking deprivation on these differential EEG characteristics? Or, more simply, this combined experimental approach would ask - how is the smoker different from the non-smoker before or after smoking? It would seem obvious then that in such a design one is increasing the amount of information output in relation to the motivational critical factors underlying smoking behaviour. Here, in order to assess the payoff of this approach, the results of two studies employing this combined research design will be presented.

The first study by Knott and Venables (1977) centered on tonic (basal) resting levels of EEG activity, with specific reference to alpha activity between 8 - 12 Hz. Non-smokers (NS) were compared with both tobacco-deprived smokers (DS) who were required to abstain from smoking for a period of 12-15 hours, and non-deprived smokers (NDS) who were required to smoke in their normal manner up until the experimental session. In order to examine the immediate effects of smoking on EEG alpha activity, a random sample of the DS and NDS groups were required to smoke 2 cigarettes (each cigarette 100mm long, yielding 1.6 mg nicotine and 21mg tar) within a ten minute period, inhaling at thirty second intervals. For control, the remaining DS, NDS and NS subjects were required to inhale air through a non-lighted cigarette for the same duration and in the same manner.   Alpha activity was recorded with silver/silver chloride disc electrodes from a unilateral right occipital - right ear placement during eyes-closed resting periods, five minutes before and 15 minutes after cigarette smoking.   The EEG signal was amplified by a Grass model 7P5 amplifier (time constant set at 0.3sec., high frequency filters at 35Hz) and the amplified signals were fed to a Precision Instrument - 6200 FM model analogue magnetic tape recorder for later off-line analysis. The EEG activity was analysed from the analogue tape by a LINC - 8 Spectrum program (Bryan, 1968) which employed the Cooley-Tukey Fast Fourier Transform algorithm. The resultant computer analysis of the data yielded two response measures - alpha amplitude and dominant alpha frequency.   Statistical analysis of pre-smoking alpha amplitude data failed to show any significant smoking effect. Significant differences were observed with dominant alpha frequency data as shown in Table 9.1.

Table 9.1 Mean dominant alpha frequencies (Hz) for non-smokers (NS), deprived smokers (DS), and non-deprived smokers (NDS) before and after tobacco (t) and no-tobacco conditions (nt).

Groups	Mean Dominant Alpha Frequencies (Hz)			
	Pre-Smoking	Post Smoking		
	3-5	3-5	8-10	13-15
NS-nt (n=9[a])	10.0	10.0	10.0	10.1
DS-nt (n=9)	9.3	9.2	9.4	9.3
DS-t (n=8)	9.3	9.8	9.9	10.0
NDS-nt (n=6)	9.8	9.7	9.8	9.8
NDS-t (n=6[a])	10.0	9.9	9.8	9.9

(a: one subject eliminated due to faulty recording)

Analysis of pre-smoking activity indicated significant differences between DS and both NDS and NS groups in that DS exhibited slower dominant alpha frequencies. No significant differences were observed between NDS and NS groups, that is they exhibited comparable EEG activity. The immediate effect of smoking two cigarettes relative to sham smoking was to produce a significant increase in dominant alpha frequency in the DS group. There was no significant time effect. If one collapses the data over time a very interesting picture emerges as shown in Figure 9.1. As stated earlier, DS showed evidence of slower alpha frequencies than both NS and NDS groups who exhibit comparable activity. The immediate effect of smoking is to increase dominant alpha frequency in DS to a level comparable to that of NS and NDS groups. One might conclude from this data then, that if NS are looked upon as a 'normative' group, then smoking as indicated in NDS and by the immediate effects of smoking in DS, tends to 'normalise' cortical activity.

The second study by Knott and Venables (1978a) centered on phasic (stimulus induced changes) EEG activity in response to visual stimulation, with specific reference to latency and amplitude components of the averaged evoked response (AER). Based on the findings that tobacco tended to normalise cortical activity, this investigation examined the hypothesis that DS would exhibit differential responsivity than NS and that smoking, as exhibited in the NDS group, would show evidence of response normalisation. Again, three groups NS, DS and NDS were examined with DS being required to abstain from smoking for 15-18 hours prior to the experimental session, and NDS were required to smoke in their usual manner up until the experimental session. Evoked responses were recorded in relation to four flash intensities ranged from 64 to 422 ft. lamberts. Each flash intensity was pseudo-randomised and presented 16 times at 5 sec. intervals. EEG activity was recorded with a Beckman biopotential silver/silver chloride miniature electrode placed at the vertex and referred to linked earlobes. The EEG signal was amplified by a Grass 7P1 amplifier (time constant set at 0.1 sec., high frequency filter at 35Hz) and the amplified signals were fed to a RACAL - Store 4 analogue FM magnetic tape recorder for later off-line analysis. EEG activity was analysed from the analogue tape by a PDP - 11/40 computer averaging system which identified three peak components of the AER for study (according to the algorithm developed by Hall *et al,* 1973a). Peak IV was a positive peak with a latency of 75-140 msec. The latency of negative Peak V ranged between 90-165 msec. and the positive Peak VI ranged between 125-250 msec. The latencies of these three peaks, and the amplitude differences between Peak IV and V, and between Peak V and VI were analysed. Statistical analysis did not yield any significant differences between Peak V and Peak VI. Significant group differences were observed however with Peak IV latency and the amplitude differences between Peak IV and Peak V. Table 9.2 presents the amplitude data. Analysis of mean amplitude values indicated DS to exhibit larger response amplitudes than both NS and NDS. No significant differences were observed between NS and NDS. A more detailed analysis however indicated significant differences to appear only for the two lowest intensities, again with DS showing greater responsivity than both NS and NDS who exhibited comparable responsiveness. Analysis of Peak IV latency values showed similar findings (Table 9.3).

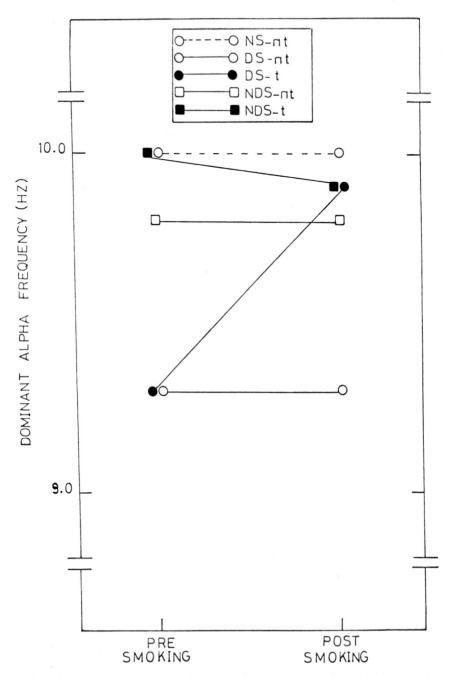

Fig. 9.1 Mean dominant alpha frequency (Hz) for non-smokers (NS), deprived smokers (DS), and non-deprived smokers (NDS) before and after tobacco (t) and no-tobacco (nt) conditions.

Table 9.2   Table of mean amplitude (μV) values for PIV-PV for four flash intensities (ft.1.) for non-smokers (NS), tobacco deprived smokers (DS) and non-deprived smokers (NDS).

Peaks	Groups	Stimulus Intensity			
		64	109	273	422
PIV – PV	NS (n=10)	8.5	5.1	7.2	8.6
	DS (n=10)	13.3	10.4	11.3	12.7
	NDS (n=10)[b]	5.5	5.8	6.5	7.8

(b: three subjects eliminated due to faulty recording)

Table 9.3   Mean latency (msec) values of peak IV for four flash intensities (ft.1.) for non-smokers (NS), tobacco deprived smokers (DS) and non-deprived smokers (NDS)

Peaks	Groups	Stimulus Intensity			
		64	109	273	422
PIV	NS (n=10)	102.1	107.8	105.8	102.7
	DS (n=10)	90.1	98.8	94.0	97.0
	NDS (n=10)[c]	115.4	113.9	114.1	113.6

(c: three subjects eliminated due to faulty recording)

Analysis of mean latency values indicated DS show faster latencies than both NS and NDS and no significant differences were apparent between NS and NDS groups. Again, a more detailed analysis indicated significant differences only at the two lowest intensities with DS showing faster latencies than both NDS and NS groups who exhibited comparable responsivity.

The payoff of these two investigations which have employed the above combined research design must of course be evaluated by their ability to isolate critical variables relevant to smoking motivation. These studies have indeed identified critical EEG parameters which differentiate non-deprived and non-smokers from tobacco deprived smokers and these findings tend to indicate that smoking has a normalising effect on cortical activity. The problem remains however in attempting to relate these findings to smoking motivation. It is important to point out here, that any theoretical attempt worth its salt must account for the fact that CNS normalisation occurred by two apparently distinctive processes. In the initial study, normalisation took place by an apparent stimulant action of smoking on dominant alpha frequency. In the final study, normalisation took place by an apparent depressant action of smoking on amplitude and latency components of the evoked response. These apparent opposing actions of tobacco smoking prevent one from adopting a simplistic arousal-oriented theory to account for the EEG findings and it would seem on this basis that the formulation of additional alternative proposals, necessitate a closer examination of the functional significance of alpha frequency and evoked responses in relation to tobacco smoking.

Dominant alpha frequency has been predominantly discussed in relation to Surwillo's (1968) information processing theory. According to the model, the latency of a response to the input of a specific stimulus to the CNS is dependent on the rate of execution of a fixed number of sequential information processing operations, and the rate of execution of each information processing operation is in turn dependent upon the rate of occurrence of electrical 'gating signals', i.e. the passing of each half wave in the EEG indicates the occurrence of a gating signal (Kristofferson 1967). Given these assumptions, the model predicts that a response always follows stimulus input after a specific number of gating signals have elapsed, and therefore, the faster the frequency of EEG, the shorter the inter-gate interval, the faster the rate of execution of operations carried out by the central processor, and hence the faster the response time. Support for this theory has been forthcoming from studies which have almost invariably reported significant positive correlations between behavioural reaction time (RT) and average period (i.e. reciprocal of frequency) of the EEG (Boddy, 1971; Surwillo, 1963, 1964a, 1971, 1974). Additional support follows from studies which have observed that the manipulation of alpha frequency (by experimental or naturally occurring processes) through photic driving (Surwillo, 1964b), carbon dioxide (Harter, 1967), biofeedback (Woodruff, 1975) and the menstrual cycle (Creutzfeldt et al, 1976), produced changes such as decreases in alpha frequency which were associated with slower RTs and vice versa.

The observation that increasing alpha frequency is associated with improved RT performance has a specific bearing on tobacco studies which have independently assessed the effects of smoking on EEG and RT. Here, tobacco-EEG studies (Lambiase and Serra, 1957; Hauser et al, 1958; Bickford, 1960; Wechsler, 1962; Ulett and Itil, 1969) have consistently shown increases in alpha frequency following smoking, and independent tobacco - RT studies have invariably reported improved efficiency of RT following tobacco smoking (Frankenhaeuser et al, 1971; Myrsten et al, 1972; Lyon et al, 1975). It is interesting to note that with respect to the Lyon et al (1975) investigation in which tobacco smoking was found to counteract the ethanol induced slowing of RT, Knott and Venables (1978b) have recently observed that tobacco smoking also prevents the ethanol induced slowing of alpha frequency.

On the above evidence and as DS exhibit slower alpha frequencies than NS, it would seem that relative to NS, DS evidence a characteristic deficit in tasks relating to the temporal organisation of behaviour. Additional support and insight into the mechanisms underlying this deficit are found in tobacco studies which have employed temporal discrimination as a response variable. Here, DS have been observed to exhibit poorer performance than NS on measures requiring temporal discrimination (i.e. estimation of two flash fusion thresholds; Tong *et al*, 1974a) and have shown improvement on temporal discrimination measures (i.e. estimation of two flash and critical flicker fusion thresholds) following smoking (Larson, Finnegan and Haag, 1950; Fabricant and Rose, 1951; Garner, Carl and Grossman, 1953; 1954; Warwick and Eysenck, 1963; Barlow and Baer, 1967; Baer, 1967). Again, as above, it is interesting to note that as Knott and Venables (1978b) have indicated anatagonistic interactions between ethanol and tobacco in relation to alpha frequency, similar effects have been observed by Tong *et al,* (1974) with respect to temporal discrimination. A possible clue to understanding the precise mechanisms underlying tobacco induced improvement in temporal discrimination is provided by Venables' (1975) discussion of interlocking factors involved in CNS discrimination of rapidly successive stimulus inputs such as is found in two flash fusion (TFF) thresholds. Though Venables cites evidence as to the role of cortical activation in improved TFF performance, additional evidence is provided which indicates that an important factor relating to efficient TFF performance is the 'rate or speed' at which the 'noise' generated by the first stimulus is dissipated by the CNS, i.e. the initial stimulus input creates noise which carries over to the second stimulus and makes the detection of the second input more difficult. Though it is conjecture here to associate slow alpha frequencies in DS with specific defective processing operations, it seems reasonable to assume that in the light of the above statements, poorer temporal discrimination in DS (relative to NS) may be a result of a slow rate of execution of information processing operations, which are specifically related to blocking, screening, filtering or to the habituation of CNS input (internal and external) which generates unwanted noise. On this basis then, the attraction of tobacco smoking would seem to lie in its ability to increase the rate at which unwanted noise is dissipated.   As the concepts of filtering and habituation have received considerable functional importance in the control of vigilance and attentional processes (Broadbent, 1958, 1971; Sokolov, 1963; Lynn, 1966; Mackworth, 1969, 1970: Pribram and McGuinness, 1975) support for the 'filtering model' would be found if investigations observed that tobacco smoking results in improved attentional performance. Indeed, such support is forthcoming in studies which have examined the effects of tobacco smoking on prolonged vigilance (Tarriere and Hartemann, 1964; Frankenhaeuser *et al,* 1971; Tong *et al,* 1977), intensive and divided attention (Leigh, Tong and Campbell, 1977) and more recently Warburton and Wesnes (1978; Wesnes and Warburton, 1978) whose investigations have observed improved vigilance/attentional performance following smoking and the ingestion of nicotine tablets. Additional behavioural evidence at the animal level is provided by Nelsen and Goldstein's (1972, 1973) data which indicated that nicotine induced improvement of selective attention performance and also reduced the frequency of inappropriate responding (to irrelevant stimulus input) as indicated by a reduction in commission errors (i.e. false positives).

In relation to the filter model being proposed, Hartley (1973), on the basis of his tobacco-signal detection data, has suggested that a possible attraction of smoking may lie in its ability to oppose the effects of external environmental noise and the resulting over-arousal in performance requiring sustained perception. This suggestion of the ability of tobacco smoking to counteract the effects of noise on human performance has received some empirical support from Tong *et al*'s (1974b) pilot investigation. Here, the effects of medium intensity noise (75dB SPL) on simple visual RTs were examined (in habitual smokers only) under tobacco (1 cigarette) and non-tobacco conditions. As shown in Figure 9.2, though non-significant

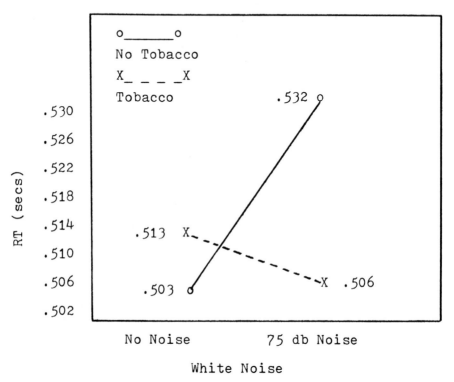

Fig. 9.2 Mean visual reaction times (seconds) of smokers (following 12-15 hours deprivation n = 12) with and without the effects of noise (75dB SPL) and tobacco (1 cigarette).

differences were observed under the no-noise condition, noise significantly increased visual RTs (i.e. decreased performance efficiency) under the no-tobacco condition. Tobacco smoking, however, significantly counteracted this noise induced decrease in performance.

Though Knott and Venables (1978a) did not discuss the above mechanisms of the proposed filtering model, the basic concept of tobacco or nicotine acting as a 'chemical stimulus filter' was employed to account for the findings that DS (relative to NS and NDS) exhibited faster latencies and larger cortical AER amplitudes to stimuli in general, and more specifically, to stimuli of low intensity. However, in view of the above discussion of the possible defective filtering processes which might accompany slow alpha frequencies, it is now within reason here to suggest that the cortical hyper-activity observed in DS is related in some manner to inefficient, or more specifically to a slow filtering capacity. This suggestion that input dysfunction results in hyper-reactive responding runs parallel to the views of Holzman (1969), McGhie (1969), Venables (1964, 1969, 1971, 1973), Lipowski (1975) and Ludwig (1975), all of whom have discussed the concept of defective filtering in relation to psychopathology. In general, the consensus of the effects of impaired ability to filter or screen out irrelevant and noxious stimuli results in a state of stimulus over-load at the cortex resulting in enhanced cortical responses and a distortion in perception characterised by an increase in perceived intensity and quality of stimulus input changes which would result in inappropriate responding and inefficient behavioural performance. This account provides a possible explanation for the observation of reduced pain thresholds (i.e. greater sensitivity to pain) observed in smokers relative to NS and the subsequent increase in pain thresholds following smoking (Nesbitt, 1973; Schachter, 1973, 1978; Seltzer *et al*, 1974). Numerous investigators have examined the psychophysiological makeup of individuals who are susceptible to stimulus overload as a consequence of an hypothesised defective CNS filtering system. Primary among these investigators is Buchsbaum (1975), whose studies have examined cortical AERs in relation to stimulus overload. Here, research has indicated that hypo-reactivity (i.e. reduced responsivity) to high intensity stimulation may be interpreted as a neurophysiological defence mechanism by which individuals who are hyper-sensitive to weak intensity stimulation, protect themselves from stimulus overload. Relative to NS, this AER response style accurately depicts the cortical reactivity of DS, and as NDS evidence comparable responsivity to NS, it would seem that tobacco smoking by increasing alpha frequency and thereby increasing filtering efficiency, induces improved screening of stimulus input and as a result alleviates the need for the protective coping mechanism described above. Though several EEG studies contradict the dual findings of increased responsiveness in DS relative to NS (Brown, 1968b) and decreased responsiveness following smoking (Hall *et al*, 1973b; Friedman *et al*, 1974), additional evidence which suggests that tobacco smoking increases filtering capacity as indicated by tobacco induced reduction in physiological responsivity is provided by studies examining such response measures as the averaged evoked response (Vasquez and Toman, 1967), alpha blocking (Friedman, Horvath and Meares, 1974), photic driving (Vogel, Broverman and Klaiber, 1977) and electrodermal responsiveness (Mangan and Golding, 1978).

   At this stage it would be absurd to suggest that the hypothesised defective filtering observed in DS (relative to NS) might be implicated as a possible predisposing factor in the initiation of smoking behaviour and any statements on this topic must await empirical research from longitudinal studies which focus directly on this point. However, it is reasonable to state, as suggested earlier, that the filtering model provides a rational working hypothesis which implicates the dysfunction of regulation to stimulus input observed in DS (relative to NS), as a possible factor involved in the maintenance of smoking behaviour. Having stated this however, it is obvious that a complete picture of its role in the maintenance of smoking requires empirical data relating to the effects of (a) tobacco withdrawal symptoms and (b) prolonged intake of tobacco on CNS on filtering capacity. In relation to withdrawal symptoms, Ulett and Itil (1969) and Itil *et al* (1971) observed EEG alterations (i.e. a reduction in alpha frequency of 1 Hz. from 10.5 Hz to 9.5 Hz) following 24 hours of tobacco deprivation, but they made no attempt to manipulate various durations of deprivation. The present author has examined some modest data in relation to EEG alpha frequency and two tobacco deprivation periods. Here, DS individuals who were required to abstain from tobacco for 12-15 hours during the initial EEG alpha - tobacco experiment, returned (along with the NS and NDS subjects) to the laboratory for two additional recording sessions (for research purposes unrelated to the specific study of tobacco deprivation) following a deprivation period of 15-18 hours.   In Table 9.4, alpha frequency data for the initial tobacco study and the addition two deprivation periods (only for subjects

Table 9.4 **Mean dominant alpha frequencies (Hz) for non-smokers (NS), deprived smokers (DS), and non-deprived smokers (NDS) during initial 13-15 hours of deprivation and two additional 15-18 hours of deprivation (each session separated by a minimum period of one week).**

Deprivation Periods	Groups		
	NS (n=9)	DS (n=13)	NDS (n=9)
13-15 (initial session	10.0	9.4	9.9
15-18 (1st session)	10.0	9.5	9.9
15-18 (2nd session)	9.9	9.4	9.8

who participated in all three sessions) are presented.   A shown, NS evidence a consistent frequency of approximately 10.0Hz, a figure which is very similar to Lindsley's (1938, 1939) 10.2Hz occipital alpha figure reported for a large group of normal adults.   DS do not exhibit any significantly marked deviation due to the extended deprivation period, and indeed the deviation of .1Hz which occurs in the first (15-18 hours deprivation) session (in a direction opposite to what one would expect) is much lower than the reported standard deviation of alpha frequency of .47Hz observed in a normal population (Lindsley and Rubenstein, 1937). Though these data represent only a minor manipulation of deviation duration (i.e. average of three hours), they do question whether the EEG alterations are due to withdrawal symptoms *per se* or are merely a return to an enduring psycho-physiological basal level which is characteristic of DS.

Brown's (1968a, 1968b, 1973) tonic EEG studies indirectly support the above notion as her data did not find significant tobacco or deprivation effects but they did indicate significant EEG characteristics existed which differentiate non-smokers from average, heavy and ex-smokers (here, non-smokers evidenced slower alpha frequencies than smokers), and they also observed that a positive relationship existed between the daily amount of smoking and degree of brain excitability. On this basis, Brown concluded that the cortical activity of smokers represents a constitutional characteristic which may be associated with a fundamental predisposition to smoking behaviour. Though the data presented might as easily be interpreted as indicating a significant effect of prolonged tobacco exposure on CNS activity, Brown directs very little discussion towards this possibility. Though subsequent correlational analysis of Knott and Venables' (1977) DS data did not yield any significant relationship between dominant alpha frequency and variables related to prolonged tobacco exposure (e.g. number of years smoking, $r = -.18$, df 11, p$\rangle$.05, number of cigarettes smoked per day, $r = -.29$, df 10, p$\rangle$.05, it is clear that additional research which examines this variable in relation to a range of deprivation periods, in light, moderate and heavy smokers is required before any definitive statements can be made with regard to the effects of prolonged tobacco exposure and CNS activity.

Up to this point, the neurophysiological mechanisms relevant to the proposed filter model have not been discussed, and although at this stage of research it is recognised that discussion is purely speculative, some recent neurophysiological research is worth mentioning. Jasper (1958) and other researchers (Demetrescu and Demetrescu, 1962) have implicated the reticular formation in controlling selective responsiveness to significant stimuli by preventing general alerting actions to all incoming stimuli and this focus parallels the findings of investigations which found significant effects of nicotine on this CNS site (Domino, 1967). However, as with recent empirical data which has focused on the role of the limbic system in the control of attention, neurophysiological investigations of nicotine action have also attributed the effects of nicotine to changes exerted by the limbic system. Here, employing electrophysiological measures, Nelsen and colleagues (Bhattacharya and Goldstein, 1970; Nelsen, Pelley and Goldstein, 1973) have provided evidence that the hippocampal limbic system is a major target area for nicotine, in that cortical activity under nicotine treatment is controlled more by the hippocampus than by the reticular formation. Based on Routtenberg's (1968) hypothesis that hippocampal activity inhibits the reticular formation, Nelsen (1974) hypothesised that the neurophysiological mechanism underlying nicotine-seeking behaviour lies in its ability to counteract inappropriate responding by the reticular formation, by its (nicotine) action on the limbic system. Support for this hypothesis was observed in their animal investigation in which nicotine treatment was found to counteract decreased performance in selective attention which was induced by electrical stimulation of the reticular formation. On this basis, these authors suggest that a possible motivation underlying smoking behaviour is its ability to reduce reticular excitation which is manifested in a hyper-stimulated anxious state inappropriate for effective behaviour and to engender what might be considered a state of useful behavioural arousal. In relation to the filter model, it is interesting to speculate here whether the often reported relaxation smoking is related to inappropriate reticular hippocampal filtering or inappropriate hippocampal limbic control of reticular filtering (or both) in DS relative to NS.

In concluding, though I have presented a rather expansive proposal to account for the tobacco-EEG data observed in the combined research designs, this is not to say that other less complex proposals are not relevant.   For example, a simpler arousal-oriented theory similar to that suggested by Schachter (1973) and Nesbitt (1973) may account for the data as follows. As implicated earlier by Knott and Venables (1977), slow dominant alpha frequencies may be looked upon as an indicator of low cortical arousal level, and according to Wilder's Law of Initial Values (1967) which holds that an inverse relation exists between 'level and response amplitude', it might well be that stimulation results in larger cortical responses in DS relative to NS, and as such DS experience these stimuli as being more intense. Tobacco smoking then increases arousal level (as indicated by higher alpha frequencies in NDS) and as such results in a reduced ceiling level, and limits the cortical response amplitudes and possibly reduces perceived intensity of stimulation.

Of course other theories may be advanced to account for the data but in the end, confirmation of any theory or set of data as being relevant to smoking motivation must await future empirical research.

References

Baer, D. (1967) Hyperventilation effects on the critical flicker frequency of smokers and non-smokers. *Journal of General Psychology,* **76**, 201-206.

Barlow, D. & Baer, D. (1967) Effect of cigarette smoking on the critical flicker frequency of heavy and light smokers. *Perceptual and Motor Skills,* **24**, 151-155.

Bhattacharya, I. & Goldstein, L. (1970) Influence of acute and chronic nicotine administration on intra- and inter-structural relationships of the electrical activity in the rabbit brain. *Neuropharmacology,* **9**, 109-118.

Bickford, R. (1960) Physiology and drug action: an electroencephalographic analysis. *Federation Proceedings,* **19**, 619-625.

Boddy, J. (1971) The relationship of reaction time to brain wave period - a re-evaluation. *Electroencephalography and Clinical Neurophysiology,* **30**, 229-235.

Broadbent, D. (1958) *Perception and Communication.* New York: Pergamon Press.

Broadbent, D. (1971) *Decision and Stress.* London: Academic Press.

Brown, B. (1968a) Brain waves in smokers. *Modern Medicine,* **36**, 40.

Brown, B. (1968b) Some characteristic EEG differences between heavy smoker and non-smoker subjects. *Neuropsychologia,* **6**, 381-388.

Brown, B. (1973) Additional characteristic EEG differences between smokers and non-smokers. In *Smoking Behaviour: Motives and Incentives,* ed. Dunn, W.L., pp. 67-81. Washington: V.H. Winston & Sons.

Bryan, J. (1968) LINC spectrum program, No. L-25. Program Library, Bethesda, Maryland: National Institute of Mental Health.

Buchsbaum, M. (1975) Averaged evoked response augmenting/reducing in schizophrenia and affective disorders.   In *Biology of the Major Psychoses: A Comparative Analysis,* ed. Friedman, D., pp. 129-142. New York: Raven Press.

Cattell, M. (1967) Introductory remarks.   Effects of nicotine and smoking on the central nervous system. In *Annals of the New York Academy of Sciences,* **142**, 1. ed. Murphree, H.

Creutzfeldt, O., Becker, P., Langestein, S., Tirsch, W., Wilhelm, H. & Wuttke, W. (1976) EEG changes during spontaneous and controlled menstrual cycles and their correlation with psychological performance. *Electroencephalography and Clinical Neurophysiology,* **40**, 113-131.

Demetrescu, M. & Demetrescu, M. (1962) Ascending inhibition and activation from the lower brain stem: the influence of pontine reticular stimulation on thalamo-cortical evoked potentials in the rat. *Electroencephalography and Clinical Neurophysiology,* **14**, 602-620.

Domino, E. (1967) Electroencephalographic and behavioural arousal effects of small doses of nicotine. A neuropsychopharmacological study. *Annals of the New York Academy of Science,* **142**, 216-244.

Dunn, W. (1973) Experimental methods and conceptual models as applied to the study of motivation in cigarette smoking. In *Smoking Behaviour: Motives and Incentives,* ed. Dunn, W.L., pp. 93-111. Washington: V.H. Winston & Sons.

Fabricant, N. & Rose, I. (1951) Effect of smoking cigarettes on the flicker fusion thresholds of normal persons. *Eye, Ear and Mouth,* **30**, 541-543.

Frankenhaeuser, M., Myrsten, A., Post, B. & Johansson, G. (1971) Behavioural and physiological effects of cigarette smoking in a monotonous situation. *Psychopharmacologia,* **22**, 1-7.

Friedman, J., Goldberg, T., Horvath, T. & Meares, R. (1974) The effect of tobacco smoking on evoked potentials. *Clinical and Experimental Pharmacology and Physiology,* **1**, 249-258.

Friedman, J., Horvath, T. & Meares, R. (1974) Tobacco smoking and the stimulus barrier. *Nature, London,* **248**, 455-456.

Garner, L., Carl, E. & Grossman, E. (1953) Effect of cigarette smoking on flicker fusion thresholds. *American Journal of Opthalmology,* **36**, 1751-1756.

Garner, L., Carl, E. & Grossman, E. (1954) Effect of cigarette smoking on flicker fusion threshold: Clinical observations on normal smokers and non-smokers. *American Medical Association Archives of Opthalmology,* **51**, 642-654.

Hall, R., Rappaport, M., Hopkins, H. & Griffin, R. (1973a) Peak identification in visual evoked potentials. *Psychophysiology,* **10**, 52-60.

Hall, R., Rappaport, M., Hopkins, H. & Griffin, R. (1973b) Tobacco and evoked potential. *Science,* **180**, 212-214.

Harter, M. (1967) Effects of carbon dioxide on the alpha frequency and reaction times in humans. *Electroencephalography and Clinical Neurophysiology,* **23**, 561-563.

Hartley, L. (1973) Cigarette smoking and stimulus selection. *British Journal of Psychology,* **64**, 593-599.

Hauser, H., Schwartz, B., Roth, G. & Bickford, R. (1958) Electroencephalographic changes related to smoking. (Abstract). *Electroencephalography and Clinical Neurophysiology,* **10**, 576P.

Holzman, P. (1969) Perceptual aspects of psychopathology. In *Neurobiological Aspects of Psychopathology,* ed. Zubin, J. & Shagass, C. pp. 144-178. New York: Grune & Stratton.

Itil, T., Ulett, G., Hsu, W., Klingenberg, H. & Ulett, J. (1971) The effects of smoking withdrawal on quantitatively analysed EEG. *Clinical Electroencephalography,* **2**, 44-51.

Jasper, H. (1958) Recent advances in our understanding of the ascending activities of the reticular system. *Reticular Formation of the Brain,* ed. Jasper, H. *et al,* London: Churchill.

Knott, V. & Venables, P. (1977) EEG alpha correlates of non-smokers, smokers, smoking and smoking deprivation. *Psychophysiology,* **14,** 150-156.

Knott, V. & Venables, P. (1978a) Stimulus intensity control and the cortical evoked response in smokers and non-smokers. *Psychophysiology,* (in press).

Knott, V. & Venables, P. (1978b) EEG alpha correlates of ethanol consumption in smokers and non-smokers, effects of smoking and smoking deprivation. *Journal of Studies on Alcohol* (under review).

Kristofferson, A. (1967) Successiveness discrimination as a two-state, quantal process. *Science,* **158,** 1337-1339.

Lambiase, M. & Serra, C. (1957) Fumo e sistema nervoso. 1. Modificazioni dell' attivita elettrica corticale da fumo. *Acta Neurologica, Napoli,* **12,** 475-493.

Larson, P., Finnegan, J. & Haag, H. (1950) Observations on the effect of cigarette smoking on the fusion frequency of flicker. *Journal of Clinical Investigations,* **29,** 483-486.

Leigh, G., Tong, J. & Campbell, J. (1977) Effects of ethanol and tobacco on divided attention. *Journal of Studies on Alcohol,* **38,** 1233-1239.

Lindsley, D. (1938) Electrical potentials of the brain in children and adults. *Journal of General Psychology,* **19,** 285-306.

Lindsley, D. (1939) A longitudinal study of the occipital alpha rythm in normal children: frequency and amplitude standards. *Journal of Genetic Psychology,* **55,** 197-213.

Lindsley, D. & Rubenstein, B. (1937) Relationship between brain potentials and some other physiological variables. *Proceedings of the Society of Experimental Biology and Medicine,* **35,** 558-563.

Lindsley, D. (1970) The role of nonspecific reticulo-thalamo-cortical systems in emotion. In *Physiological Correlates of Emotion,* ed. Black, P., pp. 147-189. New York: Academic Press.

Lipowski, Z. (1975) Sensory information input overload: behavioural effects. *Comprehensive Psychiatry,* **16,** 199-221.

Ludwig, A. (1975) Sensory overload and psychopathology. *Diseases of the Nervous System,* **36,** 357-360.

Lynn, R. (1966) *Attention, Arousal and the Orientation Reaction.* Oxford: Pergamon Press.

Lyon, R., Tong, J., Leigh, G. & Clare, G. (1975) The influence of alcohol and tobacco on the components of choice reaction time. *Journal of Studies on Alcohol,* **36,** 587-596.

Mackworth, J. (1969) *Vigilance and Habituation: A Neuropsychological Approach,* Penguin Books.

Mackworth, J. (1970) *Vigilance and Attention: A Signal Detection Approach.* Penguin Books.

Mangan, G. & Golding, J. (1978) An 'enhancement' model of smoking maintenance? *This volume.*

McGhie, A. (1969) *Pathology of Attention.* Penguin Books.

Myrsten, A., Post, B., Frankenhaeuser, M. & Johansson, G. (1972) Changes in behavioural and physiological activation induced by cigarette smoking in habitual smokers. *Psychopharmacologia, 27,* 305-312.

Nelsen, J. (1974) Neurophysiological and behavioral consequences of chronic nicotine treatment. In *Drug Addiction Vol. 3. Neurobiology and Influences on Behavior,* ed. Singh, J.M. & Lal, H. pp. 375-386. New York: Stratton Intercontinental.

Nelsen, J. & Goldstein, L. (1972) Improvement of performance on an attention task with chronic nicotine treatment in rats. *Psychopharmcologia, 26,* 347-360.

Nelsen, J. & Goldstein, L. (1973) Chronic nicotine treatment: aquisition and performance of an attention task. *Research Communications in Chemical Pathology and Pharmacology, 5,* 681-683.

Nelsen, J., Pelley, K. & Goldstein, L. (1972) Chronic nicotine treatment in rats: 2. Electroencephalographic amplitude and variability changes occurring between and within structures. *Research Communications in Chemical Pathology and Pharmacology, 5,* 694-704.

Nelsen, J., Pelley, K. & Goldstein, L. (1975) Protection by nicotine from behavioural disruption caused by reticular formation stimulation in the rat. *Pharmacology, Biochemistry and Behavior, 3,* 749-754.

Nesbitt, P. (1973) Smoking, physiological arousal and emotional response. *Journal of Personality and Social Psychology, 25,* 137-144.

Pribram, K. & McGuinness, D. (1975) Arousal, activation and effort in the control of attention. *Psychological Review, 82,* 116-149.

Routtenberg, A. (1968) The two arousal hypothesis: reticular formation and limbic system. *Psychological Review, 75,* 51-80.

Schachter, S. (1973) Nesbitt's paradox. In *Smoking Behavior: Motives and Incentives.* ed. Dunn, W.L., pp. 147-155. Washington: V.H. Winston & Sons

Schachter, S. (1978) Pharmacological and psychological determinants of smoking. *This volume.*

Seltzer, C., Friedman, G., Siegelaub, A. & Collen, M. (1974) Smoking habits and pain tolerance. *Archives of Environmental Health, 29,* 170-172.

Sokolov, E. (1963) *Perception and Conditioned Reflex.* New York: Macmillan.

Surwillo, W. (1963) The relation of simple response time to brain wave frequency and the effects of age. *Electroencephalography and Clinical Neurophysiology, 15,* 105-114.

Surwillo, W. (1964a) The relation of decision time to brain wave frequency and to age. *Electroencephalography and Clinical Neurophysiology, 16,* 510-514.

Surwillo, W. (1964b) Some observations on the relation of response speed to frequency of photic stimulation under conditions of EEG synchronisation. *Electroencephalography and Clinical Neurophysiology, 17,* 194-198.

Surwillo, W. (1968) Timing of behavior in senescence and the role of the central central nervous system. In *Human Aging and Behavior,* ed. Talland, G.A. pp. 1-35. New York: Academic Press.

Surwillo, W. (1971) Human reaction time and period of the EEG in relation to development. *Psychophysiology, 8,* 468-482.

Surwillo, W. (1974) Speed of movement in relation to period of the electroenceph-alogram in normal children. *Psychophysiology,* **11**, 491-496.

Tarriere, C. & Hartemann, F. (1964) Investigation into the effects of tobacco smoke on a visual vigilance task. *Ergonomics,* Proceedings of 2nd. I.E.A. Congress, Dortmund, 525-530.

Tong, J., Knott, V., McGraw, D. & Leigh, G. (1974a) Smoking and human experi-mental psychology. *Bulletin of the British Psychological Society,* **27**, 533-538.

Tong, J., Knott, V., McGraw, D. & Leigh, G. (1974b) Alcohol, visual discrimination and heart rate: Effects of dose activation and tobacco. *Quarterly Journal for the Study of Alcohol,* **35**, 1003-1022.

Tong, J., Leigh, G., Campbell, J. & Smith, D. (1977) Tobacco smoking, personality and sex factors in auditory vigilance performance. *British Journal of Psychology,* **68**, 365-370.

Ulett, J. & Itil, T. (1969) Quantitative electroencephalogram in smoking and smoking deprivation. *Science, N.Y.,* **164**, 969-970.

Vazquez, A. & Toman, J. (1967) Some interactions of nicotine with other drugs upon central nervous system function. *Annals of New York Academy of Sciences,* **142**, 201-215.

Venables, P. (1964) Input dysfunction in schizophrenia. In *Advances in Experimental Personality Research,* ed. Maher, B. New York: Academic Press.

Venables, P. (1969) Sensory aspects of psychopathology. In *Neurobiological Aspects of Psychopathology,* ed. Zubin, J. & Shagass, C., pp. 132-141. New York: Grune & Stratton.

Venables, P. (1971) Schizophrenia as a disorder of input processing. *Proceedings of the Academy of Medical Sciences,* U.S.S.R., **5**, 10-12.

Venables, P. (1973) Input regulation and psychopathology. In *Towards a Science of Psychopathology,* ed. Hammer, M., Sulzinger, K. & Sutton, S. New York: Wiley.

Venables, P. (1975) Signals, noise, refractoriness and storage: Some concepts of value to psychopathology. In *Experimental Approaches to Psychopathology,* ed. Kietzman, M., Sutton, S. & Zubin, J., pp. 365-380. New York: Academic Press.

Vogel, W., Broverman, D. & Klaiber, E. (1977) Electroencephalographic responses to photic stimulation in habitual smokers and non-smokers. *Journal of Comparative and Physiological Psychology,* **91**, 418-422.

Warburton, D. & Wesnes, K. (1978) Individual differences in smoking and attentional performance. *This volume.*

Warwick, K. & Eysenck, H. (1963) The effects of smoking on the CFF threshold. *Life Sciences,* **4**, 219-225.

Wechsler, R. (1962) Effects of cigarette smoking and intravenous nicotine on the brain (Abstract). *Federation Proceedings,* **17**, 169.

Wesnes, K. & Warburton, D. (1978) The effects of cigarette smoking and nicotine tablets upon human attention. *This volume.*

Wilder, J. (1967) *Stimulus and Response: The Law of Initial Value.* Baltimore, Md: Williams & Wilkins.

Woodruff, D. (1975) Relationships among EEG alpha frequency, reaction time and age: a biofeedback study. *Psychophysiology,* **12**, 673-680.

10. The effects of cigarette smoking and nicotine tablets upon human attention

KEITH WESNES AND DAVID M WARBURTON

Introduction

Attention is the process that enables the individual to ignore the vast majority of the information which emanates from the internal and external environments. Contemporary theory in psychology holds that attention is necessary because the individual has only a limited capacity to process this information. Kahneman (1973) terms the available capacity mental effort, and argues that it is applied to the performance of some tasks as opposed to others. In a similar fashion Norman (1976) postulates that the limited processing resources of the individual are applied to particular aspects of mental activity. In both of these models the limiting factor in the evaluation of environmental information is the availability of processing capacity. Thus if a number of tasks are being performed simultaneously, which together require more than the available amount of mental effort, then the performance of one or more of them will suffer. Time-based variation in the total quantity of processing capacity are accompanied by changes in physiological arousal. These theories predict that moderate increases in arousal will augment the amount of resources available to the individual.

We are interested in determining the neurochemical mechanisms controlling attention. Warburton (1975), from a consideration of a large quantity of animal experimentation, put forward the theory that by controlling electrocortical arousal, the ascending reticular cholinergic pathways are mediating the selection of stimuli from the environments. In terms of the previously descrived models of attention, Warburton has proposed that activity in cholinergic pathways determines the processing capacity of the individual. In order to investigate the possibility that human attention is controlled by cholinergic mechanisms, we have studied the attentional effect of drugs which influence cholinergic activity. In this paper we present a series of experiments in which we have attempted to measure the attentional effects of nicotine, a drug known to increase both cholinergic functioning and electrocortical arousal (Armitage and Hall, 1967), and which we thus predicted would improve attentional efficiency in our experimental situation.

Cigarette smoking and vigilance

In a vigilance task a subject is typically required to monitor a stimulus source for a brief signal which has an unpredictable and usually low probability of occurrence. It is generally observed that as the time spent performing the task increases, the probability that the observer will correctly detect the experimental signal decreases. This effect had been referred to as the vigilance decrement by many workers. It is a time-based inability to apply a constant level of mental effort to a particular task. It was decided to investigate the effects of cigarette smoking upon vigilance performance, using the Continuous Clock Task first used by Mackworth (1965), who found that the efficiency of performance of the task was sensitive to drug manipulation.

Before the first major study two small pilot studies were carried out. In the first smokers and non-smokers were tested in the continuous clock situation. The smoker group were required to smoke one inch of a king-sized filter-tipped cigarette at 15, 30 and 45 minutes into the hour-long task. The subjects were isolated in an experimental room and instructed to observe the hand of an electric clock. They were required to detect and respond to brief pauses in the otherwise continuous movement of the clock hand. It was found that the smokers improved over time while the non-smokers showed a vigilance decrement. In the second pilot study a smoking design developed by Frankenhaeuser et al, (1971) was used in which smokers are instructed to smoke 53 mm of a cigarette at twenty, forty and sixty minutes into the eighty minute experimental session. Instead of using non-smokers in this experiment, smokers were used and they were not permitted to smoke during the study; a group we shall call deprived smokers. Once again it was found that the smoker group performed more efficiently overtime than the control group.

On the basis of this encouraging data a major study into the effects of cigarette smoking upon visual vigilance was undertaken, using the same smoking design, and with both deprived smokers and non-smokers as control groups. As a partial control for the act of smoking, the two control groups were required to place one end of a pencil in their mouths for equivalent smoking periods. The signal rate was forty signals every ten minutes, the signal duration being 0.03 sec. All subjects were required to abstain from tobacco, tea and coffee for 12 hours preceding the experiment. Subjects were paid 1p for every four correctly detected signals in order to maintain their motivation during the long and boring task. The results are presented in Figure 10.1. Subjects made sufficient false alarms (false positive responses) for the data to be analysed using signal detection theory. The vertical axis represents the non-parametric index of sensitivity which was calculated from formulae presented by Grier (1971). It can be seen that the smokers maintained a constant superior level of stimulus selection compared to the two non-smoking control groups, who both exhibited decrements in performance over time. It can be seen from Figure 10.1 however that the groups differed in their levels of sensitivity, even before the smokers began their first cigarette. Consequently, a sensitivity score for the first twenty minutes was calculated and the subsequent scores were subtracted from this; making the first twenty minutes a baseline to which subsequent performance was compared. Two planned orthogonal comparisons were made between the performances of the three groups. The first comparison was between the smokers and the two non-smoking groups, while the second was between the two non-smoking groups. Using a t ratio (Kirk, 1968; p. 73), the differences of the adjusted for baseline scores between the smokers and the two control groups were found to be significant beyond the 5% level (t = 1.97, df = 27), while the

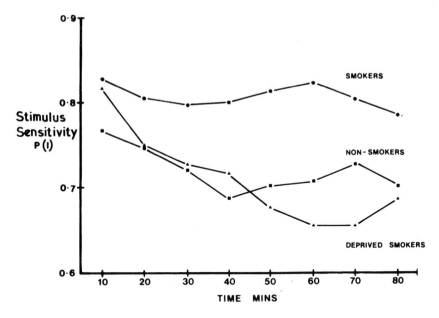

Fig. 10.1 Effects of cigarette smoking upon visual vigilance

differences between the deprived smokers and the non-smoker groups were not
found to be significant (t = 1.196, df = 27, p .3).

This study indicates that cigarette smoking in some way helps smokers to maintain
a superior level of concentration over time, when compared to either non-smokers or
other smokers not smoking. Although we would like to argue that nicotine is
responsible for the favourable action of smoking upon vigilance, the drug was only
one of a number of factors which might have influenced performance. The smokers
had not smoked for at least 12 hours before the experiment, and it is not unreasonable
to suppose that the subjects in the smoker group derived some pleasure from smoking
during the study, in contrast to the deprived smokers who knew that they would
not be able to smoke until after the session was finished. These factors may have
influenced performance, as might the various other sensory aspects of the smoking
act.

Clearly, if we wished to determine the effects of nicotine upon performance, a
more sophisticated control for the act of smoking, was needed than the oral manipulation of the blunt end of a pencil. In the next study, as an attempt to control
for the non-pharmacological aspects of smoking, a herbal cigarette which contained
no nicotine was used. In order to discover whether the beneficial effects of smoking
were specific to the visual modality an auditory vigilance task was designed.
Performance with commercially available cigarettes, having a standard nicotine
delivery of 2.1 mg was compared to that with the nicotine-free cigarettes. To
minimise variability a within subject design was employed; each subject serving in
both conditions of the experiment, and thus acting as his own control.. The same
smoking design was used as in the previous study, subjects being deprived of tobacco

and caffeine for 12 hours before the experiment, and smoking the cigarettes at twenty, forty and sixty minutes into the eighty minute task. During the experiment subjects were presented, via headphones, with one second bursts of white noise which occurred every 2½ secs. In a small proportion of these noise bursts a faint tone occurred. The subjects were required to detect and respond to those noise bursts which also contained a signal tone.

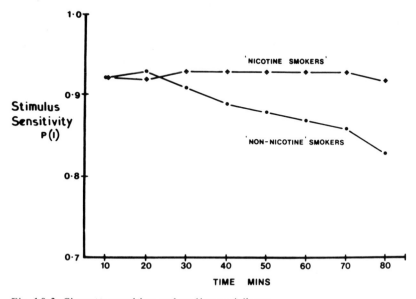

Fig. 10.2 Cigarette smoking and auditory vigilance

The results are presented in Figure 10.2. As there were no baseline differences, the performance following the first twenty minutes was compared for the two conditions. The differences in performance under the two smoking conditions was highly significant (t = 7.06, df 7, p<.0005). Thus it has been demonstrated that cigarette smoking can improve performance relative to non-smoking conditions in an auditory task as well as in a visual one. However, how far have we come towards demonstrating that nicotine was the agent responsible for the enhancement? The nicotine-free cigarettes have an unusual taste and smell, and while none of the subjects realised that the cigarettes were not made from tobacco, they could all distinguish them from the commercially available cigarette. Thus, although the subjects were going through the actions involved in smoking in the non-nicotine condition, they could differentiate the two cigarettes, which lessens the effectiveness of this control procedure to some extent. Nonetheless simply being able to differentiate the cigarettes does not necessarily imply that the subjects had different expectations of the influence of the two cigarettes upon performance.

Another method of controlling for the smoking act involves comparing the effects of various delivery cigarettes upon performance. This technique has the advantage that subjects are smoking commercially available cigarettes in all conditions of the experiment, and will thus not notice one with a peculiar taste. Furthermore several different cigarettes can be used so that the effects of a range of doses upon performance can be investigated.   It was considered worthwhile to use this procedure to determine the effects of various amounts of nicotine upon vigilance performance. Three experimental cigarettes were obtained from the member companies of the Tobacco Research Council. The cigarettes, codenamed 1, 2 and 4, had standard nicotine deliveries of 0.28, 0.7 and 1.65 mg respectively. The experimental situation was a version of the previously used Continuous Clock Task, modified so that the subjects must decide at the end of every 15 second period whether a signal occurred or not. Twelve male heavy smokers took part in the experiment, each one performing the task on three occasions, smoking different experimental cigarettes each time. As in the previous studies, during any eighty minute session the cigarettes were smoked at twenty, forty and sixty minutes after the start.

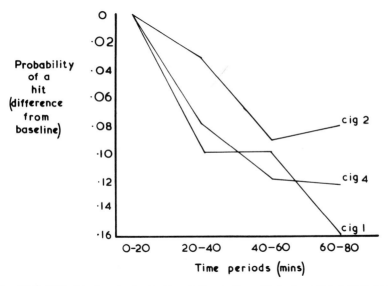

Fig. 10.3 Effects of various nicotine delivery cigarettes upon visual vigilance performance

The results are presented in Figure 10.3.   As a result of large variations in intraindividual performance between sessions, the first twenty minutes were used as a baseline against which subsequent performance was measured. Thus a positive score on the vertical axis of the figure indicates that performance has deteriorated compared to the performance during the first twenty minutes. It was predicted that cigarette 4 would produce less decrement in performance than cigarettes 1 and 2; and similarly that cigarette 2 would produce less decrement than cigarette 1. However, an inspection of the graph reveals that this prediction was not confirmed by the data.   Statistical analysis revealed that the only significant enhancement of performance is between the 0.7 mg. and the 0.28 mg. cigarettes during the first twenty minutes following baseline (Friedman Two Way Analysis of Ranks, critical difference between cigarette 2 and cigarette 1 is 10, p $<$.05).

During the experimentation the cigarette butts were collected and sent to the B.A.T. Group Research and Development Centre, Southampton, for analysis. Once the butt has been analysed for nicotine content, it is possible - knowing the filtration efficiency of the cigarette filter - to calculate the approximate amount of nicotine which has been delivered to the smoker. The results of the butt analyses are presented in another part of this volume (Warburton and Wesnes, 1978). From these data it is evident that the lower nicotine delivery cigarettes were smoked more intensively than the higher delivery cigarette. Thus on a standard smoking machine the low nicotine cigarette would be expected to deliver 0.28 mg. nicotine, while the smokers in this study received almost twice this amount. The same thing was observed for cigarette 2, whilst with cigarette 4 the smokers received roughly as much nicotine as the smoking machine would extract. Possible explanations for the individual differences in smoking behaviour are discussed elsewhere (Warburton and Wesnes, 1978). As far as the present experiment is concerned the dose range has been narrowed quite markedly, which decreases the likelihood that differences in behavioural effects would be demonstrated between the three dose levels. Furthermore the lowest dose appears to be around 0.6 mg which in itself might be sufficient to produce a significant enhancement of performance.

In this study we have investigated the effects of a smaller dose range than originally intended, as well as having compared the higher doses to a dose which may well be sufficient in itself to affect performance. The task does not seem to be sensitive enough to distinguish between these relatively small dose variations. A control situation in which subjects did not smoke might have clarified the situation, and this point will be discussed more fully in a later section.

Nicotine tablets and vigilance performance

As a rapid and easy way to deliver nicotine to the brain, cigarette smoke cannot be equalled, but from the viewpoint of psychopharmacology the quantitative aspects of this route of administration present considerable difficulties. Variations in the rate, depth and duration of inhalation of tobacco smoke make not only dose replication, but also dose quantification extremely difficult. It is also apparent from the previous discussion that it is difficult to devise a satisfactory placebo; consequently, it is not possible to be certain that nicotine is the sole agent responsible for the behavioural effects of cigarette smoking.

Another problem concerns the nature of the subject population with which workers in this field must necessarily deal. In the first place there is a good deal of evidence indicating that smokers differ from non-smokers on a number of personality characteristics (see Warburton and Wesnes, 1978). Secondly, the acute behavioural effects of a drug which is chronically self-administered by the subject population are being tested. The problem here is deciding what is the 'normal' state of the smoking population. If normality is the drug-free state then the data can be interpreted as in any psychopharmacological study. However, if the drugged state is normal then studies of the behavioural effects of cigarette smoking are comparing normal behaviour with performance after nicotine deprivation. One approach to this problem would be to determine the effects of cigarette smoking upon the performance of non-smokers. However apart from the ethical considerations involved, the unpleasant reactions which individuals demonstrate when attempting to develop a satisfactory technique would almost certainly be sufficient to mask any behavioural effects that nicotine may have.

The alternative approach which was adopted was the direct administration of nicotine. If it were demonstrated that the performance of non-smokers would benefit from nicotine, then this would strongly suggest that nicotine was having a beneficial effect upon the smokers in our previous studies, not merely restoring their performance to normal levels.

We consequently considered various techniques for directly administering nicotine to subjects. Pharmacologically, the ideal technique would be to inject it directly into the bloodstream. However subjects would find injections extremely stressful and it is likely that this would induce sufficient variance into the behavioural measures to obscure any drug effects. We chose oral administration of nicotine, favouring buccal absorption over gastro-intestinal absorption which is unsatisfactory for two reasons. Firstly, the absorption rate is determined by stomach contents, which are difficult to control and would add variability to the drug effects. Secondly, the stomach contents are acidic which slows the rate of absorption of nicotine quite dramatically. In contrast buccal absorption of nicotine is relatively rapid and the drug travels to the brain without hepatic transformation.

Nicotine tablets were prepared from a solution of nicotine free-base. A dose range was selected which was comparable to the estimated nicotine doses taken into the mouth during smoking in the previous study, i.e. 0, 1 and 2 mg. of nicotine. Initial testing of the tablets indicated that subjects could differentiate between the doses on the basis of the amount of bitterness produced in the mouth. In order to overcome this problem, a drop of Tabasco sauce was added to the placebo and the nicotine tablets giving both a bitter flavour, which was sufficient to ensure that subjects could not tell the doses apart on the basis of taste.

The absorption rates of our tablets were then tested. As nicotine markedly increases heart rate, this measure was used to determine the time taken for the nicotine to be absorbed. We administered each of our doses to a small group of subjects, using a plethysmograph to record pulse rate. The subjects were instructed to keep the tablets in their mouths for a ten minute period and heart rate measures were taken over the next 36 minute period.   As can be seen from Figure 10.4 there was a dose-dependent increase in heart rate, the peak effect for the 2 mg dose occurring ten minutes after the subjects had swallowed the tablet. This indicated that the large dose would have its peak effect twenty minutes after the subject first placed it in his mouth.

The first study with nicotine tablets was designed to determine their effects upon the vigilance performance of non-smokers, using a group of 12 subjects in which both sexes were equally represented. In order to make the study comparable to the previous ones the nicotine tablets were given to the subjects twenty, forty and sixty minutes into the eighty minute clock task. The first twenty minute period of the session was again used as a baseline against which subsequent performance would be compared. As in the previous study each subject served in each condition of the experiment. Standard counterbalancing techniques were employed for dose order effects. The heart rate study had indicated that the nicotine tablets took roughly twenty minutes to reach their peak effect, and it was consequently assumed that performance during the last forty minutes of the task would be more sensitive to the action of the drug.

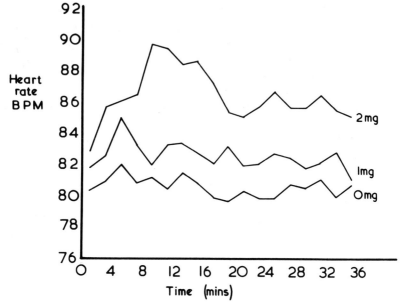

Fig. 10.4 Effects of nicotine tablets upon heart-rate

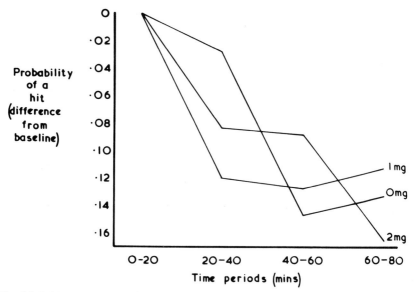

Fig. 10.5 Non-smokers, nicotine tablets and the clock test.

It is evident from Figure 10.5 that the nicotine tablets did not have any consistent effects upon performance in this task. It was predicted that performance during the last forty minutes would firstly be more efficient with the nicotine tablets than with placebo, and secondly, more efficient with 2 mg of nicotine than 1 mg. However, statistical analyses of the data revealed that these predictions were not borne out.

These data can be used to support the argument that cigarette smokers are dependent upon nicotine to function normally, and that consequently any changes in performance that have been demonstrated in previous studies have merely been restorations to normal levels, not enhancements of performance. However, the possibility remained that the nicotine tablets had produced adverse effects upon the non-smoker subjects, and that this had disrupted their attention sufficiently to counteract any beneficial effects of the drug upon performance. The experiment was run double-blind which meant that even though some subjects complained about the effects of the tablets, the experimenter had no way of relating the complaints to the dose they had received.

The next study investigated the effects of nicotine tablets upon the vigilance performance of 12 light and 12 heavy smokers, males and females again being equally represented. The light smokers smoked five cigarettes or less a day and had a smoking history of less than two years. The heavy smokers all smoked over 15 cigarettes a day and had been smoking for longer than three years. The experimental design was identical to the one used with the non-smokers. The results are presented in Figure 10.6.

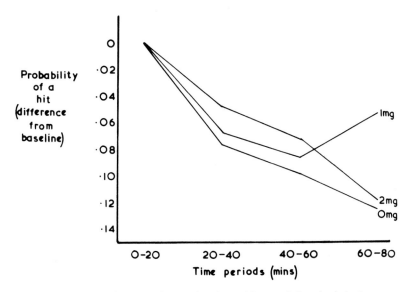

Fig. 10.6 Heavy and light smokers, nicotine tablets and the clock test.

As for non-smokers, two between-dose comparisons of the performance during the last forty minutes were made. The first comparison was between placebo and the two doses of nicotine, and the second between the two doses of the drug. Before these comparisons were tested Grubb's Test for a single outlier was carried out to determine whether the unusually large response to nicotine in one particular subject was abnormal and not related to the rest of the data. Grubb's Test revealed that this score could not have come from the same population as the rest of the data ($R = 0.561$, $p < .01$) and thus it was excluded from the statistical analyses. These analyses indicated that the difference between the placebo dose and the two nicotine doses were significant ($t = 1.927$, $df = 44$, $p < .05$), while the differences between the two doses of nicotine were not.

Thus it has been demonstrated that nicotine tablets enhanced performance relative to control. At first sight these data appear to be a validation of the argument put forward previously, that smokers require nicotine to perform normally, particularly when non-smokers in identical conditions showed no benefit from taking nicotine. However, while the nicotine-dependent argument might hold for the heavy smokers, it is hard to see how it applies to the light smokers, some of whom only smoked at weekends, usually none smoked in the mornings when the experiments were carried out, and none objected to abstaining from cigarettes during the 12 hours preceding the experiment (which was certainly not the case for the heavy smokers!). If dependence was a primary factor in determining the effects of nicotine upon performance, then one would expect heavy smokers to be affected more by nicotine than the light smokers. There was no evidence for this view, as the responsivity of the two groups to the drug could not be statistically differentiated. In conclusion, it is difficult to argue that the light smokers were dependent upon nicotine, and needed it in order to perform 'normally', although the argument can be made more convincingly for the heavy smokers.

If smokers in these studies are not dependent upon nicotine in order to perform at normal levels, how then can the absence of effect of the nicotine tablets upon non-smokers be explained? It was already been proposed that the non-smokers might have experienced adverse side effects on what was almost certainly their first direct contact with nicotine. Although there is no direct evidence in this study to support this contention, many smokers often report feelings of nausea associated with their first experiences with cigarettes, possibly due to the parasympathetic effects of nicotine. As light smokers have smoked for a period of time they will have developed a tolerance for these effects, which would ensure that their performance with nicotine was not disrupted by any side-effects. However, the question of adverse **side-effects** can only be settled by giving the subjects a debriefing questionnaire after each dose, in order to determine whether the subjects found nicotine unpleasant, and if they considered that this affected their performance. We intend to employ this technique in our future studies.

Nicotine and the Stroop effect

The Stroop test is a well established paradigm in experimental psychology in which a subject is required to name aloud the colour of the inks in which a series of colour names are printed. However, the colour names never correspond to the colour of the ink in which they are printed. Subjects find this incongruity very distracting, and take longer to complete such a list than they take to name an equivalent length list of colour blobs. The difference in time between the two conditions is termed the Stroop effect and represents the distraction caused by the incongruent colour words. We interpret this effect as a failure of the attentional process in so much as the irrelevant words are not completely ignored.

It was predicted that nicotine, by enhancing the attentional process, would enable subjects to ignore the words to a greater extent, thus reducing the Stroop effect. In order to test this prediction, the effects of 0, 1 and 2 mg of nicotine were studied upon the Stroop performance of a group of subjects comprising six smokers and six non-smokers.   As in previous studies each subject was tested with each dose on a separate occasion, the order of dose administration being balanced across subjects.

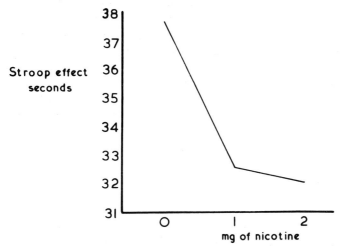

Fig. 10.7 The action of nicotine upon the Stroop effect.

It is clear from Figure 10.7 that in accordance with the prediction, nicotine reduced the magnitude of the Stroop effect in this study. The planned statistical comparison revealed that this reduction in the effect was significant ($t = 1.968$, df $= 22$, $p < .05$). No differences were found either between the effects of the two doses of nicotine upon the Stroop scores or between the responsivity of the smokers and the non-smokers to the drug.   The latter finding adds support to the argument that the smokers in our studies are not dependent upon nicotine to achieve normal levels of performance. It is interesting that in this study both smokers and non-smokers performed more efficiently with nicotine, in contrast to the differential respons-ivity observed between the two groups in the vigilance studies. This incongruity could be due to the fact that subjects took three tablets during every session of the Clock test, as opposed to one in this study.   If the non-smokers did find nico-tine tablets unpleasant in the vigilance study, it could have been a cumulative effect of taking three tablets in just over forty minutes.   Certainly none of the subjects complained about the tablets in the present study.

Cigarette smoking and rapid information processing

It has been demonstrated that smokers, in situations requiring continuous attention over extended time periods, performed more efficiently when smoking or taking

nicotine tablets when compared with the no drug condition.   It has also been demonstrated that both smokers and non-smokers are less susceptible to distraction when
taking nicotine tablets.   In order to extend the scope of the investigations a situation
was selected in which subjects are required to perform detailed processing of information presented at extremely rapid rates.   The experimental task was one that has
previously been employed to study the effects of drugs upon attention (Talland,
1966; Bakan, Belton & Roth, 1963).   In the version of the test employed here,
subjects monitored a series of numbers which were presented singly upon a TV
screen, at a rate of 100 per minute.   The subjects were required to detect series
of three consecutive odd or even numbers.   There were approximately eighty of
these triads in every ten minute period.

   In the first experiment using this task, the performance effects of cigarettes 1, 2
and 4, previously studied with the Clock task, were investigated.   This study was
performed in parallel with the clock task, and so the nicotine analyses of the cigarette
butts from that study had not been completed.   If it had been known that there was
compensation in the smoking of the lower nicotine yield cigarettes a non-smoking
control session would have been introduced into the experiment.   As it was, 23
male, heavy smokers were tested on the task, every subject performing the task with
each of the cigarettes.   The subjects performed the task for ten minutes and were
then given a ten-minute period in which to smoke the experimental cigarette.   Then
they performed the task for a further twenty minutes.   The purpose of the first
ten-minute period was to obtain a baseline level of performance against which to
compare subsequent performance.   Thus, the data for the experiment, which are
presented in Figure 10.8, are once again in the form of difference from baseline
scores for the probability of a hit (correct detection of a triad).

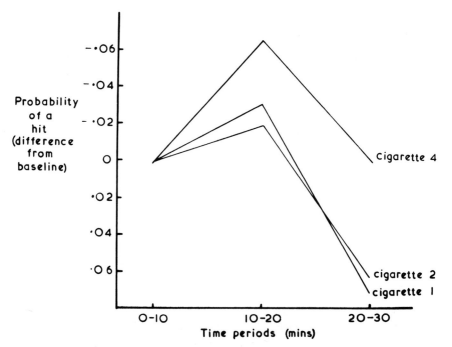

Fig. 10.8 The effects of various strength cigarettes upon rapid information processing.

While it had been predicted that performance following cigarette 4 would be more efficient that that following cigarettes 1 and 2, it had not been anticipated that performance would improve, relative to baseline, for the first ten minutes following each of the three cigarettes, as can be seen in Figure 10.8. The planned comparisons revealed that for the second ten minutes of the post-smoking period the subjects performed more efficiently after smoking cigarette 4 than after cigarettes 1 and 2 ($t = 2.037$, $df = 44$, $p < .025$). There was a similar trend for the first ten minutes of the post-smoking period which however, did not reach significance ($t = 1.355$, $df = 44$, $p < .1$). No differences were found between performance following cigarettes 1 and 2. We analysed the unexpected improvements following smoking and found that only after smoking cigarette 4 did subjects significantly improve compared to baseline ($F = 5.01$, $df = 1, 22$, $p < .05$). Thus in this study both an absolute and a relative improvement in performance have been found with the high nicotine cigarette. These data strongly suggest that this task is more sensitive than the Clock test to the differential effects of these various cigarettes upon attentional efficiency.

Next, the effects upon performance in this task of two cigarettes of differing strengths, were studied. One cigarette, codenamed 6, yielded 0.9 mg of nicotine on a standard smoking machine, while the other, codenamed 5, yielded 1. 8 mg. Both cigarettes were identical in appearance. Two control conditions were introduced into this experiment: a 'nicotine-free' smoking session, using the herbal cigarettes described earlier, and a non-smoking session. Six male and six female heavy smokers were used as subjects, each subject being tested in all four experimental conditions. The order of administration of the four conditions was balanced using a 4 x 4 Latin Square design. In the last study a practice effect was observed from session to session, and although the experimental design minimised the variance introduced by this practice, it was decided to reduce this still further by giving the subjects two twenty-minute practice sessions before they took part in the main study. The experimental procedure was identical to that used in the previous study; subjects performing the task for ten minutes, receiving the drug treatment during the next ten minutes, and finally performing the test for a further twenty minutes.

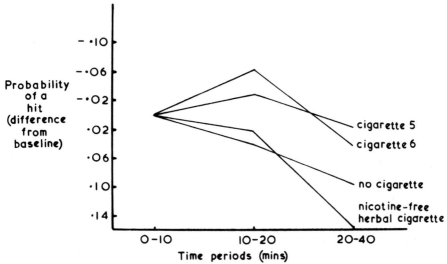

Fig. 10.9 The effects of smoking various cigarettes upon rapid information processing.

F

The data are presented in Figure 10.9.   The performance in the two tobacco smoking sessions was similar to the smoking performance in the previous study: an initial increase in efficiency which declined in the second half of the post-smoking period. In contrast, performance in the non-smoking and nicotine-free cigarette conditions showed a general decrement over the sessions.   It had been predicted that the performance in the first ten minutes following cigarettes 5 and 6 would be improved relative to baseline.   The planned comparisons revealed that the higher nicotine delivery cigarette produced a slight but insignificant enhancement ($t = 1.182$, $df = 11$, $p < .15$), while the lower delivery cigarette significantly improved performance compared to baseline ($t = 1.816$, $df = 11$, $p < .05$).

It was also predicted that performance following cigarettes 5 and 6 would be more efficient than that following the two control conditions.   This prediction was confirmed by statistical evaluation of the data which revealed that performance with these cigarettes was very significantly superior to that in the control conditions ($t = 3.219$, $df = 44$, $p < .005$).   No differences in performance were found between either the two cigarettes or the two control conditions.

In the last two studies, performance following smoking has once again been found to be more efficient compared to control conditions.   At the present time the butt analyses of the cigarettes used in these experiments have not been completed; consequently it is not yet possible to relate the performance to the actual nicotine deliveries.   However, with regard to the cigarettes smoked in the first study, the smoking profiles have been obtained from the vigilance study, in which these cigarettes were also used.   These results indicated that subjects would receive most nicotine from cigarette 4, and it was on these grounds that it was predicted that performance would be most efficient with this cigarette.   This was borne out by the data.   However without information concerning the smoking techniques subjects employed when smoking cigarettes 5 and 6, it is not possible to determine whether they received different amounts of nicotine from the two cigarettes.

The data from the nicotine-free cigarette indicate that performance following this cigarette is no better than performance following not smoking at all, suggesting that the mechanics of the act of smoking did not play a large part in the effects of smoking upon performance.

Discussion

In this paper a number of studies designed to determine the effects of nicotine upon human attention have been presented.   The general findings were that smokers performed more efficiently in the experimental situations with cigarettes or nicotine tablets than without.   We interpret these findings as representing a nicotine-induced enhancement of attentional efficiency.

The extent to which nicotine was responsible for the behavioural changes following smoking is discussed first.   It has already been pointed out that in the smoking studies it was not possible to present a control procedure which was identical to cigarette smoking in all respects except nicotine delivery.   To begin with the nicotine-free cigarettes that were used had a different taste to the experimental cigarettes.   The auditory vigilance study was carried out a number of years ago when the cigarettes were quite new on the market; consequently, none of the subjects had had any previous contact with them.   Thus while some of the subjects did find the taste unusual they did not realise that the cigarettes were not made from tobacco. However, in the recent study in which the nicotine-free cigarettes were used as a control procedure, ten of the 12 subjects were aware that the cigarettes did not contain tobacco.   Thus as well as being able to identify the nicotine-free cigarettes on the basis of taste, the subjects in this more recent study may well have had particular expectations as to the effects of these cigarettes upon performance. Similarly, in the experiments in which subjects smoked three cigarettes with varying nicotine deliveries, they were able to differentiate the cigarettes on the basis of both appearance and smoke delivery.   However, these factors appear to have had little affect upon performance.   If the inhalation of smoke (with or without nicotine) and the manipulation of the cigarette were factors which affected performance, we would have expected performance during the information processing study to have been more efficient in the nicotine-free condition than in the no smoking condition. This clearly was not the case, which suggests to us that these factors do not play a considerable part in the beneficial effects of smoking upon performance which we have observed in our studies.

Carbon monoxide delivery was another factor which was not controlled for.   However, from a consideration of the actions of carbon monoxide upon the Central Nervous System, taken together with the known behavioural effects of the gas (Guillerm, Radziszewski and Caille, 1978), we feel that it is highly unlikely that it could have improved performance in our studies.

Evidence for nicotine being the active agent in cigarette smoking comes from the studies in which the drug was administered orally and absorbed via the buccal membrane In these experiments it was demonstrated that equivalent amounts of nicotine to those which smokers typically extract from cigarettes produced enhancements of performance comparable to those produced by cigarette smoking in the vigilance and rapid information tasks.   These data strongly suggest that a significant proportion of the effects of cigarette smoking upon the performance of our experimental tasks is attributable to nicotine.   However, the possibility cannot be ruled out that they may have been some additional effects due to sensory stimulation and subjective expectations.

We would now like to consider the function of nicotine in our studies.   As mentioned earlier the possibility exists that smokers develop a tolerance to the neural effects of smoking so that they become dependent upon nicotine for normal functioning.   There are three pieces of evidence which indicate that this is not the case for the subjects in the present studies.   The first concerns the performance of non-smokers in the vigilance situations. In the first study the levels of performance of the non-smokers and deprived smokers could not be statistically differentiated. Similarly, the placebo performance of the smokers and non-smokers in the nicotine tablet study were not significantly different. These findings are contrary to those one would expect, if the smokers were performing at less than normal levels in these nicotine-free sessions. The second piece of evidence is that no differences could be found in responsivity to nicotine tablets between the heavy and light smokers. As stated earlier, the smoking habits of the light smokers would hardly suggest they were dependent upon the habit for normal functioning.   Consequently, if the heavy smokers were dependent upon smoking, differences between the two types of smoker in their responsivity to the drug would have been predicted but there was no evidence of this. Thirdly, in the Stroop test both smokers and non-smokers were found to perform more efficiently with nicotine than without; the magnitude of the enhancement being the same for both groups. We feel that these three pieces of data sufficiently rule out the possibility that the smokers in our experiments were nicotine-dependent, permitting the conclusion that the behavioural changes observed in our studies represent enhancements of performance above normal levels.

Finally we would like to argue that we are justified in inferring that the nicotine-induced increases in the quality of performance in our studies represent improvements in attentional efficiency. While this is consistent with the standard techniques in psychopharmacology for determining drug effects upon attention (Wesnes, 1977) it is possible that other aspects of behaviour were being affected by nicotine in these experiments. However it has been demonstrated that the behavioural effects of nicotine are not specific to such factors as sensory modality, type of response, task duration, meaningfulness of stimuli, and time-pressure. This makes it unlikely that another aspect of behaviour besides attention was being affected by nicotine, particularly as a high level of concentration was an essential prerequisite for efficient performance in the studies.

We feel that the arguments we have presented justify our conclusion that our data represent a nicotine-induced improvement in attentional efficiency. These data are consistent with other studies of the behavioural effects of smoking (Tarriere & Harteman, 1964; Heimstra, Bancroft & DeKock, 1967; Frankenhaeuser *et al*, 1971) and provide preliminary evidence that human attention is controlled by the ascending cholinergic reticular pathways. We have also studied the attentional effects of scopolamine, a drug which attenuates cholinergic activity and which would be predicted to disrupt attentional efficiency. In both the Clock test and the rapid information processing task scopolamine has been found to impair performance, providing further support for cholinergic involvement in human attention.

Future experimentation which we intend to carry out in our laboratory includes the monitoring of electrocortical activity during our drug studies, the determination of the effects of cholinergic drugs upon divided attention, and the evaluation of the attentional effects of substances which alter activity in other neurochemical pathways.

Acknowledgements

We are grateful to the Medical Research Council for their support of our early studies, and to the Tobacco Research Council whose financial assistance has enabled this research project to continue. We thank Jacqueline Edwards, Grant Hawkins, Bernhard Matz, Suzanne Napleton and Jon Torfi for their invaluable help with various aspects of the experimentation.

References

Armitage, A.K. & Hall, G.H. (1967) The effects of nicotine on the electro-cortico-gram and spontaneous release of acetylcholine from the cerebral cortex of the cat. *Journal of Physiology*, (London), **191**, 115-116.

Bakan, P., Belton, J.A. & Roth, J.C. (1963) In *Vigilance: A Symposium,* ed. Buckner, D.A. & McGrath, J.J., pp. 22-28. New York: McGraw-Hill.

Frankenhaeuser, M., Myrsten, A-L., Post, B. & Johannson, G. (1971) Behavioural and physiological effects of cigarette smoking in a monotonous situation. *Psychopharmacologia,* **22,** 1-7.

Guillerm, R., Radziszewski, E. & Caille, J.E. (1978) Effects of carbon monoxide on performance in a vigilance task (automobile driving). *This volume.*

Grier, J.B. (1971) Formulae for a non-parametric index of sensitivity. *Psychological Bulletin,* **75,** 424-429.

Heimstra, N.W., Bancroft, N.R. & DeKock, A.R. (1967) Effects of smoking on sustained performance in a simulated driving test. *Annals of the New York Academy of Science,* **142,** 295-306.

Kahneman, D. (1973) *Attention and Effort.* Englewood Cliffs, N.J.: Prentice-Hall.

Kirk, R.E. (1968) *Experimental Designs and Procedures for the Behavioural Sciences,* Belmont, Brockes & Cal.

Mackworth, J.F. (1965) The detectability of signals in a vigilance task. *Canadian Journal of Psychology,* **19,** 104-110.

Norman, D. (1976) *Memory and Attention.* London: Wiley

Talland, G.A. (1966) Effects of alcohol on performance in continuous attention tasks. *Psychosomatic Medicine,* **28,** 596-604.

Tarriere, C. & Hartemann, F. (1964) Investigation into the effect of tobacco smoke on a visual vigilance task. *Ergonomics,* Proceedings of the 2nd I.E.A. Congress, Dortmund, 525-530.

Warburton, D.M. (1975) *Brain, Behaviour and Drugs.* London: Wiley.

Warburton, D.M. (1978) In *Chemical Influences in Behaviour,* ed. Brown, K., Cooper, S.T. London: Academic Press (in press).

Warburton, D.M. & Wesnes, K. (1978) Individual differences in smoking and attentional performance. *This volume.*

Wesnes, K. (1977) The effects of psychotropic drugs upon human behaviour. *Modern Problems in Pharmacopsychiatry,* **12,** 37-58.

11. Effects of carbon monoxide on performance in a vigilance task (automobile driving)

R GUILLERM, E RADZISZEWSKI AND J E CAILLE

The purpose of the study was to determine at which level in the blood carbon monoxide is capable of affecting vigilance and brain electrogenesis. As a matter of fact, there is a great discrepancy of results reported in the literature. To appreciate this, it is sufficient to quote, for example, the work of Schulte (1963), Beard and Grandstaff (1970) and that of Wright, Randell and Shephard (1973). These authors have noted a performance deterioration from a COHb level of 3% and up, whereas some other authors such as Hanks (1970), Mikulka (1970), Stewart *et al,* (1973) have observed no such deterioration below 12%. As far as electrobiology is concerned, only a few investigations have been conducted. Hosko (1970) reported no deterioration of spontaneous electroencephalographic activity below a COHb level of 33%, whereas he and also Stewart *et al* (1970) described changes in visual evoked response with COHb levels greater than 15%. We have carried out an experiment in an attempt to gather additional information concerning the effects of CO on man's performance and EEG.

To avoid all laboratory constraints and the artificial nature of laboratory simulations we selected as a vigilance test nocturnal driving of a car on a circuit. This method of vigilance analysis makes it possible to avoid any training effect and it ensures good motivation on the part of the subjects.

Materials and methods

An automatic car is used to determine the precision of a long-duration drive (five hours) at night at a constant prescribed speed (60 km/h) on a closed circuit (Circuit Paul Ricard, Le Castellet, France) measuring 3.4 km. The driving precision is determined based on variations of the car from a white line drawn on the track center line: the subject has to keep the car center line on this white line for five hours.

A set of photodiodes attached to the bumper (Fig. 11.1) makes it possible to know, at every moment, the position of the car center line with respect to the white line as follows: the light emitted by small red lamps attached between photodiodes is reflected by the white line and energises the corresponding photodiode.

An automatic coding system installed within the car makes it possible to quantify the deviations and thus to estimate the driving quality objectively. This technique has been described by Caille and Bassano (1976b). To complete this system the simulation of obstacles on the road is used to determine the visual response time

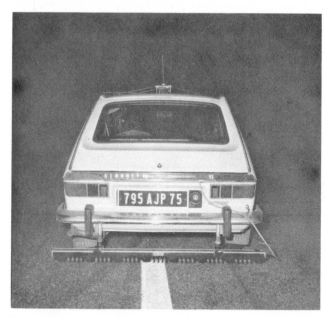

Fig. 11.1   View of the back of the car with the set of photodiodes

(VRT) of the subjects.   This simulation is carried out by means of a light that comes on randomly on the car bonnet and that the driver must switch off as quickly as possible by depressing a pedal which is near the brake pedal. Concurrently, the EEG data, which are known to reflect the activity level of some brain areas relating to vigilance, and ECG are continuously recorded.

The four parameters thus measured (driving precision, VRT, ECG and EEG) are transmitted by telemetry and recorded in a control tower, on paper and on magnetic tape for subsequent processing. The experimenters are in the control tower and can thus constantly monitor the variations of the different parameters during the test.

The experiment is carried out with eight non-smoking subjects.   Each subject has to drive the car for five hours during four non-consecutive nights so arranged as to avoid possible effects of tiredness, repetition and experimental conditions.

The experimental conditions include one night of habituation to the circuit, one reference night and two nights with COHb levels set and kept at 7 and 11% respectively.   COHb is determined with a pure-oxygen rebreathing system based on that of Sjostrand (1948) and developed by Guillerm *et al,* in 1959: partial pressures of oxygen and CO in the alveolar air are measured while they are in equilibrium with the blood (within about six minutes); this method is as reproducible and accurate as COHb determination in blood samples.

Before the test, the rapid adjustment of the COHb level to the above mentioned values is carried out within ten minutes according to a laboratory developed rebreathing technique. In order to compensate for the detoxication the COHb level is kept at the adjusted value during driving through inhalation, at regular intervals.

of a mixture of air and CO; the mixture is so designed as to require short periods of inhalation: five or ten minutes; to disturb the subject as little as possible this readjustment is carried out only every hour by means of a light and low resistance mouth respirator (Fig. 11.2) connected to the bottle containing the mixture of air and CO which is located on the back seat of the car. Orders are given to the subject by radiotelephone.

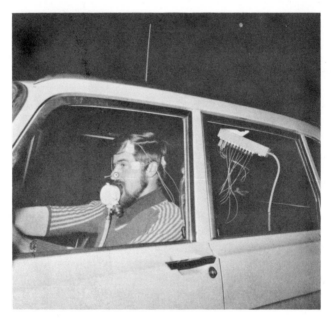

Fig. 11.2 Experimental conditions during adjustment of the COHb level

A thirty - minute break was made after three driving hours to allow the subjects to relax and, if need be, to go to the lavatory; we took advantage of this break to check COHb levels.

Results

COHb levels
The COHb values obtained after adjustment, during the break and after the five-hour test are presented in Table 11.1. Results indicate that the COHb levels on the whole are satisfactory throughout the period of five hours.

Driving precision
The values (arbitrary units) shown on the graph correspond to deviations from the mean. In any case the time history of the driving performances is the same: there is an improvement during the first hour followed by a gradual deterioration; after the relaxation break, the performance variations are similar but they occur in a much

Desired COHb	Initial level	Control after 3 hrs.	Final level
7%	8.2% (±0.19)	7.23% (±0.26)	7.34% (±0.20)
11%	12.15% (±0.61)	11.4% (±0.38)	11.03% (±0.34)

Table 11.1   Results of the obtained COHb levels after adjustment (mean of eight subjects ± s.e.)

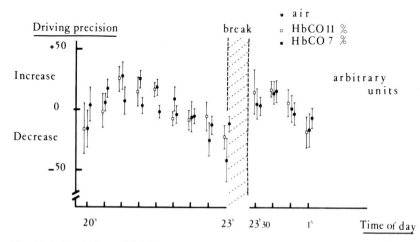

Fig. 11.3   Variation of driving precision. The data shown correspond to deviations from the mean (mean of eight subjects ± s.e.)

shorter time. Such variations clearly denote an effect of tiredness. It becomes evident and this is proved statistically, that the COHb levels of 7 and 11% cause no significant changes in the driving precision.

Visual reaction time
Changes are relatively mild on the whole and VRT is not significantly affected by COHb levels of 7 and 11%.
In any case, after relative stability during the first hour, there is a slight increase in the VRT which reveals a gradual building up of tiredness.

EEG
A small and non-significant deterioration of the cortical activity is observed during driving, independent of experimental conditions; such a deterioration results in a synchronisation of the alpha waves the frequency of which is reduced by less than 0.5 Hertz (Table 11.2).

F*

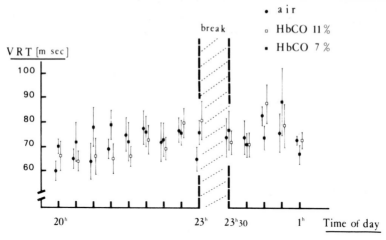

Fig. 11.4 Variation with time of visual reaction time during a five hour car ride
(mean of eight subjects $\pm$ s.e.)

| | | α – waves frequency | |
COHb level	Before	During 5 hour car ride	After
0	9.7 ± 0.1	9.5 ± 0.1	9.3 ± 0.1
7%	9.5 ± 0.1	9.3 ± 0.1	9.2 ± 0.1
11%	9.7 ± 0.1	9.4 ± 0.1	9.6 ± 0.1

Table 11.2 α–wave frequency (mean of eight subjects $\pm$ s.e.) before, during and
after five hour car ride.

Heart rate

The data show a significant decrease in heart rate (10 beats/min.; p = .001) during
the five hours of driving, independent of the experimental situation; this decrease
denotes a gradual building up of tiredness probably combined with the circadian
rhythm.

The presence of carbon monoxide in the blood causes no significant changes in heart
rate, at most a slight increase with COHb levels of 7 and 11% during the second part
of the test.

Discussion

This study attempted to answer the question of whether there are carbon monoxide
effects on performance in man. The analysis of our results suggests the absence of
effects of subacute carbon monoxide intake at COHb levels of 7 and 11% upon the
psychomotor performance. These results conflict with several other studies which

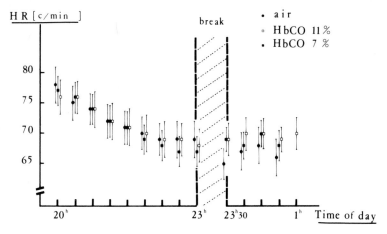

Fig. 11.5 Variation with time of heart rate during a five hour car ride (mean of eight subjects $\pm$ s.e.)

reported performance decrements with COHb levels below 5% (Beard and Wertheim, 1967; Wright *et al*, 1973). However it can be said that other research groups and in particular Stewart *et al*, (1973) studying the same parameters failed to find any decrements below 12% and that 'Beard was unable to reproduce his original findings when using a double blind procedure' (cited by Stewart, 1975). Finally, Ray and Rockwell (1970) have shown a decrement in driving performance with COHb levels up to 8% but they used only three subjects which we consider insufficient. For this reason we used eight subjects and were therefore able to perform better statistical analyses on the data. Our results agree well with those of McFarland (1973) who did not observe any decrement of the ability to drive motor vehicles with COHb levels of 6, 11 and 17%.

It is known that the effects of carbon monoxide and its toxicity are the result of tissue hypoxia caused by the inability of the blood to carry sufficient oxygen. The absence of significant effects on psychomotor performances and EEG at levels of 7 and 11% suggests that hypoxia is not sufficient to induce variations of neuronal metabolism. This is consistent with the case of hypobaric hypoxia where more important oxyhaemoglobin desaturation is required to affect vigilance and brain electrogenesis. Finally, it is possible that during acute and subacute carbon monoxide exposures, there is an efficient mechanism of compensation of the decrease in oxygen transport capacity of the blood by an increase of cerebral blood flow (MacMillan, 1975).

Under all experimental conditions, we observe a gradual deterioration of the operational behaviour and of the cortical activity; this denotes a gradual building up of tiredness which clearly shows the realistic aspect of the test as well as the functional value of the measured parameters. These results must be compared with the results obtained with the same technique by Caille and Bassano (1976a) when studying the effects of depriving regular smokers of tobacco. These results have shown that the deprivation of tobacco in extraverted subjects (selected for their well-modulated brain activity) results in a deterioration of the operational behaviour and in a synchronisation of cortical structures. Smoking one cigarette makes it possible to return to the normal level of brain activity. To explain these variations a subsequent experiment carried out in the laboratory with smokers deprived for 24 hours has shown that the effects of inhaling nicotine alone (by inhalation of aerosols in the form of bitartrate) in equal quantity to that contained in one cigarette are for the most part similar to those of the entire cigarette (internal report, not published).

All our results (effect of carbon monoxide; effect of depriving smokers of tobacco; effect of inhaling nicotine) show that the effect of nicotine contained in the smoke seems to be more important than that of carbon monoxide. This conclusion is of significant practical importance especially as regards the beneficial effect of smoking on driving performance in normal smokers with a COHb level not greater than 11%.

Acknowledgement

We thank P. Caille for his technical assistance.

References

Beard, R.R. & Grandstaff, N. (1970) Carbon monoxide exposure and cerebral function. In Biological effects of carbon monoxide, ed. Coburn, *Annals of the New York Academy of Sciences,* **174,** 385-395.

Beard, R.R. & Wertheim, G.A. (1967) Behavioural impairment associated with small doses of carbon monoxide. *American Journal of Public Health,* **57,** 2012-2022.

Caille, E.J. & Bassano, J.L. (1976a) La cigarette dans le champ cerebral. *Psychologie Médicale,* **8,** 893-908.

Caille, E.J. & Bassano, J.L. (1976b) Le geste du fumeur dans une tache de vigilance monotone. *Psychologie Médicale,* **8,** 631-638.

Guillerm, R., Badré, R., Dupoux, J., Porsin, M. & Colin, B. (1959) Sur une méthode d'évaluation de l'oxycarbonémie à partir des concentrations d'oxyde de carbone mesurées dans l'air alvéolaire. *Revue de Médecine Navale,* **14,** 237-259.

Hanks, T.T. (1970) Human performance of a psychomotor test as a function of exposure to carbon monoxide. In Biological effects of carbon monoxide, ed. Coburn. *Annals of the New York Academy of Sciences,* **174,** 421-424,

Hosko, M.J. (1970) The effect of carbon monoxide on the visual evoked response in man. *Archives of Environmental Health,* **21,** 174-180.

MacMillan, V. (1975) Regional cerebral blood flow of the rat in acute carbon monoxide intoxication. *Canadian Journal of Physiology and Pharmacology,* **53, 644-650.**

Mikulka, P. (1970) The effect of carbon monoxide on human performance. In, Biological effects of carbon monoxide, ed. Coburn. *Annals of the New York Academy of Sciences,* **174,** 409-420.

McFarland, R.A. (1973) Low level exposure to carbon monoxide and driving performance. *Archives of Environmental Health,* **27,** 355-359.

Ray, A.M. & Rockwell, T.H. (1970) An exploratory study of automobile driving performance under the influence of low levels of carboxyhaemoglobin. In,

Biological effects of carbon monoxide, ed. Coburn. *Annals of New York Academy of Sciences,* **174**, 396-408.

Schulte, J.H. (1963) Effects of mild carbon monoxide intoxication. *Archives of Environmental Health,* **7**, 524-530.

Sjostrand, T. (1948) A method for the determination of carboxy-haemoglobin concentrations by analysis of the alveolar air. *Acta Physiologica Scandinavica,* **16**, 201-210.

Stewart, R.D., Peterson, J.E., Baretta, E.D., Bachand, R.T. & Hosko, M.J. (1970) Experimental human exposure to carbon monoxide. *Archives of Environmental Health,* **21**, 154-164.

Stewart, R.D., Newton, P.E., Hosko, M.J. & Peterson, J.E. (1973) The effect of carbon monoxide on time perception. PB 232-544. Rep. CRC APRAC-CAPM 3-68, pp. 1-50. Springfield: NTIS.

Stewart, R.D. (1975) The effect of carbon monoxide on humans. *Annual Review of Pharmacology,* **15**, 409-423.

Wright, G., Randell, P. & Shephard, R.J. (1973) Carbon monoxide and driving skills. *Archives of Environmental Health,* **27**, 349-354.

12. Effects of cigarette smoking on human performance

ANNA-LISA MYRSTEN AND KARIN ANDERSSON

Whatever motive the smoker might have for lighting his cigarette it is reasonable to assume that he expects to gain some rewarding effects. He may claim that smoking brightens him up, makes him concentrate better, or relieves him from tension and anxiety.

Considering the pharmacological effects of tobacco smoking it seems to be well established that it induces an increase in cortical and autonomic arousal (Kershbaum *et al,* 1966; Ulett & Itil, 1969). In other words, smoking leads to a state which should logically be experienced as heightened alertness, but which is just as often referred to as relaxation or sedation. Various psychological explanations have been offered of the paradoxical effect of smoking (e.g. Schachter, 1973).

In a number of studies on smoking motivation interest has been focused on relationships between smoking habits and arousal level in the individual (e.g. Frith, 1971). This approach, which is based on observations regarding both subjective and physiological effects of smoking, has been adopted by scientists within different research areas. Experimental psychology has mainly been concerned with the question whether the known pharmacological effects of smoking on general arousal are accompanied by observable changes in performance efficiency as well as in mood and wakefulness.

A concept of an activation or arousal continuum underlying motivational and behavioural phenomena was early recognised by theorists in this field and has since received convincing support from results obtained in both human and animal studies. The frequently described inverted-U relationship between activation and performance, suggesting that optimum level of arousal varies with the complexity of the task, is now too well-known to require any further mention.

In the context of stress research the concept of arousal has been of basic importance when accounting for the deleterious influences of both overstimulation and understimulation. When studying this topic experimentally various means have been used for manipulating the arousal level and examining the consequence of the induced changes.

Sophisticated experimentation within the field of learning and memory has paid attention to the influence of arousal-inducing factors in the external situation, such as social interference and noise as well as to the characteristics or demands of the task. However, the use of pharmacological agents for varying arousal has not been practiced to any greater extent in learning experiments.

Smoking, arousal and performance

The aim of this paper is to present some results obtained in experimental studies concerned with effects of tobacco smoking on physiological and psychological functions. The research work has been carried out along three main lines involving (1) Immediate effects of smoking on sensorimotor and cognitive functions, (2) Interactions of smoking with alcohol effects, and (3) Symptoms and reactions during smoking deprivation.

Our experimental design requires a special comment, since we have used habitual smokers as subjects, who have been tested under smoking and non-smoking conditions. To set up the necessary control conditions is always connected with certain problems. Using smokers in a control condition where they are deprived of smoking can undoubtedly give rise to justified criticism. Similar objections could of course be raised against making non-smokers smoke. We have tried to manage these difficulties by not accepting heavy smokers as subjects and, furthermore, by conducting the experiments in the morning (before lunch) when the need to smoke should not be too strong in light and moderate smokers. These precautions have not, however, been taken in the deprivation studies, which have included all categories of smokers.

Our basic assumption has been that there exists a more or less consistent relationship between an individual's arousal level and his actual performance in different kinds of tasks. This being our starting point we have used both simple and more complex tests and have also explored the influence of factors in the experimental setting. As indicator of physiological arousal heart rate fluctuations have been used - in some studies also catecholamine excretion.

Effects of smoking on sensorimotor functions

Our first study dealt with effects of smoking during a prolonged reaction-time task (Frankenhaeuser *et al*, 1971). Fig. 12.1 illustrates performance during the eighty minute test period, when the subjects were isolated in a test chamber responding to light stimuli. It can be seen that the reaction times increased during the course of the test period when the subjects were deprived of smoking. When they were allowed to smoke while performing the test they were able to maintain their efficiency at an even level.

The heart rate data, shown in Fig. 12.2 indicate that the initial values were almost identical in the two conditions. Only small fluctuations were obtained in the non-smoking condition, while there was a marked increase in heart rate after smoking, persisting during the entire test period.

Adrenaline output was considerably higher when the subjects had smoked, 7.3 ng/min as compared to 3.3 ng/min in the non-smoking condition. According to the self-reports the subjects felt more alert, less restless, and more relaxed when smoking, which reflects the often claimed subjective effects - stimulating as well as calming.

We have referred to this relatively early study to give an idea of our experimental model using three sets of data. The results in terms of physiological, behavioural and subjective activation point in the same direction, i.e. that smoking raised the general arousal and thus counteracted the gradual decrease in efficiency, which typically occurs in a boring, monotonous situation.

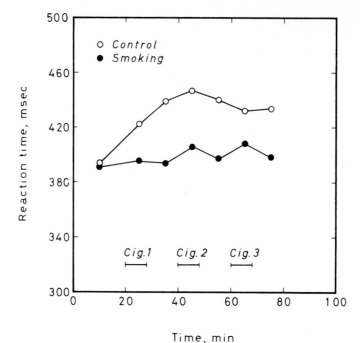

Fig.12.1 Successive mean scores in visual-reaction time in a control condition and a smoking condition.   The first point represents the mean of two 'pre-cigarette' measures. (From Frankenhaeuser *et al*, 1971).

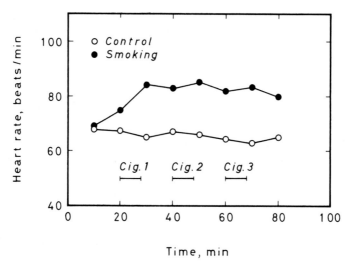

Fig. 12.2 Successive measures of heart rate in a control condition and a smoking condition.   The first point represents the mean of two 'pre-cigarette' measures. (From Frankenhaeuser *et al*, 1971).

An interesting finding was obtained when this study was replicated using the same reaction-time test, though performed under more stressful conditions. It was again found that performance improved after smoking not only in relation to the non-smoking scores but also in comparison to the pre-smoking level (Myrsten *et al*, 1972). Heart rate showed the characteristic pattern induced by smoking, but adrenaline excretion was not influenced. As the adrenaline level in the non-smoking condition was found to be fairly high, it could be argued that the experimental situation was in itself sufficiently stressful to bring about an increase in excretion rate. Under these circumstances smoking produced no further adrenaline increases. This phenomenon has been observed also in later studies. Therefore, heart rate seems to be a more suitable indicator of cigarette-induced arousal changes than adrenomedullary activity, because of its great susceptibility to effects of smoking.

The results may be interpreted in terms of the inverted-U relationship between arousal and behavioural efficiency. When simple tasks are involved, as those used here, an increase in arousal can facilitate performance. It is obvious that the stimulant effects of cigarette smoking - in both experimental settings - raised the general arousal to a level where the subjects could maintain better standards of efficiency.

A later study, aimed at comparing the effects of a 15-hr smoking deprivation on different cognitive abilities, showed that performance in the complex tasks was significantly inferior in the smoking condition as compared to the deprivation condition, whereas there were no differences between conditions with regard to the simple perceptual tests (Elgerot, 1976). It is suggested that the combined effects of smoking and work induced an arousal level, at which the subjects were too 'excited' to perform at their best on the complex tasks.

Effects of smoking on learning and memory

Results obtained in earlier studies on learning and arousal agree that high arousal during learning leads to improved ultimate memory, but are suggestive of contradictory opinions as regards immediate recall (Kleinsmith & Kaplan, 1963; Berlyne *et al*, 1966). In these investigations high-arousal states have been induced by white noise and high-arousal words. Convincing results from animal studies also point to a consolidation of the memory trace following nicotine administration. It was therefore considered of interest to examine whether or not nicotine administered through tobacco smoking would influence the human learning process.

In the first study in this series verbal rote learning was followed under two different conditions - smoking nicotine cigarettes and smoking nicotine-free cigarettes (Andersson & Post, 1974). Fig. 12.3 demonstrates that pre-smoking scores nearly coincided in the two conditions and also that immediately after the first nicotine cigarette there was a drop in learning score (nonsense syllables) as compared to the period following the first nicotine-free cigarette. However, after the second cigarette the two curves described almost the same time course, although there was a slight improvement during the last two trials in the nicotine condition.

With regard to physiological arousal the two treatments elicited completely different patterns. Heart rate increased after the first nicotine cigarette to a level which was significantly higher than after the nicotine-free one. The responses to smoking were less marked after the second cigarette and the differences were no longer significant. Thus, the first nicotine cigarette led to a marked increase in arousal and a concomitant decrease in learning. At the time of the second cigarette, however, the differences in arousal level between the two conditions were less accentuated and there were no longer any differences in performance.

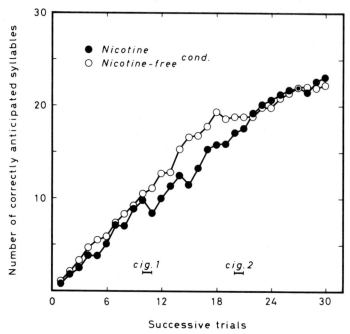

Fig. 12.3 Mean number of correctly anticipated syllables on a verbal rote learning task in a nicotine and a nicotine-free condition. (From Andersson & Post, 1974).

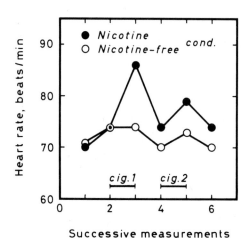

Fig. 12.4 Mean heart rate at successive measurements in a nicotine and a nicotine -free condition. (From Andersson & Post, 1974).

These findings fit in well with Walker's consolidation theory postulating that consolidation of the memory trace is accompanied by a temporary inhibition of recall, serving to protect the memory trace against disruption (e.g. Walker & Tarte, 1963). Under circumstances of high arousal, the increased non-specific neural activity will produce a more intense consolidation, leading to improved ultimate memory but also to a less acceptable trace in short-term memory. Viewing our results from this angle, the impaired performance after the first nicotine cigarette may thus be attributed to an intensified consolidation process with simultaneous inhibition of immediate recall. The data so far supported the first part of Walker's theory.

To explore the second part of the theory, i.e. whether later recall following high-arousal learning would be improved, a new experiment was conducted in which the same memory task was used. Now smoking and non-smoking conditions were compared. The results confirmed those obtained in the previous study, in that the cigarette-induced arousal was accompanied by a significant impairment in serial-learning performance. When recall was tested later the picture was reversed, perform-ance being better in the smoking condition than in the non-smoking condition (Andersson, 1975). These findings, implicating different effects of smoking on short-term and long-term memory, provide additional support for Walker's theory.

The adverse effects of smoking on short-term memory are also applicable to alternative interpretations, suggesting that arousal level regulates the flow of incoming stimuli. According to Easterbrook a state of high arousal leads to increased selec-tivity of attention, which implies that the individual will leave out peripheral stimuli and concentrate on the relevant ones (Easterbrook, 1959).

Another study dealt with the aspect of attention by examining the role of selec-tive attention during cigarette-induced arousal (Andersson & Hockey, 1975). The memory test used consisted of 'relevant' and 'irrelevant' information. The subjects were instructed to concentrate on serial recall of Swedish words (relevant information) presented one at a time. Each word could appear in any of four corners of the slide (irrelevant information). Recall of location of the words served as a measure of incidental learning. Fig. 12.5 shows, firstly, the percentage of words recalled in correct order and irrespective of order, and, secondly, the percentage of correct locations of total number of recalled words. It can be seen that the two groups did not differ with regard to the relevant task, but also that smoking significantly reduced irrelevant information. The results imply that attentional processes are affected by cigarette smoking in the same way as by other arousal-increasing events. Easterbrook's hypothesis, proposing that the range of cues are reduced in states of high arousal, was supported by these findings. The increased selectivity of attention might be subjectively interpreted by the smoker himself as an improved ability to concentrate when smoking.

Interactions of smoking with alcohol effects
Another line of research has been concerned with alcohol/tobacco interactions, which have been studied both during acute intoxication and during the hangover phase. We shall restrict our account to findings obtained during the intoxication phase.

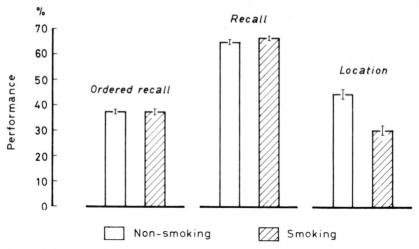

Fig. 12.5 Means and standard errors for the percentage of words recalled in correct order (Ordered recall) and irrespective of order (Recall) as well as the percentage of correct locations of the total number of recalled words (Location) in a smoking and non-smoking session. (From Andersson & Hockey, 1975).

The experiments were conducted in a relaxed social atmosphere, the subjects and experimenters having dinner together (Andersson *et al*, 1977). Alcohol was consumed as mixed beverages in an amount corresponding to 1.43 g alc/kg body weight. During the course of the meal the subjects smoked six cigarettes and in addition nine cigarettes during the remaining part of the evening. In the non-smoking sessions they received the same treatment except for the cigarettes.

It was found that the interaction was rather complex, being synergistic for some of the functions studied and antagonistic for others. In Fig. 12.6 it is seen that cigarettes and alcohol combined produced relatively higher peripheral arousal than alcohol alone, as reflected in adrenaline excretion and heart rate. Motor coordination, measured by tests of hand steadiness and standing steadiness, was more impaired after the joint administration of alcohol and cigarettes than following alcohol without smoking.

The most interesting result was that performance in reaction-time tasks and in mental arithmetic tasks was significantly better with cigarettes, which indicates that smoking counteracted the depressant effects of alcohol. The subjects described themselves as being more alert and relaxed when they were allowed to smoke - thus referring to both sedative and stimulant effects of the cigarettes. The fact that they considered themselves less talkative, less tired, and more able to concentrate at the same time as they showed better performance points to a sobering-up effect of smoking. In other words, when the subjects smoked they achieved a level of activation that was more adequate for efficient functioning.

Effects of smoking deprivation
The data presented so far have been used to illustrate effects of smoking, but might just as well demonstrate effects of short-term tobacco abstinence. The results have

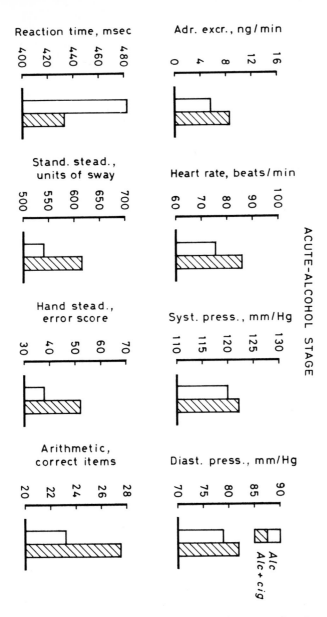

Fig. 12.6 Mean values of measurements of adrenaline excretion, heart rate, blood pressures, reaction time, standing steadiness, hand steadiness, and arithmetic performance, obtained during an alcohol and an alcohol+cigarette condition. (Andersson *et al*, 1977).

referred to comparisons between a smoking situation and a non-smoking situation in which light and moderate smokers have participated. But as we have argued earlier, non-smoking may be regarded as an exceptional condition for habitual smokers, the effects of which are likely to increase with duration of withdrawal.

We have made systematic studies of symptoms and reactions in habitual smokers, who have been deprived of smoking for several days. In one study 14 police officers volunteered to abstain from smoking for five days, during which time they kept diaries on their subjective reactions, their smoking desire, and their activities (Myrsten, Elgerot & Edgren, 1977). The most frequent symptoms reported were sleep disturbances, depressions, anxiety, irritation, and difficulties in concentrating. To study changes in physiological arousal urine samples for analysis of catecholamine excretion were collected almost daily during a 15-day period including the deprivation days. Psychological tests were performed on three occasions, before, at the end of and after the deprivation period. The test data were compared to corresponding values from a matched control group, comprising smoking colleagues of the same age and with similar smoking habits as the abstaining subjects. Fig. 12.7 illustrating catecholamine excretion during the three test days, show that the time pattern differed in the two groups. The excretion rates of both adrenaline and noradrenaline decreased successively from the first to the third test day in the control group, which reflects these subjects' habituation to the experimental situation. In the abstaining group adrenaline excretion was considerably lower on the second test day, when the subjects had been deprived of smoking for four days, than on the first day which preceded the smoking cessation and on the third day when they had taken up smoking again. Noradrenaline excretion decreased slightly from the first to the second test day, but showed a marked rise on the third day. As regards performance in the psychological tests there were no signs of deteriorating efficiency in the abstainers, which they themselves had expected.

In general the results show that a sudden break of a long-lasting smoking habit may induce rather pronounced changes and disturbances in both physiological and psychological functions. It should be emphasised that the subjects were highly motivated to take part in the experiment. During this period they attended courses at the police school and therefore lived far away from their homes and working places. The fact that they attended classes together made them experience a strong backing from each other, which certainly must have helped them to accomplish the difficult task.

A later study, in which school teachers participated as subjects, was less successful. These subjects, who at first had shown great interest in the project, later changed their attitudes - they 'forgot' to give urine samples and omitted to keep diaries. Expressions of irritation and hostility were frequent and the subjects stated that they had difficulties when associating with their colleagues during coffee and lunch breaks. It is obvious that this group of subjects had greater difficulties in abstaining from smoking than the previous group, which might be due to the fact that they, at the time of the experiments, lived and worked under their ordinary circumstances. As the smoking habit seems to be closely linked to a person's social life, a break of the habit would most probably affect his relations to friends and colleagues.

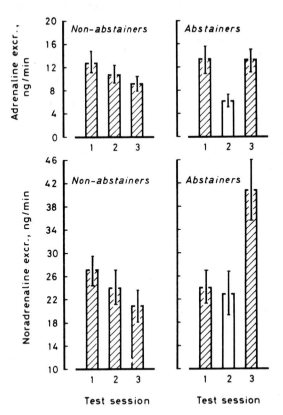

Fig. 12.7 Mean values for adrenaline and noradrenaline excretion in the abstaining group and the non-abstaining group, obtained on the test days during Smoking period 1, Abstinence period, and Smoking period 2. (From Myrsten *et al*, 1977)

Concluding remarks

The data reviewed in this paper show that cigarette smoking induces an increase in physiological arousal which is often accompanied by changes in mental efficiency. Judging from the self-reports the effects at the psychological level are conceived as both alerting and calming.   Our subjects generally stated that smoking increased their alertness and improved their ability to concentrate at the same time as it made them feel relaxed and at ease.

The relative importance of pharmacological and psychological factors in maintaining the smoking habit has been extensively discussed in various contexts (e.g. Jarvik, 1970).   The heightened state of arousal induced by smoking is compatible with the view that people smoke to achieve stimulation and excitement, but contradicts the idea that a great number of smokers use the cigarettes to obtain a sedational effect. However, it is most likely that an increase in arousal makes a person feel more confident in his ability to cope with the task set and thus relieved from tension and anxiety, even if his actual performance might not be improved. Moreover, the ritual of lighting and handling a cigarette may induce a state of relaxation under conditions of stress and strain. As for the frequent claim that smoking favours the ability to concentrate a possible explanation may be offered by the fact that the cigarette-induced arousal seems to be associated with increased selectivity of attention, which gives the smoker the impression of focusing his attention on relevant rather than on irrelevant aspects of the task.

Assuming that the habitual smoker has an almost constantly increased arousal it would be expected that, when he is suddenly deprived of smoking, the arousal drops below his 'normal' level, which in turn may affect mood and wakefulness. This was in fact what was found in our deprivation studies, the results of which suggest that the unpleasant symptoms which are often associated with smoking cessation, may, at least partly, be attributed to the lowering of physiological arousal level.

Acknowledgements

The studies reviewed in this paper have been supported by grants from the Swedish Tobacco Company (Project No. 7505) and the Swedish Cancer Society (Project No. 623) as well as by grants to Professor Marianne Frankenhaeuser from the Swedish Medical Research Council (Project No. 997 and 2371).

References

Andersson, K. (1975) Effects of cigarette smoking on learning and retention. *Psychopharmacologia,* **41**, 1-5.

Andersson, K. & Hockey, G.R. (1975) Effects of cigarette smoking on incidental memory. *Reports from the Department of Psychology, University of Stockholm.* No. 455.

Andersson, K., Hollstedt, C., Myrsten, A.-L. & Neri, A. (1977) The influence of tobacco smoking on the acute-alcohol and the post-alcohol stage. *Blutalkohol,* **14**, 366-380.

Andersson, K. & Post, B. (1974) Effects of cigarette smoking on verbal rote learning and physiological arousal. *Scandinavian Journal of Psychology,* **15**, 263-267.

Berlyne, D.E., Borsa, D.M., Hamacher, J.H. & Koenig, I.D.(1966) Paired associate learning and the time of arousal. *Journal of Experimental Psychology,* **72**, 1-6.

Easterbrook, J.A. (1959) The effect of emotion on cue utilisation and the organisation of behaviour. *Psychological Review,* **66**, 183-201.

Elgerot, A. (1976) Note on selective effects of short-term tobacco abstinence on complex versus simple mental tasks. *Perceptual and Motor Skills,* **42**, 413-414.

Frankenhaeuser, M., Myrsten, A.-L., Post, B. & Johansson, G. (1971) Behavioural and physiological effects of cigarette smoking in a monotonous situation. *Psychopharmacologia,* **22**, 1-7.

Frith, C.D. (1971) Smoking behaviour and its relation to the smoker's immediate experience. *British Journal of Social and Clinical Psychology,* **10**, 73-78.

Jarvik, M.E. (1970) The role of nicotine in the smoking habit. In *Learning Mechanisms in Smoking,* ed. Hunt, W.A., pp. 155-190. Chicago: Aldine.

Kershbaum, A., Bellet, S., Jiminez, J. & Feinberg, L.J. (1966) Differences in effects of cigar and cigarette smoking on free fatty acid mobilisation and catecholamine excretion. *Journal of American Medical Association,* **195**, 1095-1098.

Kleinsmith, L.J. & Kaplan, S. (1963) Paired associate learning as a function of arousal and interpolated interval. *Journal of Experimental Psychology,* **65**, 190-193.

Myrsten, A.-L., Elgerot, A. & Edgren, B. (1977) Effects of abstinence from tobacco smoking on physiological and psychological arousal levels in habitual smokers. *Psychosomatic Medicine,* **39**, 25-38.

Myrsten, A.-L., Post, B., Frankenhaeuser, M. & Johansson, G.(1972) Changes in behavioural and physiological activation induced by cigarette smoking in habitual smokers. *Psychopharmacologia,* **27**, 305-312.

Schachter, S. (1973) Nesbitt's paradox. In *Smoking Behaviour: Motives and Incentives.* ed. Dunn, W.L., pp. 147-155. Washington: V.H. Winston & Sons.

Ulett, G.A. & Itil, T.M. (1969) Quantitative electroencephalogram in smoking and smoking deprivation. *Science,* **164**, 696-970.

Walker, E.L. & Tarte, R.D. (1963) Memory storage as a function of arousal and time with homogenous and heterogenous lists. *Journal of Verbal Learning and Verbal Behaviour,* **2**, 113-119.

13. The absorption of carbon monoxide from the conducting airways of the human lung

GORDON CUMMING, ANDREW R GUYATT AND MICHAEL A HOLMES

Interest in carbon monoxide has two principal aspects, firstly the possible adverse effects of this gas on health, and secondly its use to study the process of gas exchange in the lung.

This paper, is concerned principally with the second aspect, in particular with the mechanism of carbon monoxide uptake during smoking, studying the absorption of carbon monoxide in people who do not inhale. We have therefore investigated whether there is any uptake of carbon monoxide from the conducting airways, and in order to appreciate what is implied by this latter term, it is necessary to review some recently developed concepts in respiratory physiology.

As fresh gas flows into the lungs during inspiration down the branching airways its forward velocity diminishes progressively since the summed area of cross section increases rapidly. At a certain point the linear forward velocity due to bulk flow becomes equal to the velocity of gas movement due to thermal diffusion and this point is defined by $\frac{dS}{dx} = \frac{\dot{V}}{D}$ where $\frac{dS}{dx}$ is the rate of increase of cross sectional area with respect to distance, $\dot{V}$ is the gas flow rate into the lungs and D is the molecular diffusion coefficient.

At the equilibrium point therefore, where bulk flow and diffusion result in equal velocities, there is established a gradient of concentration which is stationary in the airways, fresh gas enters this interface without displacing it and diffuses through it to enter the alveoli. The position of this stationary interface clearly depends upon tidal volume and breathing frequency, but in anatomical terms is likely to be in the respiratory bronchioles. The volume demarcated by the sum of all the standing interfaces and the lips defines the conducting airways, whilst that volume peripheral to the interfaces constitutes the gas mixing zone.

The question to be answered by this paper is whether measurable absorption of carbon monoxide occurs proximal to the stationary interface, through the mucosa of the buccal cavity and bronchi. Since it is known that carbon monoxide is absorbed in the gas mixing zone, some device is also required to indicate whether any of the inspired carbon monoxide has entered this zone.

The principle of the method employed is to introduce into the tidal volume a bolus of known volume of carbon monoxide (0.3% concentration) at a point which may be predetermined so that the bolus may enter the gas mixing zone completely or may remain entirely upstream of the stationary interface. Following expiration the volume of carbon monoxide recovered may be measured and by difference the volume absorbed is found. The problem is complicated however by the possibility that some of the carbon monoxide may enter the gas mixing zone, being both physically diluted and subsequently absorbed at alveolar level. Accordingly, we have incorporated in the bolus an inert marker gas, argon, as customarily used in the single breath transference test. Any reduction in the expired volume of this gas will indicate that some of the bolus has reached the gas exchanging part of the lung and moreover it allows a correction to be made for dilution.

In order to implement this experimental design several technological developments were called for. The first was a rapid analyser for carbon monoxide, since it is necessary to analyse events within a single breath, and an instrument with a response time of 100 ms. is appropriate. Infra-red devices are useful but have in general response times of several seconds but a new instrument developed by Beckman has appropriate characteristics and measures up to 0.5% CO. There must also be a simultaneous measurement of argon and for this a mass spectrometer is called for. Since carbon monoxide has a mass/charge ratio of 28, identical to that for molecular nitrogen it is not possible to measure carbon monoxide in the lungs by conventional techniques using mass spectroscopy.

An alternative, which we have been exploring, but which has not been used in the present work is to use the stable isotope of carbon ^{13}C, which gives a mass charge ratio of 29. At this point in the spectrum there is a small contribution from $^{14}N^{15}N$ but this is readily corrected for, so that the mass spectrometer can be used for all the gases, with the consequent advantages of having similar characteristics for each signal. The cost of such a gas mixture however normally precludes its use.

The second development used in a recent study although not in the pilot work mostly discussed here was a valve which could be operated by a signal from a spirometer and which would introduce a bolus of gas mixture incorporating argon and carbon monoxide of a known size and at a known point in inspiration. This device was made with a series of electromagnetically operated poppet valves, actuated by a sensing device operated by an electrical signal from a wedge spirometer in a "bag-in-a-box" system. The device was used by having one inspiratory bag containing air and a second one containing the argon/carbon monoxide mixture. During a normal inspiration of one litre the subject first inspired air and after either 700, 800 or 900 ml. of air the valve switched and this was followed by 100 ml. of gas mixture, followed again in the first two instances by air to bring the total inspiration up to one litre. In the pilot study a similar manoeuvre was done by manually altering a tap during inspiration to give a bolus, though of course this could not be done with the same precision. Thus the gas mixture could be inspired into the conducting airways, or deeper into the gas mixing zone, and its volume is precisely known.

During the succeeding expirate it is then necessary to measure the quantity of argon and carbon monxide which is recovered, thus permitting a measurement of the quantity of gas retained within the lung.

In both studies the data were first recorded using an analogue FM tape recorder from which they could be recovered at analysis. In order to measure gas volumes it is necessary to compare simultaneous records of gas concentration and volume or flow. Since there is a delay time for both gas analysers, representing the dwell time within the sample line, this must be corrected for before analysis, and this is done electronically or by the digital computer. We have analysed the present data by producing analogue records from the tape, both on a strip recorder to demonstrate the time course of each study, and on an X-Y plotter to compare the gas concentration and inspired or expired volume for each gas, from which the various gas volumes could be read directly.

In later work we intend to use digital computation, as is done routinely in this laboratory for other studies. Here each channel of information is sampled at 30 ms intervals, to give a table of digital values, the flow column is then moved backwards an appropriate amount, (normally four values to allow for a delay time of 100 ms). relative to the gas concentration columns making them synchronous. The instaneous gas concentrations are then multiplied by the instaneous flow rates to yield the instaneous gas flux. These various gas fluxes are then summed in each expiration and where necessary inspirations, to give respective gas volumes.

In the present study when the volume of indicator gas expired is equal to that inspired no demonstrable absorption has occurred. When there is less expired than inspired, this may result either from loss by transfer to the blood, or from mixing into the lung gas which remains behind after a normal expiration. The former may be distinguished from the latter by an increase above unity of the argon (carbon monoxide ratio in expired gas). These two differing fates of inspired tracer permits the definition of that volume in the airways where significant absorption begins, and from what has been said earlier it will be clear that this is distal to the stationary interface.

In the pilot study, done without breath-holding, there was no appreciable uptake of carbon monoxide in male smokers when the bolus was given in the last 120 ml. of inspiration, i.e. was confined to the large airways. The results in females were similar but much less clear cut, probably due to difficulties resulting from the smaller lung volumes of these subjects which made these manual tests harder to perform. A preliminary look at the later study shows the same results, though with prolonged breath-holding some loss of carbon monoxide may occur due to diffusion in the gaseous phase from the large airways into the gas exchanging parts of the lung.

Further studies are in progress to apply these techniques to the measurement of carbon monoxide transference, utilising direct measurements of dead space for the gas, rather than the indirect methods necessary so far, due to the slow response times of conventional carbon monoxide analysers.

14. The analysis of smoking parameters: inhalation and absorption of tobacco smoke in studies of human smoking behaviour

ROGER G RAWBONE, K MURPHY, M E TATE AND S J KANE

Introduction

An earlier conference on Smoking Behaviour, held in 1972, dealt exclusively with the question 'what are the motivational mechanisms sustaining cigarette smoking behaviour?', considering this from both the psychological and pharmacological points of view. During that conference it was suggested by Armitage (1973), however, that an important question, frequently inadequately considered, was that of (nicotine) dosage. Ashton and Watson had shown in 1970 that the human smoker can and does adjust the dose (of nicotine) he takes into the mouth by adjusting the size of his puffs and the rate at which he puffs when smoking. Furthermore, as Armitage stated, the smoke can be inhaled very deeply, moderately deeply, slightly or not at all. Since that time many reports have considered questions which relate to how people smoke and to the smoke uptake and retention, but, apart from a study by Guillerm and Radziszewski (1975), there have been no published studies exploring the range of techniques available and their application in the study of such questions.

This paper will describe techniques which may be used to answer the questions 'How do people smoke?' and 'What is the smoke uptake and retention?'; it will explore some of the relationships between smoke uptake and smoke retention and finally describe the results of experiments to study differences between habitual middle tar and habitual low tar smokers and to study the effects of switching between middle and low tar products.

'How do people smoke?'

In the analysis of this question we are concerned with the physical smoking profile. The dose of tobacco smoke constituents available to the smoker will depend upon the cigarette specification (Table 14.1). However, for any given cigarette, it is the smoking profile which will affect how much of the dose is delivered to the smoker and how much is absorbed.

Table 14.1 Factors determining the characteristics of a cigarette product.

Cigarette Specification

i) Filler - Tobacco based
    Additives
    Diluents / Substitutes
ii) Configuration
iii) Wrapper
iv) Filter - Type
    Ventilation
v) Misc. - Pressure drop....

Quantitative measurements of the smoking profile which can be made are the number of cigarettes smoked, cigarette butt length, puff parameters (puff volume, puff duration, number of puffs and inter-puff interval) and the inhalation pattern.
'What is the smoke uptake and retention?'
Here we are trying to quantify the smoke uptake and dose absorbed as a result of the smoking profile. Most approaches to this question attempt to estimate the dose of tobacco smoke from an analysis of certain smoke components or their markers - commonly carbon monoxide or nicotine. It should be noted however that carbon monoxide is a measure of the gas/vapour phase of the smoke whilst nicotine is a reflection of particulate matter and it is possible that these two phases of the tobacco smoke behave differently in terms of their pulmonary distribution and absorption.

Carbon monoxide may be measured in the blood or in exhaled air whilst nicotine is usually measured in the blood or in the urine. A somewhat different approach is the estimation of nicotine intake from that retained in the cigarette butt.

Measurement of puff parameters

Method
Puff parameters can be obtained from measurements of the pressure drop across a small resistance inserted between the cigarette and the smoker. In this situation, when there is air flow during puffing, the pressure drop created across the resistance will be related to the gas flow. The relationship will depend upon whether the airflow is turbulent, when the flow rate will be proportional to the square root of the pressure drop, or laminar, when the flow will be directly proportional to the pressure drop. In either case puff volume can be derived by integration of the flow signal against time and puff and interpuff intervals can be measured directly.

Specialised cigarette holders have been designed incorporating devices to produce a pressure drop with either turbulent flow (orifice plate) or, as used in the present experiments, laminar flow (filter insert). Both types of device have their advantages and disadvantages but it is not appropriate to discuss these in detail in this paper. It is necessary, however, to outline some of the problems associated with the filter insert type of holder as employed in the studies to be described. The holder is shown in Fig. 14.1. It contains a replaceable 6mm cellulose acetate filter across which the pressure drop can be measured using a differential pressure guage. The assumption is that this pressure drop is linearly related to the flow of gas through it, i.e. that the flow is laminar and

$$Q = Kp \qquad -(1)$$

where Q is the flow rate, p is the pressure drop and K is a constant. Fig. 14.2 shows the pressure drop versus flow relationship of the holder for air over the range of flows found during normal smoking. It can be seen that the relationship is curvilinear indicating that the basic assumption regarding flow derivation is not correct. Nevertheless, the degree of curvature is relatively slight and the overall error introduced in computing puff volume from the flow signal is accordingly small.

This relationship between pressure and the flow has been obtained by drawing air through the filter holder at room temperatures. The exact relationship between

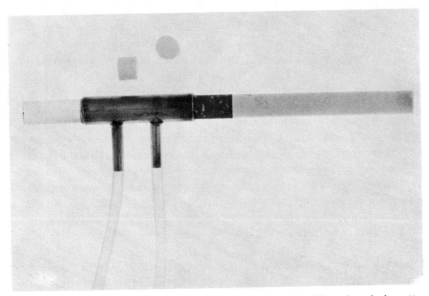

Fig. 14.1 The filter insert cigarette holder with a king-size filter tipped cigarette. Two of the 6mm cellulose acetate filter inserts, across which the pressure drop is measured during smoking, are shown alongside the holder.

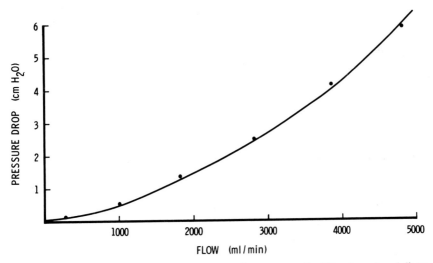

Fig. 14.2 The relationship between pressure drop across the filter insert and flow of air through the holder over a range of flows found during normal smoking.

the pressure drop and laminar flow is given by the equation of Hagen-Poiseuille:

$$Q = \frac{\pi p\, r^4}{8\, nl} \qquad\qquad -(2)$$

where r is the radius of the device, l is the length of the device and n is the viscosity of the gas.

Although therefore flow may be proportional to pressure drop the constant in equation (1) is dependent upon the viscosity of the gas which in its turn will be influenced by temperature. In the present situation therefore any calibrations of the filter holder should be carried out using tobacco smoke at the temperatures found in mainstream smoke. Measurement of the temperature within the filter insert during normal smoking is not constant, rising during puffing and falling between puffs. An overall rise of about 6°C has been recorded smoking to approximately 8mm from the cigarette filter, after which the temperature rises steeply. An evaluation of the characteristics of the filter insert holder using tobacco smoke at a temperature 3-5°C above that of ambient air was found to give results within 3% of those using air.

There is one further question which has to be considered when using the filter insert holder - does the deposition of tobacco smoke condensate within the filter insert, which inevitably occurs during smoking, affect its characteristics? In practice no differences could be detected in the pressure drop versus flow relationships of filter inserts studied before and after the smoking of a cigarette through the holder. It should be noted that when performing butt nicotine analysis (*vide infra*) the filter insert should be included to take into account the condensate (nicotine) deposited within it. The analyses described indicate that the filter-insert holder, calibrated with air at room temperature, gives an approximation of the flow rate and hence the volume of tobacco smoke passing through it as a cigarette is smoked. The filter insert requires renewing for each cigarette smoked and the calibration should thus be performed before each study. As the derived flow signal is only being used to calculate the puff volume, calibration can more readily be carried out by passing a series of known volumes through the holder and recording the appropriate signal. As a final check of the system a volume calibration of the filter holder was performed using both air and tobacco smoke when, over a range of volumes (10-60ml), the results were within 5% of each other.

This technical evaluation enables the limitations of the calibration procedures and the precision of our measurements to be known. However, one must then consider the effect on the puff parameters of smoking with such a holder. There is the intro-duction of the holder changing the weight and feel of the cigarette; the added dead space (1.6ml) with stagnation of smoke between puffs affecting taste; and the added draw resistance caused by the filter insert. The latter is in fact relatively small when compared to an unventilated king size filter-tipped product as shown in Fig. 14.3 but may become of importance with different product designs.

In addition to these factors there are the differences in smoking pattern which may result from a subject being studied in an experimental situation. This is discussed by Comer and Creighton (1978) but our own observations, relating to butt analyses (*vide infra*), would confirm significant differences in the smoking profile between individuals smoking without the cigarette holder in a relaxed atmosphere to smoking with the holder in an experimental laboratory situation.

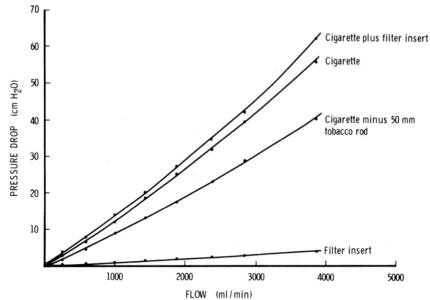

Fig. 14.3 The relationship between pressure drop and air flow across a king size filter-tipped cigarette and across the cigarette plus filter insert. The relationship for the filter insert (see Fig. 14.2) and the cigarette minus 50mm tobacco rod are also shown for comparison.

Comparison of measured puff parameters with standard machine smoking parameters
Despite the limitations of the modified cigarette holder described in measuring puff volume, direct measurements of puff duration and interpuff interval can be accurately made. We have measured all these parameters in twenty subjects during the smoking of 100 cigarettes covering a range of product types. Analysis of the average result for each cigarette gives an overall mean puff volume of 47.5ml (standard deviation (S.D.) $\pm$ 6.42ml), mean puff duration of 2.28 sec (S.D. 0.3 sec) and mean interpuff interval of 35 sec (S.D. 9.2 sec). The 95% confidence intervals for the means of our data are puff volume 44.96-50.04ml, puff duration 2.16-2.40 sec and interpuff interval 31.27-38.53 sec and for each of these parameters the mean result is thus significantly different from the standard (T.R.C.) machine smoking parameters of one 35ml puff of 2 sec duration with an interpuff interval of 58 secs.
  It is not only possible, using the modified cigarette holder, to make quantitative measurements of puff parameters but one may also observe the puff flow profile. In any individual, this profile tends to remain constant and a classification of smokers on the basis of their puff flow profile has been proposed (Adams, 1966).

Measurement of inhalation

Method
Depth of inhalation has been measured by recording movements of the chest wall using a mercury strain gauge chest pneumogram. This consists of a thin, elastic-walled tube containing mercury which is held under tension across the upper part of the

anterior chest wall by a strap passing around the subject.   As the chest expands with inhalation the mercury-filled tube is stretched, thus changing its length and cross-sectional area, and hence its electrical resistance. This change in electrical resistance can be displayed on a recording device. In order to relate the change in resistance to a change in lung volume a calibration must be performed simultaneously measuring the chest pneumogram deflection and lung volume changes. The lung volume changes can conveniently be recorded at the mouth using a spirometer. It will be apparent that this calibration must be carried out each time the chest pneumogram is applied to or adjusted on a subject and must therefore be performed at the beginning of each smoking study.

   A typical calibration for one subject study is shown in Fig. 14.4 where the linear regression line for volume change versus pneumogram deflection is shown both over a large volume range (0-5 litres) and a smaller volume range (0-2 litres) as might be expected in smoking studies.

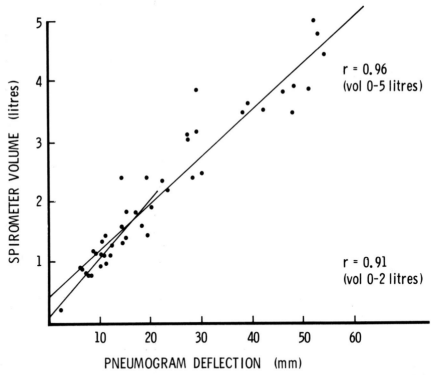

Fig. 14.4 The chest pneumogram calibration from one subject study. Correlations between the pneumogram deflection and simultaneous measurement of lung volume changes as measured by spirometry at the mouth. The correlation coefficients and linear regression lines are shown over the total (0-5 litre) volume range and a smaller (0-2 litre) volume range as might be found in smoking studies.

In all experimental studies we have performed, the correlation coefficient, over the range 0-2 litres for the calibration procedure, has been greater than 0.90.

Comparison of measured inhalation with a subject's subjective assessment
This technique for evaluating inhalation may be used to investigate whether a person's subjective analysis of his inhalation correlates with the volume of gas which he actually inhales.

In a preliminary study, 15 subjects have been presented with a 140mm analogue scale with the extremes 'do not inhale' to 'inhale maximally'. They were asked 'to place a mark along the line in a position between the two extremes which corresponds as closely as possible to the way in which you smoke'. As a validity check subjects answered this question on two occasions with an intervening period of at least 24 hours. Analysis of the data using a paired t test gave a mean difference of -1mm with a standard deviation of the difference of 19mm (p=0.9, N.S.).

Subjects then smoked a cigarette with the chest pneumogram in position and the mean smoke inhalation volume for that cigarette calculated. The results of the relationship between the analogue scale recording and the mean inhaled volume are shown in Fig. 14.5.

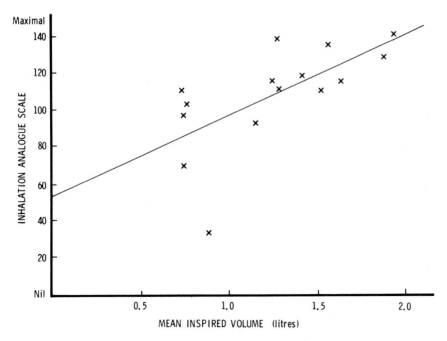

Fig. 14.5 Comparison between a subjective measurement of inhalation as recorded on an analogue scale, and an objective measurement of inhalation - the mean inhaled volume as measured from the chest pneumogram. The linear regression line for the data (r=0.65, p <0.01) is shown with its extrapolation, indicating that the intercept is not zero.

An apparent linear relationship exists over the range of inhalation studied (r=0.65, p <0.01). There are however few observations over the lower range of subjective inhalation and the linear regression line for the data does not, as shown, extrapolate towards the origin. It would therefore seem likely that a linear relationship does not hold good over the full range of inhalation.   It is over the lower range of inhalation, not covered in this experiment, that much interest lies - do people who state that they are non-inhalers really not inhale when smoking?

It may be argued that the actual inhalation volume should not be expected to correlate with a measure of subjective inhalation because what is regarded as a minimal inhalation in a 'large' subject may be regarded as a maximal inhalation in a 'small' subject. In order to correct for this the mean inhaled-smoke volume of each subject has been related to their vital capacity, this being used as a measure of lung 'size'. The result was surprising and is open to speculation for it was found that in all cases the mean inhaled volume was approximately 25% of the vital capacity (26% $\pm$ 3 (S.D.)).

Smoke exposure index

As in the case of the puff flow profile the chest pneumogram trace will give a qualitative indication of the form of the inhalation.   Two examples are shown in Fig. 14.6; in the first of these the subject has taken a deep inhalation with immediate exhalation whilst in the second example a more shallow inhalation is followed by a period of breathholding prior to subsequent exhalation.

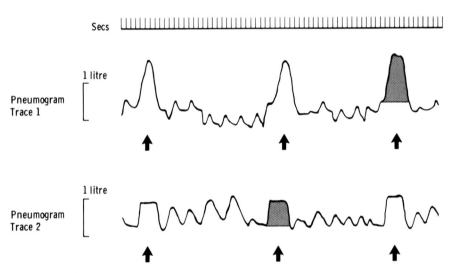

Fig. 14.6 Two examples of the chest pneumogram tracing showing different patterns of inhalation. In each example the inhalation of tobacco smoke is indicated by the arrows and, for one inhalation, the area from which the smoke exposure index is calculated has been shaded.

The exposure of the lungs to tobacco smoke during smoking will thus not only depend upon the depth of inhalation of the smoke but also on the time which this smoke remains in the lungs. In order to take this into account a smoke exposure index has been derived from the chest pneumogram trace by summing the area under the curve for each inhalation of smoke. The areas were measured by planimetry and representative examples are indicated in the traces shown in Fig. 14.6.

The relationship between puff and inhalation profiles

Derivation of the puff flow profile and the inhalation profile have been described separately but useful information may be gained by combining these techniques. In Fig. 14.7 are shown two examples.

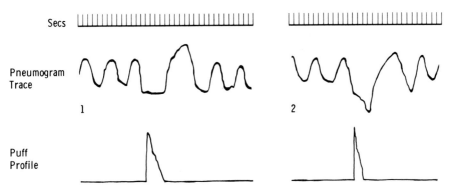

Fig. 14.7 The pneumogram tracing and the puff flow profile from two smokers during normal smoking to illustrate: i) the relationship of the puff to the inhalation and ii) the pattern of chest wall movement during puffing and preceeding the inhalation of smoke.

The time relationships of puffing from the cigarette and inhalation of the smoke can be studied when it is observed that the puff is taken into the mouth from the cigarette before being inhaled into the lungs. This has important implications in terms of dose exposure for it means that the whole of the smoke bolus is potentially available to be taken deeply into the lungs at the beginning of inhalation rather than being distributed throughout the total inhaled volume of air.

Recording both puff and inhalation profiles it is also possible to note any gross movements of the chest wall during puffing. In the majority of subjects studied the pattern shown in the first example of Fig. 14.7 is observed where virtually no movement of the chest wall takes place. However, in a few subjects, most notably smokers of high tar products, there is an apparent active exhalation following the puff prior to the subsequent inhalation. This is shown in example 2 Fig. 14.7. The implication of this pattern of smoking is that the bolus of tobacco smoke has been blown from the mouth and very little, if any, is available at the subsequent inhalation (presumably this is also the pattern in cigar smokers).

Measurement of carbon monoxide

Method

Tobacco smoke contains carbon monoxide and studies have shown that the venous carboxyhaemoglobin saturation (HbCO%) of 'inhaling' cigarette smokers is significantly higher than that of non-smokers. Measurement of venous carboxyhaemoglobin, with the necessity of obtaining a blood sample by finger prick or venepuncture, was not considered satisfactory for (large scale) studies in a 'normal' population. It was therefore decided to measure carbon monoxide in mixed expired air and to derive the partial pressure of carbon monoxide in alveolar air using the Bohr equation.

This equation is based upon the law of conservation of matter which, for this example, states that the volume of carbon monoxide in any expired breath (fractional concentration of carbon monoxide x tidal volume) equals the volume coming from the alveoli plus the volume coming from the dead space. Substituting and rearranging the equation will give the fractional concentration of carbon monoxide in alveolar air (F_ACO):-

$$F_ACO = \frac{V_T.Fe\ CO - V_D.Fi\ CO}{V_T - V_D} \qquad -(3)$$

where FeCO is the fractional concentration of carbon monoxide in mixed expired gas, FiCO is the fractional concentration of carbon monoxide in inspired gas, V_T is the tidal volume and V_D is the dead space.

   The details of the method have been published in detail elsewhere (Rawbone, Coppin and Guz, 1976) where it is also shown that the results for alveolar carbon monoxide partial pressure obtained correlate with the simultaneous measurement of venous HbCO% (HbCO% = 240 P_ACO (mmHg) - 0.26; r = 0.96; p <0.001).

A comparison of alveolar carbon monixde between smokers and non-smokers and the changes in alveolar carbon monoxide occurring during the day with smoking
As an initial evaluation of the technique the alveolar carbon monoxide partial pressure (P_ACO) was measured at random times throughout the day in 35 non-smokers and 35 smokers. The smokers, who had not smoked for at least twenty minutes prior to study, were unselected on the basis of cigarette consumption or tar yield of their regular brand. The results are shown in Fig. 14.8 as a simple histogram.

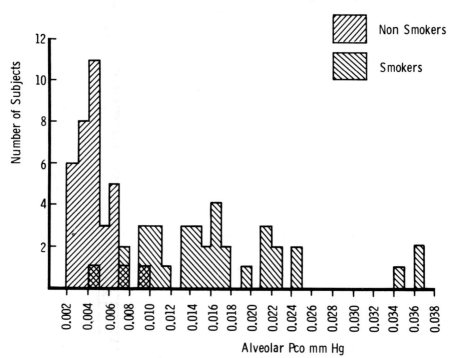

Fig. 14.8 Histogram showing the distribution of alveolar carbon monoxide partial pressure in smokers and in non-smokers.

Non-smokers fell within a relatively narrow range (mean P_ACO 0.004 mmHg; S.D. 0.002 mmHg) whilst the range for smokers was much greater (mean P_ACO 0.016 mmHg; S.D. 0.008 mmHg). The two populations are significantly different (unpaired t test, $p < 0.001$).

In order to evaluate the suitability of the technique for more detailed studies of smoking behaviour the changes in P_ACO with smoking were followed over a 12-hour period in two volunteer, regular smokers of ten to twenty middle tar cigarettes per day. Neither subject had smoked for at least 12 hours prior to the commencement of the study period during which they were allowed to smoke without restriction. Both smoked the same brand of cigarette which yielded 25mg carbon monoxide/ cigarette under standard (TRC) machine smoking conditions. Before smoking each cigarette and exactly 15 minutes after, measurements of P_ACO were obtained and the results, from both subjects are shown in Fig. 14.9. It can be seen that the P_ACO increases with each cigarette smoked (mean increase 0.0036 mmHg, subject A; mean increase 0.0027 mmHg, subject B) and fell between smoking. The overall pattern in both subjects is a rise in P_ACO during the early part of the day with a tendency for the level to plateau after 14.00 hours. In subject B, who was asked to chain-smoke four cigarettes at the end of the study period, there was a further increase in the level of P_ACO.

Cigarette butt nicotine analysis

The characteristics of a filter cigarette can, by machine smoking the product using standard (TRC) smoking parameters, be defined in terms of the measured mainstream smoke nicotine and a derived filter retention efficiency. The filter retention efficiency is calculated from measurements of the mainstream smoke nicotine and the filter nicotine:

$$\text{Filter retention efficiency (F)} = \frac{N_R}{N_S + N_R} \qquad -(4)$$

where N_R is the filter nicotine and N_S is the mainstream smoke nicotine.

If it is assumed that the filter retention efficiency is a constant for any given product specification then, knowing the amount of nicotine retained in the filter after human smoking, it is possible to estimate the amount of nicotine presented to the smoker (mainstream smoke nicotine).

$$N_S = \frac{N_R (1 - F)}{F} \qquad -(5)$$

Once the amount of nicotine presented to the smoker has been determined, an index of the way in which the cigarette has been smoked may be obtained by calculating the ratio of the smoker's mainstream smoke nicotine value to the mainstream smoke nicotine measured on machine smoking. We have called this the nicotine compensation ratio which, because it relates the smokers value to the standard machine smoking figure, may be compared both between subjects and across product types.

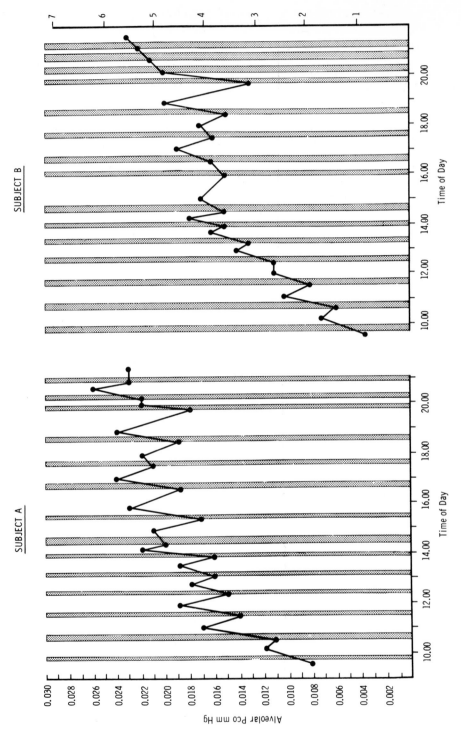

Fig. 14.9 Variations in alveolar carbon monoxide partial pressure with cigarette smoking throughout a 12-hour period in two subjects (A and B). The vertical bars indicate periods of cigarette smoking.

A comparison between the increment in alveolar carbon monoxide and butt nicotine analysis

Two indicators of a subject's 'dose of tobacco smoke' have now been described - measurement of the increment in alveolar carbon monoxide from smoking a single cigarette reflects the 'dose' absorbed whilst the derivation of mainstream smoke nicotine reflects the 'dose' presented to the subject.   It is of interest to compare these two measurements. Forty-seven subjects took part in a study where each was asked to chain-smoke five cigarettes.   Carbon monoxide measurements were made before and 15 minutes after the smoking period and each subject's cigarette butts were collected and pooled for nicotine analysis, in this way minimising errors due to analytic technique.   Both the increment in carbon monoxide and the nicotine presented to the smoker have been related to machine smoked values to allow inter-subject and inter-product comparisons and the results are shown in Fig. 14.10 as a scattergram.

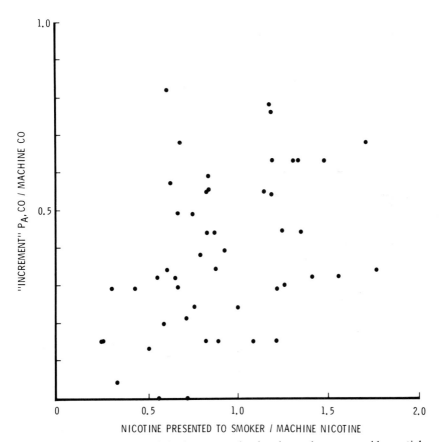

Fig. 14.10 A scattergram of the increment in alveolar carbon monoxide partial pressure/machine smoked carbon monoxide yield versus the derived nicotine presented to the smoker/machine smoked nicotine value (nicotine compensation ratio) in 48 subjects ($r=0.28$, $p > 0.05$).

G*

It can be seen that there is no significant relationship between the two measurements (r=0.28, p 0.05).

The 'dose' of tobacco smoke presented to the smoker (as measured by butt nicotine) is not therefore equal to or even proportional to the 'dose' of tobacco smoke absorbed by the smoker (as measured by the carbon monoxide increment) and the major factor in determining the differences is probably related to inhalation of the smoke from the mouth into the lungs.

The relationship between the alveolar carbon monoxide increment and the smoke exposure index

If inhalation is the major determinant of differences between the 'dose' of tobacco smoke presented to a subject during the smoking of a cigarette and the 'dose' absorbed during smoking, then a relationship might be expected between the smoke exposure index (reflecting the depth of inhalation of smoke and the time which this smoke remains in the lungs) and the increment in alveolar carbon monoxide (reflecting the 'dose' of smoke absorbed).

Habitual middle tar smokers
In Fig. 14.11 the carbon monoxide increment has been plotted against the smoke exposure index for ten habitual middle tar smokers smoking one cigarette of their usual brand.

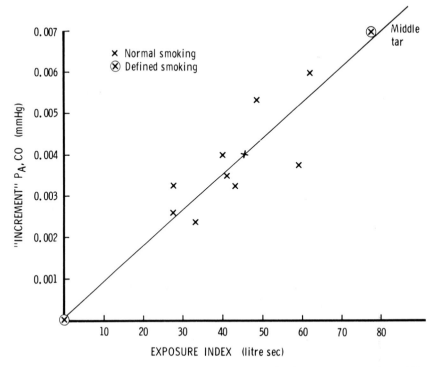

Fig. 14.11 The relationship between the increment in alveolar carbon monoxide partial pressure and the smoke exposure index in habitual middle tar smokers. x, normal smoking; ⊗, defined smoking either with maximal inhalation and breathholding or no inhalation.   The linear regression line for all measurements is shown (r=0.96, p<0.001).

There is an apparent linear relationship between these two measurements (r=0.65, p<0.05). In order to define the relationship further the range of inhalation was extended by instructing one subject to smoke with deep inhalation and breathholding, and three subjects to smoke without inhalation. When these defined-smoking measurements are added to the measurements obtained on normal smoking the linear regression line is as shown in Fig. 14.11 and the correlation coefficient for the data is 0.96 (p<0.001).

It should be noted that when there is no inhalation there is no measurable increment in carbon monoxide suggesting no significant buccal absorption; this is different to the situation found with nicotine when absorption through the buccal mucosa can be readily demonstrated.

Habitual low tar smokers

A similar linear relationship between the increment in alveolar carbon monoxide and the smoke exposure index to that found in middle tar smokers has been demonstrated in five habitual low tar smokers (r=0.94, p<0.05). The linear regression line is shown with the data in Fig. 14.12.

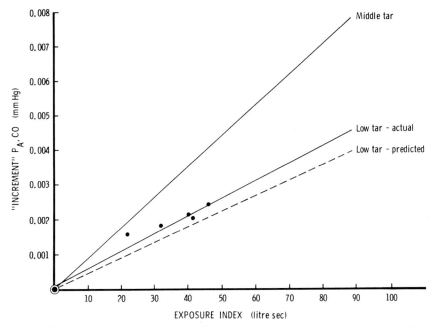

Fig. 14.12 The relationship between the increment in alveolar carbon monoxide partial pressure and the smoke exposure index in habitual low tar smokers. •, normal smoking; ◉, defined smoking without inhalation. The linear regression line for the measurements is shown (r=0.94, p<0.05) together with the predicted regression line - see text. For comparison the linear regression line of middle tar smokers is shown.

A comparison between habitual middle tar smokers and habitual low tar smokers

Inhalation

Fig. 14.12 shows, in addition to the linear regression line for low tar smokers, the regression line for the middle tar smokers previously discussed and shown in Fig. 14.11. These two lines are significantly different at the 5% level.

The significant relationships between the increment in carbon monoxide and the smoke exposure index for both middle and low tar smokers is perhaps surprising, for within each tar group there is a range of products of differing carbon monoxide yield. More important however, is the implication of the demonstrated relationship, that all smokers of the same product type inhale an amount of carbon monoxide which falls within relatively narrow limits, such that the inhalation pattern is the major determinant of the carbon monoxide increment. Although the 'dose' of tobacco smoke presented to smokers differs widely from subject to subject, the 'dose' inhaled and available for absorption tends towards a constant.

If, in Fig. 14.12, the slope of the middle tar regression line is set to represent the relationships between inhalation pattern and rise in alveolar carbon monoxide for an average middle tar product containing 20mg carbon monoxide per cigarette, then the relationship for an average low tar product, which contains 10mg carbon monoxide, can be predicted. The predicted line for such a product is as shown in Fig. 14.12 and it is not significantly different from the actual line obtained from habitual low tar smokers ($p > 0.05$). Furthermore, as can be seen from Figs. 14.11 and 14.12, the values for the smoke exposure index of the middle tar smokers overlap the values for the low tar smokers and statistically there is no difference between the two groups ($p > 0.05$). One must therefore conclude that there is no difference between the inhalation patterns of habitual middle tar and habitual low tar smokers, and, at any given level of smoke exposure index, differences in carbon monoxide increment can be accounted for by the differences in carbon monoxide content of the different product types.

Alveolar carbon monoxide increments

In the previous studies investigating the relationships of alveolar carbon monoxide increments with the smoke exposure index, subjects were studied at random times during the working day. It is possible that the increments in carbon monoxide with smoking may show a changing pattern, other than random variation, during the day. In order to investigate between-product differences therefore, measurements of carbon monoxide were made in relation to the first cigarette of the day. Nine middle and nine low tar smokers were studied before and after their first cigarette of the day on three separate days over a period of three weeks. The results are shown in Table 14.2 as the mean group levels.

Table 14.2 The mean alveolar carbon monoxide partial pressures before and after smoking the first cigarette of the day in groups of habitual middle and low tar smokers.

	Middle Tar Group	Low Tar Group	Level of Significance
Pre smoking level (mmHg)	.0063 $\pm$ .000669	.0068 $\pm$ .001045	NS
Post smoking level (mmHg)	.0094 $\pm$ .000840	.0086 $\pm$ .001085	NS
Increment (mmHg)	.0031 $\pm$ .000328	.0017 $\pm$ .000371	$p < .01$

Mean $\pm$ Standard error   NS not significant

The increment in carbon monoxide for the group of middle tar smokers is significantly higher than that for the group of low tar smokers ($p < 0.1$); the magnitude of this difference is approximately two-fold which is as predicted from the average carbon monoxide deliveries of the two product groups.

More interesting however is the observation that the pre-smoking level of carbon monoxide in the two groups of subjects is the same. This might be accounted for by the approximation of initially different values to within the limits of measurement capability as the levels of carbon monoxide decay exponentially during the night (period of no smoking). The other possibility to be considered is that, despite the fact that middle and low tar smokers appear to smoke on average in an identical way, they eventually plateau at the same average level of carbon monoxide. This may be a reflection of differences in cigarette consumption or pattern of smoking, modification of smoking parameters during the day or the influence of carbon monoxide back pressure from the blood which increases as the day progresses.

Smoking parameters

As a separate study of habitual middle tar and habitual low tar smokers, cigarette butt length, butt nicotine and puff parameters were measured.

Seven middle tar and five low tar smokers entered the study and response parameters were recorded twice in each subject with an intervening period of seven days. Puff parameters, butt length and filter nicotine values were all derived from the smoking of a single cigarette on each of the two occasions. For the present analysis the mean value from the duplicate measurements in each subject have been used to calculate the group statistics on which analyses have been performed using the unpaired t test. The results are shown in Table 14.3

Table 14.3 Puff parameters, butt nicotine and butt length in groups of habitual middle and low tar smokers.

Test	Low Tar Smokers N = 5	Middle Tar Smokers N = 7	Level of Significance
Puff duration secs	1.74 ± 0.028	1.92 ± 0.205	NS
Puff interval secs	43.6 ± 5.430	38.8 ± 4.873	NS
Number of puffs	9.8 ± 1.07	10.9 ± 0.77	NS
Nicotine to smoker mg/cig	0.53 ± 0.033	0.78 ± 0.052	$p < .001$
Nicotine compensation ratio	0.70 ± 0.043	0.70 ± 0.047	NS
Tobacco butt length mm	12.1 ± 2.081	10.2 ± 0.856	NS

Mean level ± standard error
NS not significant

No significant differences are apparent between the middle and low tar smokers for puff parameters, butt length or the way in which the cigarettes have been smoked as judged from the nicotine compensation ratios. There is a significant difference in the amount of nicotine presented to the smokers but this is merely a reflection of the differences in nicotine yield of the two product groups.

Habitual middle tar and habitual low tar smokers

Both the studies of inhalation patterns and smoking parameters presented would appear to suggest that there are no differences between habitual middle and low tar smokers in the way in which they smoke and inhale their respective products. Differences in carbon monoxide, nicotine and presumably tar presented to smokers are merely a reflection of the differences between the products and not modified by smoking. This conclusion would appear to be contrary to a lot of published experience but such studies are predominantly switching studies where middle tar smokers are studied smoking low tar products and vice versa, comparisons being made between the two sequential smoking periods.

Cigarette switching studies

Smoking parameters

An experiment to examine the effects on smoking parameters of subjects switching from middle to low tar cigarettes was conducted in nine habitual middle tar smokers. The original experimental design was for the subjects to smoke their own middle tar product for the first two weeks of the study and then switch to a defined low tar product for four weeks. Following this second period, on a low tar product, subjects were expected to switch back to their middle tar product for the third study period which would last a further four weeks. During the study however, at the completion of the second period, five subjects declined to switch back to their original middle tar product, electing to remain at the low tar level. This is presumably a reflection of the bias of subjects volunteering for such smoking studies! As a consequence, the original study population consists of two potentially different groups and for the analyses presented here these groups have been treated separately. Group A are those subjects who, in the third period, switched back to their original middle tar product (n=4) whilst group B are those subjects who elected to remain on the low tar product (n=5).

Response measurements were obtained weekly during the ten week study period. Smoking parameters were recorded from the smoking of a single cigarette, butt length and butt nicotine analyses were the average from a 24 hour butt collection and cigarette consumption was the mean daily consumption from a weekly record. For the summary results presented the mean response for all subjects in each of the two groups is given for each of the three smoking periods. Examination for differences between the groups has been carried out using the unpaired t test.

Table 14.4 presents the results from Group A where subjects have switched back to the middle tar product for the final smoking period. There are no significant differences for any parameter between the first and third smoking periods when subjects were smoking the middle tar products. The nicotine compensation ratio would indicate however that the low tar product is being significantly 'oversmoked' when compared to the middle tar product and from the puff parameters this would seem to be the result of taking larger puff volumes. Despite this 'oversmoking' of the low tar product, compensation, in terms of nicotine, is not complete. Although the decrease in nicotine presented to the smoker is not significant when switching to the low tar product, there is a significant increase when switching back to middle tar in the third

Table 14.4   A comparison of smoking parameters between the three stages of a cigarette switching study. Subjects in Group A (n=4) who switched back to a middle tar product for the final smoking period.

		Experimental Stage			Level of Significance		
		1 Middle Tar	2 Low Tar	3 Middle Tar	1 v 2	1 v 3	2 v 3
Puff Duration	secs	2.1 $\pm$ 0.17	2.4 $\pm$ 0.10	2.4 $\pm$ 0.09			
Puff interval	secs	32.1 $\pm$ 4.92	34.1 $\pm$ 3.65	37.0 $\pm$ 2.30			
Puff number		10.0 $\pm$ 1.07	10.2 $\pm$ 0.66	9.4 $\pm$ 0.46			
Puff volume	cc	44.1 $\pm$ 3.94	53.3 $\pm$ 2.85	46.3 $\pm$ 2.31	p $<$ .05		p $<$ .05
Nicotine to smoker	mg/cig	0.96 $\pm$ 0.081	0.83 $\pm$ 0.029	1.00 $\pm$ 0.031			p $<$ .001
Nicotine compensation ratio		0.79 $\pm$ 0.078	1.00 $\pm$ 0.035	0.84 $\pm$ 0.034	p $<$ .01		p $<$ .01
Tobacco butt length	mm	8.1 $\pm$ 0.52	7.7 $\pm$ 0.60	7.3 $\pm$ 0.50			
Cigarette consumption daily		25.3 $\pm$ 2.96	25.8 $\pm$ 1.44	29.9 $\pm$ 2.09			

Mean level $\pm$ standard error

Table 14.5 A comparison of smoking parameters between the three stages of a cigarette switching study. Subjects in Group B (n=5) who elected to remain on a low tar product for the final smoking period.

		Experimental Stage			Level of Significance		
		1 Middle Tar	2 Low Tar	3 Low Tar	1 v 2	1 v 3	2 v 3
Puff duration	secs	2.1 ± 0.20	2.2 ± 0.10	2.5 ± 0.12		$p < .05$	
Puff interval	secs	37.1 ± 4.3	34.3 ± 4.60	34.7 ± 4.90			
Puff number		9.3 ± 0.54	10.1 ± 0.64	10.5 ± 0.84			
Puff volume	cc	41.0 ± 2.88	48.2 ± 2.50	52.1 ± 3.24	$p < .05$	$p < .01$	
Nicotine to smoker	mg/cig	1.07 ± 0.024	0.89 ± 0.023	0.88 ± 0.032	$p < .001$	$p < .001$	
Nicotine compensation ratio		0.88 ± 0.018	1.08 ± 0.029	1.07 ± 0.039	$p < .001$	$p < .001$	
Tobacco butt length	mm	8.4 ± 0.78	8.8 ± 0.65	9.8 ± 0.96			
Cigarette consumption	daily	23.8 ± 1.86	27.0 ± 1.60	25.4 ± 1.00			

Mean level $\pm$ standard error

period of the study.   No changes in butt length or cigarette consumption were noted.

In Table 14.5 are shown the results of subjects in Group B who elected to remain on low tar products.   There are no significant differences for any parameter between the second and third smoking periods when subjects were on the low tar product. As in Group A the nicotine compensation ratio is significantly higher after switching to the low tar product, suggesting some attempt to compensate but again, as shown by the nicotine dose, this compensation is not complete.   As before puff volume would appear to be an important factor in compensation and there are no significant changes in butt length or cigarette consumption.

This study would confirm other reports in that changes in smoking parameters are demonstrable when subjects *switch* to products in a different tar group - there is some attempt to maintain the 'dose' of smoke at a constant level.

Inhalation

In addition to the above study we have had the opportunity of looking at the inhalation pattern in one subject smoking products from different tar groups. The subject is a habitual middle tar smoker and measurements of carbon monoxide increment and smoke exposure index were made on two consecutive days whilst he smoked his normal brand of cigarette. The results are shown in Fig. 14.13 where it can be seen that there is good agreement between the two sets of observations.

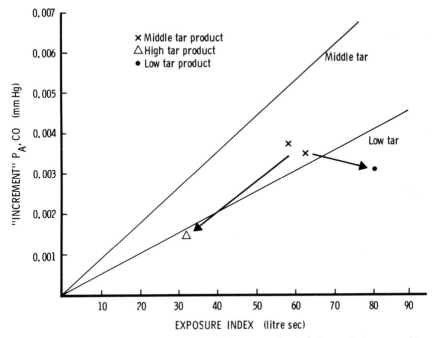

Fig. 14.13 The relationship between the increment in alveolar carbon monoxide partial pressure and the smoke exposure index for a habitual middle tar smoker smoking his normal product (x), and low tar product (●) and a high tar product (△). For comparison the linear regression lines of middle and low tar smokers are shown.

On a third occasion the subject was given a low tar product to smoke and, as indicated, there was an increase in exposure index with a marginal fall in carbon monoxide increment. This result parallels the results obtained from the measurements of smoking parameters outlined above and might suggest an attempted compensation. The results are also in agreement with the previously defined relationships of carbon monoxide increment and exposure index for the different product groups.

On another occasion the subject was given a high tar product to smoke. In this situation the results, as shown, are not as one might have expected; the exposure index decreased as one might have predicted but the carbon monoxide increment unexpectedly showed a dramatic fall. Furthermore, considering the carbon monoxide yield of the product, the rise in alveolar carbon monoxide was well below that which one would have predicted from the carbon monoxide increment - exposure index relationships as previously discussed. Observation of the chest pneumogram tracing offered an explanation for this discrepancy in that the pattern observed was that demonstrated in example 2 of Fig. 14.7 with an apparent active exhalation prior to the first inhalation following the puff. The only other time that this pattern has been observed was in one habitual high tar smoker who has been studied and he consistently showed this feature in his smoking.

The reason for this unusual pattern of smoking must be in terms of an organoleptic response, a topic which has been little discussed in relation to smoking behaviour. The middle tar habitual smoker switching to the high tar product commented spontaneously on the taste and strength of the cigarette such that he found it difficult to inhale. Such organoleptic factors may however not only be relevant when considering the changes in smoking pattern on switching to or smoking a product in a higher tar category but may also be important, in contributing to the changing parameters observed, when switching to a lower tar product. If middle tar smokers are asked to comment when given a low tar product they frequently indicate the products to be unsatisfactory in terms of their strength and taste.

Conclusions

In this paper, we have attempted to outline some of the available techniques for the analysis of smoking parameters and cigarette smoke absorption, and described their application in a wide ranging series of studies.

We may attempt to summarise the act of smoking in terms of the parameters discussed as follows:

1. There is no correlation between the 'dose' of tobacco smoke presented to the smoker (estimated from butt nicotine analysis) and the amount of smoke absorbed by the smoker (measured by increments in alveolar carbon monoxide levels).

2. There is a significant correlation between the amount of smoke absorbed by the smoker and the smoke exposure index derived from the volume and time periods of inhalations following the puffing of a cigarette.

It will thus be realised that the 'dose' of tobacco smoke absorbed by the subject is not simply the product of the 'dose' of smoke presented to the smoker and the smoke exposure. Rather it is equal to the product of the 'dose' of smoke inhaled and the smoke exposure where the 'dose' inhaled tends to be a constant and represents the 'dose' of smoke presented to the smoker modified by factors which are not clearly defined.

With regard to differences in the act of smoking between smokers of different product types we have seen that for habitual smokers of middle and low tar products there are no demonstrable differences and the dose of cigarette smoke presented to a smoker is dependent upon the cigarette specification. Differences in absorption of smoke inhaled are dependent upon the pattern of inhalation but for any given inhalation pattern differences in smoke absoprtion are again dependent upon the cigarette specification.

In switching studies there is some evidence that subjects adjust their smoking to maintain a constant 'dose' of cigarette smoke but, whilst this may be true, the possibility of changes due to organoleptic factors has not been ruled out. Whatever the cause of the observed modifications to the smoking profile it would be important to ascertain whether these persist or are relatively short lived.

The broad approach to the analysis of smoking taken in this paper has perhaps challenged some widely held concepts and certainly raised a large number of questions which will require further study. One overriding question, however, which must be posed is whether this type of study can be justified at all? The answer must be 'yes' for the current yardsticks available for measuring success in providing a low risk product are smoke chemistry screening and the results of bio-testing in animals, based on standard smoking parameters. As we have seen the smoker can and may modify these parameters and hence modify the quality and/or the quantity of smoke when smoking a particular product.

We need to know the extent of such modifications in order to attempt, in the short term, to predict long term morbidity response rather than await the results of long term epidemiological studies. In any event, in the final analysis, the yardstick for judging the relative risk factor of different smoking products must be the human response.

Acknowledgement

We thank Professor A. Guz, Department of Medicine, Charing Cross Hospital Medical School for providing facilities for technique development. We are grateful to the Editor of Clinical Science and Molecular Medicine for his permission to publish Fig. 14.8 and Fig. 14.9.

References

Adams, P.I. (1966) Measurements on puffs taken by human smokers. *20th Tobacco Chemists Research Conference.* Winston-Salem, N.C.

Armitage, A.K. (1973) Some recent observations relating to the absorption of nicotine from tobacco smoke. In *Smoking Behaviour: Motives and Incentives,* ed. Dunn, W.L. pp. 83-92. Washington: V.H. Winston & Sons.

Ashton, H. & Watson, D.W. (1970) Puffing frequency and nicotine intake in cigarette smokers. *British Medical Journal,* **3,** 679-681.

Comer, A.K. & Creighton, D.E. (1978) The effect of experimental conditions on smoking behaviour. *This volume.*

Guillerm, R. & Radziszewski, E. (1975) A new method of analysing the act of smoking. *Annals du Tabac,* **13**, 101-110.

Rawbone, R.G., Coppin, C.A. & Guz, A. (1976) Carbon monoxide in alveolar air as an index of exposure to cigarette smoke. *Clinical Science and Molecular Medicine,* **51**, 495-501.

15. The effects of nicotine-enhanced cigarettes on human smoking parameters and alveolar carbon monoxide levels

P J DUNN AND E R FREIESLEBEN

Introduction

In recent publications (e.g. Rawbone, Coppin and Guz, 1976a, b, Wald *et al*, 1975, Wald and Howard, 1975), levels of carbon monoxide determined from alveolar air and/or from blood as carboxyhaemoglobin have been used as an index of exposure to tobacco smoke. These techniques have been employed to distinguish between populations of smokers and non-smokers, and to assist in the prediction of the development of disease associated with cigarette smoking. In instances where frequent sampling is required, analysis of alveolar air is favoured over the measurement of blood carboxyhaemoglobin because of the ease of obtaining samples and of the simpler analytical procedures involved. For these reasons, this technique was used in an attempt to learn more about the relationship between levels of CO and nicotine delivered by cigarettes and their corresponding effects on human smoking patterns and alveolar CO levels.

Studies conducted by Russell *et al*, (1973, 1975) and Guillerm *et al*, (Guillerm and Radziszewski, 1975, Guillerm and Broussolle, 1975), have shown a relationship between body CO levels and nicotine intake and it has been suggested that smokers modify their smoking to regulate nicotine intake. One could speculate from this finding that a change in inhalation (duration, depth or frequency) is one means of 'smoke compensation' i.e. a smoker would unconsciously inhale cigarette smoke of higher nicotine concentration to a lesser extent, resulting in a lower body CO level, all other factors in cigarette design being equal (e.g. draw resistance and CO delivery). This study was therefore directed towards testing the foregoing assumption by monitoring alveolar CO levels and smoking parameters when smokers were presented with a cigarette of different nicotine delivery.

Method

Subjects

From the in-house staff, four heavy smokers of filter cigarettes, delivering 1.0 mg. nicotine under standard smoking conditions, volunteered to be monitored for their smoking patterns as well as for CO uptake for every second or third cigarette smoked through five working days. These subjects, three women and one man, all with sedentary type jobs, were chosen such that smoke monitoring was easily arranged within their working environment. Also, with the more stable and higher body resting CO levels associated with this relative inactivity, any change in body CO level which might occur as a result of differences in cigarette construction may be more readily observed.

Procedure

With a Teflon cigarette holder, attached by flexible plastic tubing to a Sanborn transducer (Hewlett-Packard Model 270), a differential pressure was recorded across the
cigarette during smoking. With no additional resistance in the mouthpiece, these
smoking patterns of pressure drop (reported in the Tables as maximum puffing effort,
MPE) were recorded on a Moseley multi-speed strip-chart recorder such that number
of, interval between and duration of puffs were obtained for each smoking. In addition,
the estimated area under each pressure drop curve gave a measure of relative smoke
volume. (True volume measurements would have necessitated the placement of an
added resistance in the mouthpiece from which the differential pressure, and thus
velocity could have been obtained). The effect of the cigarette holder on the smoking
patterns was thought to be small, and would in any case be consistent for all products
smoked.

The technique for collection of alveolar air comprised rebreathing of lung exhalate
into a laminated plastic bag, following the format of Hansen *et al* (1972). Alveolar
CO concentrations, expressed as ppm, were determined gas chromatographically on
the lung exhalates following the procedure of Grieder and Buser (1971), with few
alterations. The 'before smoking' CO samples were collected immediately before the
commencement of cigarette smoking and the 'after smoking' CO samples were collected
three minutes after the termination of smoking. Mouth nicotine levels were estimated
indirectly using standard filter efficiency data and individual butt nicotine determinations (Willits *et al,* 1950).

After each smoker had accustomed himself to the mouthpiece and the presence of
the recording instrumentation, he was monitored over a five day period while smoking
his regular cigarette. He then smoked the experimental cigarette for an acclimatisation
period of three days before undergoing monitoring for the following five days.

The experimental cigarette was equivalent in all respects to the regular (control)
cigarette except for the addition to the tobacco prior to cigarette manufacture of
sufficient nicotine citrate in aqueous solution to increase the smoke nicotine yield
by 30%. With the addition of this salt, no change was observed in smoke pH, perhaps
indicating that the subjective properties were not grossly altered.

In Table 15.1 are listed the cigarette specifications and the smoke yields obtained
under standard machine smoking conditions for the two cigarettes studied.

Observations and discussion

The human smoking data as well as changes in alveolar CO concentration for each of
the four smokers with the two different cigarettes (094 and 410) are presented in
Table 15.2. The data for subjects 1 and 2 are averages for every third cigarette smoked,
and for subjects 3 and 4, every second cigarette smoked during five consecutive working
days. This format was required due to the limitations of time available for smoke
monitoring and CO analyses.

For the parameters describing the puffing characteristics of the smokers, it will be
noted that large differences were found amoung the four smokers, even with the same
type of cigarette. Similarly, the amounts of nicotine taken into the mouth differed
considerably from smoker to smoker. The large standard deviations reflect how widely
each smoker altered his smoking habits to satisfy his particular needs.

Table 15.1 Product data for cigarettes* studied

Cigarette identification	094 (control)	410
Cigarette length (mm)	72	72
Filter Type	CA**	CA**
Filter Pressure Drop *** (cm H_2O)	2.5	2.5
Total Cigarette Pressure Drop (cm H_2O)	9.6	9.6
Nicotine Delivery (mg/cigarette)	1.01	1.32
Total Particulate Matter (mg/cigarette)	19.9	21.4
CO Delivery (mg/cigarette)	22.4	21.2
Filter Efficiency (%)	22.4	22.4

*   Cigarettes were conditioned (60% RH and 22°C) and smoke yields obtained under standard machine smoking of one 35 ml puff of two seconds duration taken once per minute to a 30 mm butt length.

** Cellulose acetate

*** Pressure drop in cm of water determined at a velocity of 1050 cc/min.

In Table 15.3 the directions of change as well as levels of significance for this product change are noted. The changes in butt length, puff number, duration, and relative effort (MPE) were within 10% of the normal cigarette with one exception (not statistically different). Likewise there was little change in relative volume per puff or per cigarette.

In spite of the lack of consistency in change of some of the parameters of smoking habits measured, the CO resting levels (alveolar CO levels before) were lower for all four smokers when smoking the experimental cigarette with the 30% higher nicotine delivery. The decrease ranged from 10% to 47% and averaged 27% for the four subjects. These differences are illustrated graphically in Figures 15.1 - 15.4 for the respective smokers.

Because of fluctuations in body resting CO levels caused by changes in overnight metabolism and variations in smoking early in the day, it appeared that a daily equilibrium may be established some time after the eighth cigarette (11:00 - 11:30 a.m.). For this reason alveolar CO resting levels after this time were averaged and subjected to statistical analyses. Analyses of variance showed that the CO resting levels found with the nicotine enhanced cigarettes were significantly lower, relative to the control at greater than the 95% level for each of the four smokers and at greater than the 99% level for all but smoker number 4. Since similar levels of significance were found

Table 15-2 Human smoking data and alveolar CO concentrations

Subject No.	1		1		2		2		3		3		4		4	
Cigt. Identif'n	094		410		094		410		094		410		094		410	
	Ave.*	S.D.	Ave.*	S.D.	Ave.*	S.D.	Ave.*	S.D.	Ave.*	S.D.	Ave.*	S.D.	Ave.*	S.D.	Ave.*	S.D.
Butt Length (mm)	25.5	3.0	26.3	2.9	19.2	2.0	21.1	1.7	24.9	3.4	25.5	2.2	22.7	2.7	25.4	3.0
Puff No.	8.9	0.9	9.4	1.5	12.5	1.7	12.7	1.4	9.2	1.9	8.3	1.5	8.3	0.8	8.5	1.0
Average Interval Between Puffs (sec)	36.8	8.5	47.9	14.9	40.2	9.8	41.0	9.9	55.6	23.3	**69.7**	24.1	60.0	9.8	55.3	8.7
Average Puff Duration (sec)	2.01	0.17	2.02	0.15	1.42	0.14	1.44	0.10	1.30	0.14	1.32	0.10	1.60	0.20	1.70	0.15
Average Rel. MPE (chart units)	67.6	7.2	69.0	8.5	49.6	4.4	50.2	7.8	50.5	5.5	49.7	6.2	48.4	6.3	49.2	8.0
Ave. Rel. Volume/ Puff (calculated)	67.9	8.2	69.7	9.2	35.2	3.3	36.1	6.1	32.8	5.3	32.8	4.6	38.7	5.4	41.8	6.3
Ave. Rel. Volume/ Cigt. (calculated)	605		655		440		459		301		272		321		355	
Mouth Nicotine/ Cigt. (mg.)	2.56	0.45	2.01	0.31	3.25	0.73	2.25	0.38	1.59	0.35	1.73	0.35	2.04	0.35	2.08	0.38
Alveolar CO level before (ppm)	27.6	6.2	19.2	6.4	28.9	9.7	15.3	4.9	28.2	9.0	22.6	8.1	22.1	7.6	19.8	5.4
Alveolar CO level after (ppm)	30.8	6.5	21.9	6.3	34.0	9.6	18.3	5.4	35.2	10.9	29.6	8.8	32.1	9.7	29.8	8.5
CO uptake (ppm)	3.2	2.4	2.7	1.7	5.1	3.4	3.0	1.7	7.0	5.4	7.0	3.5	10.0	4.5	10.0	4.9
Total Daily Cigt. Consumption	39		50		42		41		19		21		24		23	
Total Daily Mouth Nicotine Intake (mg)	99.8		100.5		136.5		92.3		30.2		36.3		48.9		47.8	
Total No. of Cigts. Monitored	34		35		35		35		44		30		42		30	

* Average of all cigarettes monitored during the working hours of 5 consecutive days.

Table 15.3 Differences in smoking parameters (Level of significance: 0.01) 094/410

Subject No.	1	2	3	4
Butt Length (mm)	NC	I	NC	I
Puff No.	I*	NC	NC	I*
Ave. Interval Between Puffs (sec.)	I	NC	I*	D*
Ave. Puff Duration (sec.)	NC	NC	NC	I*
Ave. Rel. M.P.E. (Charts Units)	NC	NC	NC	NC
Ave. Rel. Volume/Puff (Calculated)	NC	NC	NC	I*
Mouth Nicotine/Cigt. (mg)	D	D	NC	NC
Alveolar CO Level Before (ppm)	D	D	D	D*
Alveolar CO Level After (ppm)	D	D	D	NC
CO Uptake (ppm)	D	NC	NC	NC
Total Daily Cigarette Consumption	I*	NC	NC	NC

* Level of significance: 0.1   I: increase   NC: no change   D: Decrease

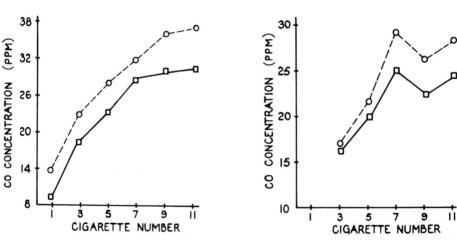

Figs. 15.1 - 15.4 Alveolar resting CO levels for the respective smokers throughout the working day. Level O   094 (Control); □ 410;

with the data collected over the entire working day, this may indicate that equally valid estimates of alveolar CO levels may be obtained by sampling within this shorter time period.

Although it may be speculated that these lower body resting CO levels may have resulted from a decrease in CO uptake (difference in alveolar CO concentration before and three minutes following cigarette smoking), such a decrease was observed for only smokers 1 and 2 while the other two smokers showed no change in body CO uptake. Since both cigarettes deliver almost equivalent amounts of CO by standard machine smoking, changes in smoking patterns and/or inhalation are likely to be responsible for the lower body resting CO levels. As most of the smoking parameters for the two cigarettes seldom differed by more than 10%, it would appear that this lower CO level was due to changes in inhalation patterns (assuming no extreme changes in body metabolism or cigarette consumption for any of the smokers, during the course of the study).

The possibility that the smokers inhaled less smoke from the experimental cigarette (410) because of decreased subjective acceptability, can be ruled out because a panel of 12 smokers, including the four involved in this study, found it to be slightly more acceptable (p. = 0.90) on the basis of reduced irritation and improved taste quality.

When the four smokers were given the cigarette of higher nicotine delivery, the changes in mouth nicotine were quite inconsistent. Subjects 1 and 4 appeared to achieve the same total daily mouth nicotine intake from each of the two types of cigarettes but they were not consistent with regard to inhalation patterns, as reflected by alveolar CO uptake. Subject No. 2 smoked the same number of each type of cigarette, but a reduction in inhalation was reflected in a 41% decrease in CO uptake with a 32% decrease in mouth nicotine intake, while smoking the nicotine enhanced cigarettes. Subject No. 3 increased his daily mouth nicotine intake by approximately 20% but showed no change in CO uptake (i.e. inhalation), with the 410 cigarette.

With the lack of correlation of nicotine intake and CO uptake, for each smoker, the smoking parameters measured in this study do not consistently reflect nicotine compensation. Alveolar CO levels, however, may be a reliable indicator of inhalation and as they were lower for all four subjects, one may conclude that the higher nicotine deliveries of the 410 cigarettes caused the smokers to reduce to varying degrees the amounts of smoke actually inhaled. This lends some support to Russell's hypothesis of compensation for nicotine (Russell, 1976) but it would be unwise to draw such a conclusion based on this experiment alone.

Conclusions

From this preliminary study there appears to be no direct relationship between the cigarette smoke yield of CO obtained under standard smoking conditions and the actual alveolar uptake of CO during smoking. The alveolar resting levels of CO were significantly lower for all smokers when cigarettes of unchanged CO yield but 30% higher nicotine yield were smoked. Although two of the four smokers appear to duplicate total daily nicotine intake with the two different cigarettes smoked, this apparent regulation of mouth nicotine is not complemented by observed changes in CO uptake.

The smokers did not compensate for the 30% increase in nicotine delivery by significantly altering puff number, interval, duration or butt length. As well only small differences in puffing effort and relative volume were recorded with this cigarette change. No decrease in total daily cigarette consumption was noted with the increased nicotine availability.

With the nicotine enhanced cigarette, all smokers reduced, to varying degrees the amount of smoke inhaled, as evidenced by the lower alveolar CO resting levels. This greater availability of nicotine to the smoker may be, as suggested by Russell (1976) an effective means of reducing the intake of tar and CO. This study is being continued with a larger panel of smokers.

Acknowledgement

The technical assistance of Miss Cecile Letourneau and Mrs. Ninon Gauthier is gratefully acknowledged.

References

Grieder, K. & Buser, H. (1971) Gaschromatographische bestimmung von kohlenmonoxid in der ausatmungsluft und im blut, *Beiträge zur Tabakforschung,* **6**, 36-40.

Guillerm, R. & Broussolle, B., (1975) Resultats au plan respiratoire de la substitution d'une cigarette a fumée peu irritante à la cigarette habituelle chez de grands fumeurs, *Le Poumon et Le Coeur,* **31**, 277-281.

Guillerm, R. & Radziszewski, E. (1975) Une nouvelle méthode d'analyse de l'acte du fumeur. *Annales due Tabac,* 101-110, Paris: SEITA.

Hansen, O., Wilke, H., Malorny, G. & Goethart, M. (1972) Absorption and release of carbon monoxide during breathing of low CO concentrations by smokers and non-smokers. *Staub-Rheinhaltung der Luft,* **32**, 43-46.

Rawbone, R.G., Coppin, C.A. & Guz, A. (1976a). Carbon monoxide in alveolar air as an index of exposure to cigarette smoke. *Clinical Science and Molecular Medicine,* **51**, 495-501.

Rawbone, R.G., Coppin, C.A. & Guz, A. (1976b) A simple method for the estimation of carbon monoxide in alveolar air and its application in epidemiological studies in smoking. *European Journal of Clinical Investigation,* **6**, 320.

Russell, M.A.H. (1976) Low-tar medium-nicotine cigarettes: a new approach to safer smoking. *British Medical Journal,* **1**, 1430-1433.

Russell, M.A.H., Wilson, C., Patel, U.A., Cole, P.V. & Feyerabend, C., (1973) Comparison of effect on tobacco consumption and carbon monoxide absorption of changing to high and low nicotine cigarettes. *British Medical Journal,* **4**, 512-516.

Russell, M.A.H., Wilson, C., Patel, U.A., Feyerabend, C. & Cole, P.V. (1975) Plasma nicotine levels after smoking cigarettes with high, medium and low nicotine yields. *British Medican Journal,* **2**, 414-416.

Wald, N. & Howard, S. (1975) Smoking, carbon monoxide and arterial disease. *Annals of Occupational Hygiene,* **18**, 1-14.

Wald, N., Howard, S., Smith, P.G. & Bailey, A. (1975) Use of carboxyhaemoglobin levels to predict the development of diseases associated with cigarette smoking. *Thorax,* **30**, 133-140.

Willits, C.O., Swain, M.L., Connelly, J.A. & Brice, B.A. (1950) Spectrophotometric determination of nicotine, *Analytical Chemistry,* **22**, 430-433.

16. The effects of a reduced draw resistance cigarette on human smoking parameters and alveolar carbon monoxide levels

P J DUNN

Introduction

Numerous studies have been carried out investigating the changes in smoking habits when smokers were given cigarettes of higher and/or lower smoke delivery. These results indicate that smokers adjust the intensity (puff number, butt length, puffing effort, volume, duration) with which they smoke (Creighton and Lewis, 1978a, Adams, 1976), alter daily cigarette consumption (Russell *et al*, 1973; Goldfarb, Jarvik and Glick, 1970; Frith, 1971), or vary the depth of inhalation (Dunn and Freiesleben, 1978; Russell *et al*, 1975) with the different smoking product. Each of these changed smoking parameters has been presented as evidence of a form of compensation to regulate body nicotine intake.

Since it has been reported that a smoker may vary nicotine uptake by a factor of as much as 100 with either his normal smoking product or with one of totally different delivery depending solely on the depth of inhalation (Harke, 1970), the changes noted for the more easily measurable smoking parameters mentioned above, may become meaningless relative to this inhalation factor. Questionnaires relating to the degree of inhalation are interesting (Schmidt, 1977), but experience has proven that such studies are not always in agreement with CO analyses used to indicate inhalation depths (Wald *et al*, 1975).

In a previous communication from this laboratory (Dunn and Freiesleben, 1978) the technique of estimating CO concentrations in exhaled air was used on a limited number of smokers as an estimate of smoke inhalation. This work showed that when a nicotine enhanced cigarette was smoked, no nicotine regulation was apparent from butt nicotine data relative to the normal cigarette, but there was in fact a lesser degree of inhalation as evidenced by a significant decrease in lung CO concentrations in exhaled air. Although both cigarettes compared in the previously mentioned study had equivalent unlit draw resistance, the ease of availability of the added nicotine caused no change in the maximum puffing efforts of the smokers to obtain a satisfying mouthful of smoke.

A recent study using cigarette-smoking baboons (Rogers, 1977) has suggested that a low draw resistance cigarette allows for greater inhalation. Higher blood CO levels were found with the cigarette of lower draw resistance despite significantly fewer puffs having been taken from it. It was decided therefore to investigate the effects of cigarettes of equivalent nicotine delivery but of changed draw resistance on smoking parameters, mouth nicotine intake and alveolar CO levels of heavy cigarette smokers.

Subjects and method

Seven heavy smokers of a popular medium delivery cigarette available in Canada volunteered from the in-house staff to participate in this comparative study. Monitoring took place within the usual working environment such that normal smoking, aside from the addition of the mouthpiece could be followed. Laboratory personnel were not included in the study to avoid any possible prejudice by panel members. Smoking parameters and alveolar CO levels were monitored following the same techniques outlined previously (Dunn and Freiesleben, 1978). It was only after acclimatisation to the smoking instrumentation and the smoking products that smoking data were collected. Each smoker was monitored for smoking patterns and alveolar CO resting levels three times per day for five working days. Monitoring commenced after 10:30 a.m. such that each smoker had already smoked at least six cigarettes.

Alveolar air samples were collected not only before the smoking of each of the cigarettes monitored by the smoking instrumentation but also before each succeeding cigarette through the working day. Thus with this greater number of samples, a better estimate of daily resting CO levels could be ascertained. In addition the butts of these cigarettes smoked through the working day were collected for butt length and nicotine determination.   In this way a better estimate of the changes in smoking habits, relative to these two parameters was available without the somewhat obtrusive monitoring instrumentation.

The physical parameters and smoke deliveries of the two brands compared in this study are listed in Table 16.1.   The experimental cigarette was made with the same tobacco blend as the control but a variation of paper type and filter construction resulted in a decrease of approximately 30% in draw resistance and standard CO delivery.

Table 16.1 Product data for cigarettes studied

Cigarette Type	589-1 (Control)	442
Cigarette Length (mm)	72	72
Filter Type	C.A. *	C.A.
Filter Pressure Drop (cm H_2O at 1050 cc/min)	7.0	3.3
Total Cigarette P.D. (cm H_2O at 1050 cc/min)	13.5	9.5
Nicotine (Mainstream Smoke) (mg/cigarette)	0.87	0.88
TPM (Mainstream Smoke) (mg/cigarette)	16.5	15.3
CO (mg/cigarette)	24.8	17.7
Filtration Efficiency %	43.3	21.4
Paper Porosity	Low	High

* Cellulose Acetate

Observations and discussions

The directions of change and levels of significance for the smoking parameters and alveolar resting CO levels when the smokers switched from their normal (589-1) cigarette to the cigarette of 30% reduced draw resistance (442) are illustrated in Table 16.2.

Table 16.2 Differences in smoking parameters (Level of Significance: 0.01) 589-1/442

I: increase
D: decrease
NC: no change

Subject No.	1	2	3	4	5	6	7
Butt Length	NC	NC	NC	NC	D	NC	D
Puff Number	I	NC	NC	D	NC	NC	D
Ave. Interval Between Puff	D	NC	NC	NC	I	NC	I
Ave. Puff Duration	D*	D*	D*	D	D	D	D
Ave. Rel. M.P.E.	I	I	I	I	I	I	NC
Ave. Rel. Volume/ Puff (Calculated)	I*	I*	I	I*	I	I	NC
Mouth Nicotine/Cigt.	I	I	I	I	I	I	I
Alveolar CO Level	D	D**	D	D	D	D	D
Total Daily Cigt. Consumption	NC	NC	NC	NC	NC	NC	NC

  * Level of Significance: 0.10
 ** Level of Significance: 0.20

The results of the panel, trained to assess cigarettes subjectively, indicated a marginal preference for the control cigarette (589-1) on the basis of less impact and irritation. This cigarette was felt to provide better taste, though the 442 cigarette yielded more taste.

As estimated from butt nicotine analyses there was a 77% increase in mouth nicotine levels for both types of cigarettes when the smokers were being monitored by the smoking instrumentation. These changes in nicotine levels were not accounted for by any significant change in average butt length, though not surprisingly, more variation in butt length occurred when the smokers were not being monitored. Despite the effect of the monitoring procedure (i.e. mouthpiece) it is believed that comparison of the smoking parameters is valid because the percentage differences found between the two types of cigarettes were similar regardless of whether or not the smokers were being monitored.

When the smokers switched to the cigarette of reduced draw resistance, overall there were no trends or significant changes with regard to butt length, puff number or interval between puffs. The smokers, however, took puffs of 9.5% shorter duration and of 20% greater effort which resulted in an increase of 28% in relative velocity (calculated) with this product change. An average increase in relative volume per puff of 9% was observed for six of the seven smokers studied. An increase of 7% in total relative volume per cigarette was noted for five of the seven smokers as a result of changes in puff number.

These changes in smoking parameters resulted in a significant increase of 56% in mouth nicotine intake. A similar increase in CO delivery to the mouth would be anticipated since there is a linear relationship between CO/nic. delivery and puff volume (Creighton and Lewis, 1978b). Assuming that no changes in inhalation patterns occurred, an average increase in alveolar resting CO levels of 10% above that of the normal cigarette would be anticipated, after correcting for the difference in CO deliveries as given by standard machine smoking. Despite the substantial increase in nicotine to the mouth with the cigarette of lower draw resistance, the alveolar resting levels decreased by an average of 16% which is markedly (29%) less than the level predicted using mouth nicotine as an indicator of total smoke concentration. This difference is quite possibly due to all smokers inhaling less deeply with the increased nicotine concentration in the mouth. These results are not unlike the decrease in lung CO levels observed when smokers were given cigarettes of increased nicotine achieved through the addition of the citrate salt (Dunn and Freiesleben, 1978).

The ease of availability of nicotine with the cigarette of lower draw resistance (more nicotine per unit effort) did not cause a decrease in total amount of smoke taken from the cigarette; in fact the smokers appeared to show increased effort when smoking this cigarette. Although no downward trend in this effort was observed throughout the total smoking observation period, it is unknown whether, over a longer period of time, there may be a reduction in mouth nicotine intake to the previous level. Despite this increased mouth nicotine intake there was no significant change in total daily cigarette consumption.

An equivalent trial study with smoker No. 5 had been carried out for a seven-day period, one year prior to the investigation with the group of seven smokers. At that time a similar increase in mouth nicotine intake was found along with a corresponding decrease in alveolar CO levels. A similar change in puffing effort was noted with the product change and like the most recent study, no other significant changes in smoking parameters were found.

Conclusions

The tendency to regard the easily measurable smoking parameters such as total daily cigarette consumption, butt length, nicotine content, puff number, volume or effort as indicators of amount of smoke inhaled, can be most misleading. Based upon the observations in this experiment as well as the previously reported study using nicotine enhanced cigarettes, it is apparent that the smoker can vary quite extensively his inhalation patterns and that this inhalation characteristic is the major factor controlling the amount of smoke received in the lungs. Hence, in experiments designed to measure how a smoker responds to cigarettes of different types, or to cigarettes smoked under different experimental (e.g. more stressful) situations, it is essential to have an estimate of inhalation such as measurements of carbon monoxide in the exhaled breath.

Acknowledgement

The technical assistance of Miss Cecile Letourneau and Mrs. Ninon Gauthier is gratefully acknowledged.

References

Adams, P.I. (1976) Changes in personal smoking habits brought about by changes in smoke yield. *Proceedings of the Sixth International Tobacco Scientific Congress,* Tokyo. 102-108.

Creighton, D.E. & Lewis, P.H. (1978a) The effect of different cigarettes on human smoking patterns. *This volume.*

Creighton, D.E. & Lewis, P.H. (1978b) The effects of smoking pattern on smoke deliveries. *This volume.*

Dunn, P.J. & Freiesleben, E.R. (1978) The effects of nicotine enhanced cigarettes on human smoking parameters and alveolar CO levels. *This volume.*

Frith, C.D. (1971) The effect of varying the nicotine content of cigarettes on human smoking behaviour. *Psychopharmacologia,* **19**, 188-192.

Goldfarb, T.L., Jarvik, M.E. & Glick, S.D. (1970) Cigarette nicotine content as a determinant of human smoking behaviour. *Psychopharmacologia,* **17**, 89-93.

Harke, H.-P. (1970) Zum problem des 'Passiv-rauchens'. *Münchener medizinische Wochenschrift,* **112**, 2328-2334.

Rogers, W.R. (1977) The effect of cigarette type and blood carbon monoxide level: studies with the cigarette smoking baboon. *American Review of Respiratory Disease,* Supplement **115**, 158.

Russell, M.A.H., Wilson, C., Patel, U.A., Cole, P.V. & Feyerabend, C. (1973) Comparison of effect on tobacco consumption and carbon monoxide absorption of changing to high and low nicotine cigarettes. *British Medical Journal,* **4**, 512-516.

Russell, M.A.H., Wilson, C., Patel, U.A., Feyerabend, C. & Cole, P.V. (1975) Plasma nicotine levels after smoking cigarettees with high, medium and low nicotine yields. *British Medical Journal,* **2**, 414-416.

Schmidt, F. (1977) Defused cigarettes - slogan or reality, *World Smoking and Health,* **2**, 35-38.

Wald, N., Howard, S., Smith, P.G. & Bailey, A. (1975) Use of carboxyhaemoglobin levels to predict the development of diseases associated with cigarette smoking. *Thorax,* **30**, 133-140.

H

17. Pharmacological and psychological determinants of smoking

S SCHACHTER

The gist of the anti-smoking campaign is simply 'Quit and if you can't or won't quit, switch to a low-nicotine, low-tar cigarette'. With the backing of the American Cancer Society, the Royal College of Physicians and the Public Health Service, this message pervades the mass media and appears responsible for the tedious competition among tobacco companies for the safest cigarette, the search for an acceptable tobacco -free cigarette stimulated by the British government and taxation policies such as that of New York City which taxes cigarettes by nicotine and tar content in an apparent effort to use economic muscle in order to help the smoker help himself. Though no one has bothered to make explicit the premises on which such policy is based, it appears reasonable to guess that, in part, the low nicotine and tar compaign is based on the notion that cigarette smoking stems from a variety of psychological, sensory and manipulative needs which can probably be as well satisfied with a low as with a high nicotine cigarette.

The possibility that this campaign may perversely be increasing the health hazards of smoking has been raised by Domino (1973), Russell (1974a) and others who point out that there is evidence, after all, that nicotine is addicting. To the extent that the smoker is an addict, he is probably smoking to keep nicotine or one of its active metabolites at some optimal level. If, then, the heavy smoker does switch to low nicotine brands, he may very well end up smoking more cigarettes and taking more puffs of each. He will in the process of regulating nicotine probably get the same amounts of nicotine and tar and unquestionably get more of the combustion products, such as carbon monoxide which appears to be at least as much of a medical villain as tar or nicotine for it is implicated in the increased risk to smokers of arterio-sclerosis, ischaemic heart disease, fetal damage and so on (Larson, Haag and Silvette, 1961; US Surgeon General's Report, 1972). If this shift in level of smoking is permanent, the net effect of switching to low nicotine cigarettes should be to increase the dangers of smoking. From this point of view, the concerned smoker should smoke high, not low, nicotine cigarettes.

Since almost everyone would agree that cigarette smoking involves both pharma-cological and psychological determinants there does seem to be some support for either position. Whether rationality dictates the recommendation of a low or a high nicotine cigarette depends, of course, on the relative importance of the pharmacological versus the psychological needs satisfied by smoking.

On the gratifications of smoking

Almost any smoker can convince you and himself that there are major psychological components to smoking. They will convince you that smoking calms them; that it helps them work; that they smoke more at a party and so on. In short, smoking serves some psychological function; it does something positive for the smoker and this is the reason he smokes. This emphasis on the functional properties of smoking is at the heart of virtually every serious psychological attempt to understand smoking. Presumably nicotine or tar or some component of the act of smoking is so gratifying that despite the well-publicised dangers the smoker is unwilling to give up the habit. Undoubtedly the ultimate eulogy of the act is Marcovitz's suggestion (Marcovitz, 1969) that 'as a psychological phenomenon, smoking is comparable to the ritual of the Eucharist. There the communicant incorporates bread and wine and in so doing symbolically introjects the Lord Jesus Christ. This is a conscious process, with the hope of identification, of attaining some of the attributes of Jesus. Similarly, the smoker incorporates the smoke introjecting in an unconscious fantasy some object which will confer on him its magic powers.' (p. 1082). Among these magic powers, smoking serves to 'delimit the body image in the quest for the sense of self,' to 'relieve the unconscious fear of suffocation' and as 'proof of immortality'. Though no one has matched Marcovitz's panegyric, almost all attempts to account for the habit have assumed that it does something positive for the smoker - an assumption that is shared by the smoker himself for numerous studies indicate that heavy smokers report that cigarettes relax them or stimulate them, put them at ease, give them something to do with their hands, and so on. In short, for both the psychologist and the smoker, the act of smoking is functional; it does something for the smoker and this is the reason he smokes. In this paper, I shall concentrate on one of the presumed motivations for smoking. Smokers widely report that they smoke more when they are tense or anxious and they also report that smoking calms them. Smoking, then serves a respectable psychological function and this presumably is one of the motivations for and explanations of smoking under stress.

Before worrying through interpretations of these facts, let us make sure that they are facts. Firstly, does smoking increase with stress? The available evidence indicates that indeed it does, if the stress is fairly intense. In two almost identical experiments (Schachter et al, 1977b; Schachter, Silverstein and Perlick, 1977), my associates and I manipulated stress within the context of experiments presumably designed to measure tactile sensitivity. In high stress conditions, such sensitivity was measured by the administration, sporadically over an experimental hour, of a series of intense, quite painful shocks. In low stress conditions, the shocks were a barely perceptible tingle. Between the testing intervals, the subjects, all smokers, were free to smoke or not as they pleased. In both studies, the subjects smoked considerably more in high than in low stress conditions.

Turning to the effects of smoking on stress, we ask next does smoking reduce stress? The answer appears to be that it depends upon how you look at it. Silverstein (1976) attempted to answer the question by measuring how much electric shock a subject was willing to take within the context of a study of tactile perception. The procedure required that electrodes be attached to a subject's fingers, that he be exposed to a series of shocks of gradually increasing voltage and that he report when he could first feel the shock, next when the shock first became painful and finally when the shock became so painful that he could no longer bear it. Silverstein assumed that the more anxious the subject, the less pain he would be willing to tolerate. There were four experimental groups -- smokers who smoked either high or low nicotine cigarettes during the experiment or who did not smoke at all during this time and a group of non-smokers who did not smoke.

The results of this experiment are presented in Figure 17.1. The ordinate plots the number of shocks the subjects endured before calling it quits. It is clear that smokers take more shocks when they are smoking high nicotine than when smoking low nicotine cigarettes than when not smoking. Given this pattern one has a choice of interpretations: either nicotine decreases anxiety or lack of nicotine increases anxiety. The choice of depends, of course, on the position of the group of non-smokers who, as can be seen in Figure 17.1 take virtually the same number of shocks. as smokers on high nicotine. It would appear then that smoking is not anxiety reducing but, rather, that no smoking or insufficient nicotine is for the heavy smoker, anxiety increasing.

Precisely the same pattern of results emerges in a study of irritability conducted by Perlick (1977). Within the context of a study of aircraft noise, subjects, watching a television drama, rated how annoying they found a series of simulated over-flights. During the experiment, heavy smoking subjects were permitted *ad lib* smoking of high nicotine cigarettes in one condition, of low nicotine cigarettes in another condition and were prevented from smoking in a third condition. Finally, there was a control group of non-smokers. The results are presented in Figure 17.2 where it can be seen that smokers on high nicotine cigarettes are markedly less irritated. by this series of obnoxious noises than are smokers restricted to low nicotine cigarettes or prevented from smoking. However, these high nicotine smokers are neither less nor more irritated than the group of non-smokers. Again it would appear that smoking doesn't make the smoker less irritable or vulnerable to annoyance, not smoking or insufficient nicotine makes him more irritable.

This same pattern is characteristic of psychomotor as well as emotional behaviour. Heimstra, Bancroft and DeKock (1967) examined the hypothesis that smoking facilitates driving performance by comparing *ad lib* smokers, deprived smokers and non-smokers in a six-hour simulated driving test. On a variety of measures of tracking and vigilance, *ad lib* smokers do neither better nor worse than non-smokers but do markedly better than deprived smokers.

Again and again, then, one finds the same pattern - smoking doesn't improve the mood or calm the smoker or improve his performance when compared with the non-smoker. *   However not smoking or insufficient nicotine makes him considerably

*There is of course, an alternative interpretation of this consistent pattern. Rather than indicating withdrawal, it is conceivable that people who become smokers are by nature more frightened of shock more irritated by noise and worse drivers than people who never become smokers, and that for such people smoking is indeed calming and does improve psychomotor performance. Though nothing short of a longitudinal study could unequivocally settle the matter, it should be noted that there have been formidable number of studies that compared smokers and non-smokers on virtually every personality dimension imaginable. Smith (1970) in his review of this literature concludes that the *only* variables which, with reasonable consistency, discriminate between smokers and non-smokers are extraversion and anti-social tendencies. And even on these variables the differences are quite small.

THE EFFECTS OF NICOTINE ON TOLERANCE OF SHOCK

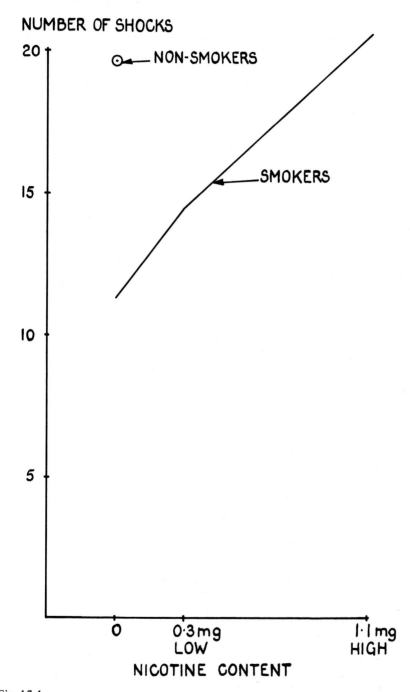

Fig. 17.1

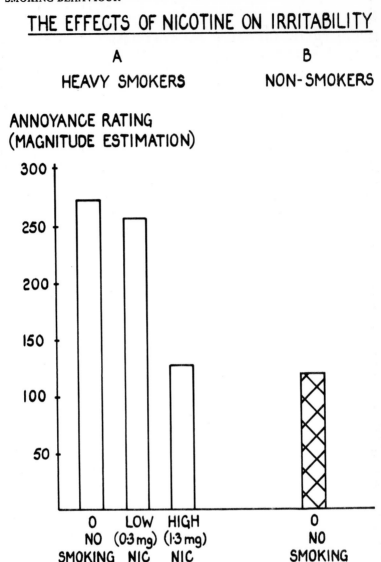

THE EFFECTS OF NICOTINE ON IRRITABILITY

A
HEAVY SMOKERS

B
NON-SMOKERS

ANNOYANCE RATING
(MAGNITUDE ESTIMATION)

Fig. 17.2   NICOTINE MANIPULATION

worse on all dimensions. Given this persistent fact, how then, to account for the fact that the smoker smokes more when he is stressed? One can, obviously, account for the generally debilitating effects of no or low nicotine by assuming that the deprived smoked is in withdrawal but this assumption alone cannot account for the effects of stress on smoking rate unless one assumes that stress, in some fashion, depletes the available supply of nicotine. And this hypothesis, of course can account for this pattern of data only if it is the case that the smoker, an addict, is smoking to keep nicotine at a constant level.

Another way of phrasing this same conclusion is that the heavy smoker gets nothing out of smoking. He smokes only to prevent withdrawal. I freely admit that this is a perverse conclusion to reach about a habit that is quite as costly and universally pervasive as smoking but the existing data for humans don't encourage any other conclusion. Though my colleagues and I have found occasional hints that smoking may do something for the smoker when compared to the non-smoker (Silverstein, 1976) in general these differences have been quite small. In addition, Heimstra (1973) has presented tentative evidence that smokers may have somewhat less mood fluctuation than non-smokers and there have been numerous studies (Larson et al, 1961) suggesting that smoking may affect one or another psychomotor or mental ability but in general these have all been small effects and inconsistent from study to study. It should be noted, however, that almost all studies of the matter have used long-time, heavy smokers as subjects. It may be that in the early stages of the smoking habit, there are indeed major gratifications and effects, that the smoker gradually adapts to these effects and by the time smoking no longer does anything for him he is thoroughly addicted.

Nicotine as addiction

Though almost everyone would probably agree that cigarette smoking, with nicotine or some nicotine metabolite as the active agent, is addicting, the evidence in support of this assumption is puzzlingly inconsistent. On the assumption that one manifest-ation of addiction is the regulation of nicotine intake, studies of the matter have either pre-loaded subjects with varying amounts of nicotine or have manipulated the nicotine content of the available cigarettes and measured the effects on smoking. There have been at least ten such studies on human subjects with results varying from no indication of regulation to one study which appears to indicate exquisitely precise control of nicotine intake. At one extreme, Finnegan, Larson and Haag (1945) and Goldfarb, Jarvik and Glick (1970) supplied subjects with several weeks' worth of cigarettes of varying nicotine content and checked daily cigarette consumption. Though both studies did find some subjects who regulated - i.e., smoked substantially more low than high nicotine cigarettes - the groups of subjects as a whole failed to demonstrate regulation. In sharp contrast, Ashton and Watson (1970), observed subjects smoke high and low nicotine cigarettes under controlled conditions and found evidence of precise regulation in that their subjects puffed considerably more at low than at high nicotine cigarettes and, via this mechanism, extracted almost the same amount of nicotine from the two kinds of cigarettes. Between these extremes Frith (1971) and Russell et al (1973) find reasonably good evidence of nicotine regulation and at least five studies (Herman, 1974; Jarvik, Glick and Nakamura, 1970; Johnston, 1942; Kozlowski, Jarvik and Gritz, 1975; Lucchesi, Schuster and Emley, 1967) have found a tendency for smokers to regulate nicotine intake but, at best, crudely and imprecisely.

Though there is probably no single, simple reconciliation of this spectrum of diverse results one suggestion may partially account for the general failure to find conclusive evidence for the precise regulation that might be expected from the addiction hypothesis. There are smokers who don't inhale; there are smokers who simply toy with the habit smoking an occasional cigarette at parties and meetings and, most importantly, there are undoubtedly many smokers, sensitive to the health hazards, who deliberately inhibit smoking by such devices as imposing an upper limit on daily consumption, scheduling smoking, restricitng smoking to particular occasions and so on -- all devices intended to lower consumption and which would tend to mask such behavioural manifestations of addiction as tracking nicotine content. To the extent that such people are subjects in studies of regulation, one should expect that the manipulation of level of nicotine would have weak effects on smoking behaviour.

In an attempt to eliminate such subjects, Schachter (1977) deliberately selected a group of subjects who satisfied the following criteria:

a. By self-report, the subject currently smoked at least a pack a day and had smoked at this level for many years.

b. By self-report, the subject was trying neither to cut down or limit his smoking.

c. If the subject had every attempted to quit, he reported great difficulty and suffering.

d. By self-report, the subject exhibited 'regular' smoking behaviour, i.e. smoked about the same amount each day, began smoking in the morning and continued regularly throughout the day, etc.

The salient characteristics of each of these subjects are presented on the left side of Table 17.1 where it can be seen that they all had smoked a pack or more a day for at least twenty years. For the course of the experiment these subjects agreed to smoke only the experimenter's cigarettes and on alternating weeks each subject was presented with cartons of specially prepared and packaged cigarettes which delivered either 1.3 mg of nicotine per cigarette or 0.3 mg of nicotine per cigarette. At bedtime, the subjects noted the number of cigarettes smoked.

Obviously, there was an inherent and deliberate circularity in the design of this study. I was simply asking, do smokers who appear to be addicted by one set of criteria (behavioural self-description), behave in an addicted fashion on a totally independent criterion (nicotine regulation)? The effects of the nicotine manipulation are presented on the right side of Table 17.1. Obviously, the manipulation had a strong

Table 17.1 The effects of nicotine content on smoking

Subject Characteristics					Smoking Behaviour Cigs/day on:		
Subject	Age	Sex	No. yrs. a serious smoker	No. cigs/day self report	Low (0.3 mg) Nic	High (1.3 mg) Nic	% Increase High Nic to Low Nic
J.A.	52	F	30	30	31.25	21.50	+45.3
S.S.	37	F	22	40	55.00	40.50	+35.8
R.R.	38	F	19	40	42.50	30.75	+38.2
R.S.	43	F	27	20	22.75	20.00	+13.8
D.R.	47	F	29	40-45	70.75	58.75	+20.4
R.A.	50	M	40	30	30.25	26.25	+15.2
J.E.	52	M	33	33	48.00	44.25	+ 8.5
Mean	45.6		28.6	33.6	42.93	34.57	+25.3

and consistent effect on these long-time heavy smokers for each of them smoked more low than high nicotine cigarettes. One the average, there was a 25% increase (p<.01) of smoking accompanying the manipulations of nicotine content.

It does appear, then, that heavy, long-time smokers do regulate nicotine. Given that the manipulation involved a four-fold difference in nicotine content while smoking increased only 25%, it would appear to be at best crude and imprecise regulation. There is, however, reason to believe that nicotine regulation is considerably more precise than these data suggest. First, several studies (Ashton and Watson, 1970; Herman, 1974; Schachter *et al*, 1977b) report that smokers puff more at low than at high nicotine cigarettes — clearly a mechanism for increasing nicotine intake. Second, given the range of nicotine content in this study precise regulation was virtually impossible. For example, a subject who normally smoked two packs a day of 1.3 mg nicotine cigarettes would have to smoke almost nine packs a day of our low nicotine cigarettes to get his customary dose of nicotine. Under these circumstances, virtually any theory of addiction would predict withdrawal for the subjects on low nicotine cigarettes. Though unfortunately no systematic provision was made in this study to measure withdrawal, there is dramatic anecdotal evidence that the subjects who were the worst regulators in this study were in states of marked irritability and explosive emotionality while on the low nicotine cigarettes. Supporting this observation, Perlick (1977) and Silverstein (1976) have both demonstrated experimentally that heavy smokers on low nicotine cigarettes are markedly more anxious and irritable than such smokers on high nicotine cigarettes.

It does appear, then, that heavy smokers do adjust smoking rate so as to keep nicotine at a roughly constant level. To account for this fact, one may suppose that there is an internal machine of sorts — one which detects the level of nicotine and regulates smoking accordingly. To begin consideration of the nature of such a regulator let us review some of the basic facts about the metabolic fate and excretion of nicotine. As summarised by Goodman and Gilman (1958):

'Nicotine is chemically altered in the body, mainly in the liver but also in the kidney and lung. The fraction of nicotine which escapes detoxication is completely eliminated as such in the urine along with the chemically altered forms. The rate of excretion of the alkaloid is rapid and increases linearly with the dose. When the urine is alkaline, only one fourth as much nicotine is excreted as when the urine is acid; this is explained by the fact that nicotine base is reabsorbed from an alkaline urine.' (page 622).

The effects of the acidity of the urine on the rate of excretion of unchanged nicotine suggests, given the fact that smokers regulate nicotine intake, that the pH of the urine may affect the rate of smoking. Whether an effect of any consequence is to be anticipated, however, depends on the proportion of unchanged nicotine which is excreted. One can make reasonably accurate estimates from the work of Beckett and his associates. Beckett, Rowland and Triggs (1965) have shown that subjects who smoke twenty cigarettes a day excrete an average of 1.0μg nicotine per minute under normal conditions, 5.0μg nicotine per minute when the urine was made acidic by the oral administration of ammonium chloride and 0.1μg/min after oral administration of the alkaliser sodium bicarbonate. In another study, Beckett and Triggs (1967) have demonstrated that smokers whose urine has been maintained acidic excrete in unchanged form about 35% of known quantities of nicotine that have been administered either by intravenous injection, inhalation of nicotine vapour or smoking. Putting these facts together, it appears reasonable to estimate that the proportion of nicotine which will be excreted in unchanged form will vary with the manipulated acidity of the urine as follows:

urine is:	% nicotine excreted
acid	35
normal	7
alkaline	<1

Obviously the exact proportions will vary with the precise pH of the urine. However, one thing seems clear: given the quite low proportion of unchanged nicotine which is excreted under normal or placebo conditions, increasing the alkalinity of the urine can at best have trivial effects on plasma level nicotine while increasing the acidity of urine can potentially have substantial effects. If then, one assumes first, that changes in urinary pH are reflected in circulating nicotine and second, that the amounts smoked vary with changes in plasma level nicotine, it should be expected that experimentally increasing the acidity of the urine will increase the amounts smoked.

To test this guess, Schachter, Kozlowski and Silverstein (1977) manipulated urinary pH by, in alternate weeks, administering to a group of 13 smokers substantial daily doses of placebo or of the acidifying agents vitamin C (ascorbic acid) and Acidulin (glutamic acid hydrochloride). The subjects were given cartons of their favourite cigarettes and kept count of the amount they had smoked each day of the study. The effects of these manipulations on smoking are presented in Table 17.2 where it can be seen that acidification is accompanied by increased smoking. During the period they were taking either of two different acidifying agents, subjects smoked 20% more cigarettes than during the time they were taking a corn starch placebo.

It should be specifically noted that in keeping with the magnitude of the pharmacological effects this 20% increase is not a large experimental effect. On the basis of our estimation of nicotine excretion one would expect, at best, roughly a 30% increase

Table 17.2 The effects of vitamin C, Acidulin and placebo on cigarette smoking

Condition	Cigarettes smoked per day	Mean % change from placebo
Vitamin C	26.7	+19.8
Placebo	23.1	--
Acidulin	28.1	+20.9
Comparison	p value	
Vitamin C vs Placebo	<.05	<.05
Acidulin vs Placebo	<.01	<.01

in smoking with even a strongly effective acidifying manipulation which ours was not. It seems clear that of the body's two chief mechanisms for disposing of nicotine, enzymatic breakdown and urinary excretion of unchanged nicotine, the urinary excretion route plays by far the lesser role in the confirmed smoker. Nevertheless acidification does affect smoking behaviour and this finding raises the possibility that it may be useful to invoke this bit of pharmacological machinery in order to understand some of the presumed psychological and situational determinants of smoking rate. Conceivably, events that stimulate smoking may do so via their action on urinary pH.

To learn if this guess had any merit as a possible explanation of the stress-smoking relationship, Schachter et al (1977b) examined the effects of a variety of academic stressors on pH. In one study, subjects urinated immediately before an obviously stressful event such as delivering a Colloquium lecture or taking Ph.D. examinations. And, for control purposes, these same subjects urinated at precisely the same time on routine, non-stressful days. The results are presented in Table 17.3 where it can be seen that for nine of ten subjects, the urine is considerably more acidic on stress than on control days.

Precisely the same pattern is manifest in another study of the effects of stress (Schachter et al, 1977b). Nine of the twenty members of an undergraduate seminar

Table 17.3 The effects of academic stress on urinary pH

| Subject | pH on: | | Stress-Control |
	Stress Day	Control Day	
	A. Colloquium Talk		
E.G.	5.50	6.35	-0.85
H.T.	5.70	5.95	-0.25
M.C.	6.70	6.90	-0.20
H.K.	5.50	6.20	-0.70
S.S.	5.40	6.45	-1.05
	B. Ph.D. Oral Defense		
E.D.	5.40	7.10	-1.70
A.L.	6.00	6.20	-0.20
	C. Ph.D. Comprehensive Examination		
B.S.	5.85	5.80	+0.05
I.S.	5.20	5.70	-0.50
D.P.	5.40	5.70	-0.30
All subjects (mean)	5.67	6.24	- .57

were assigned to read highly technical material and prepare 10-15 minute oral reports for class. The remaining students were simply expected to listen to the reports. All of the students urinated shortly before class. For the reporters pH averaged 6.01 and for the listeners 6.67 (p .05). Before a control class, pH was identical for the two groups of students.   It does appear that stress, at least of the sort endemic to academic life, acidifies the urine, — a finding which at least encourages the exploration of a pharmacological interpretation of smoking behaviour.

To review the line of argument so far: it has been widely reported that smoking increases with stress and that smoking is calming.   These observations appear to go hand in hand and to support the assertion that nicotine or tar or some component of the act of smoking is anxiety reducing.   The experimental facts are peculiarly at variance with this interpretation.   Smoking does increase with stress but smoking smokers are no more or less calm than a control group of non-smokers.   They are, however, considerably calmer than groups of smokers who are prevented from smoking or permitted to smoke only low nicotine cigarettes.   This fact can be interpreted as indicating that smoking isn't anxiety reducing but that not smoking or insufficient nicotine is anxiety increasing.   In effect, the smoker smokes more during stress because of budding withdrawal symptoms and not because of any psychological property of nicotine or of the act of smoking.   Such an interpretation is plausible if one assumes that the smoker smokes in order to keep nicotine at some constant level and that there is something about the state of stress that depletes the body's supply of nicotine. A variety of studies have been described which, via the effects of urinary pH on the rate of nicotine excretion, suggest a biochemical mechanism that could account for this set of facts.

Though this elegant juxtaposition of facts makes almost irresistable the conclusion that the smoker's mind is in the bladder, obviously we are hardly yet in a position to rule out psychological explanations of smoking.   Though 'anxiety reduction' seems, by now, a particularly unsatisfactory explanation of the stress-smoking relationship, innumerable other purely psychological explanations are still conceivable. Ferster (1970), for example, has attempted to explain the relationship in these terms:

'With the increase in emotional symptoms there is frequently a major cessation in most of the ongoing repertoire the person might engage in.   With such a temporary decrease in the frequency in most of the items in a person's repertoire, the relative importance of even the minor reinforcers increases enormously.   Thus the relative position of smoking in the entire repertoire is increased considerably when other major items of the repertoire are depressed.   Smoking becomes something to do when no other behaviour is appropriate'.   (page 99).

In short, though the effect of pH on nicotine elimination is a well established pharmacological fact, it may have little, if anything, to do with the effects of stress on smoking for it is certainly conceivable that stress, with or without accompanying pH changes, will affect smoking rate.   In order to learn if pH changes are a necessary and sufficient explanation of the stress-smoking relationship, it is clear that we must experimentally pit the mind against the bladder and this Schachter, Silverstein and Perlick (1977) attempted to do in an experiment which independently manipulated stress and the pH of the urine.   If it is correct that pH changes are a necessary part of the machinery, we should expect more smoking in high than in low stress conditions when pH is uncontrolled and no difference between the two conditions when pH is experimentally stabilised.   If, on the other hand, pH changes are irrelevant to the smoking-stress relationship, there should be more smoking in high than in low stress conditions no matter what the state of the urine.

In this study, too, stress was manipulated by use of electric shock. The experiment already described on the effects of stress on smoking (Schachter *et al,* 1977b) was replicated with one major modification — in one pair of conditions the high or low stress manipulation began fifty minutes after the subjects took a placebo; in the other condition it began fifty minutes after subjects had taken 3g. of bicarbonate of soda — an agent virtually guaranteed to quickly elevate urinary pH and for a time to stabilise it at highly alkaline levels. In Table 17.4, we note first the effects of the manipulation on urinary pH.   Examining first the two placebo conditions, it will be noted that pH decreases in the High Stress condition (p = .02) and tends to increase

Table 17.4   The effects of the manipulations on urinary pH

Condition	N	Mean pH:			No. of subjects whose pH:		
		Pre-stress	Post-stress	Pre-post	Decreased	Stayed same	Increased
High Stress-Placebo	12	6.00	5.83	-0.17	8	3	1
Low Stress-Placebo	12	5.99	6.13	+0.14	4	1	7
High Stress-Bicarbonate	12	6.08	7.44	+1.36	0	0	12
Low Stress-Bicarbonate	12	6.20	7.01	+0.81	2	1	9

in the Low Stress condition.   In the two bicarbonate conditions, in sharp contrast, pH increases markedly from the beginning to the end of the experiment and the stress manipulation has had absolutely no effect on pH.

Next we note that on a variety of self-report measures, the manipulation of stress was highly successful in both the placebo and bicarbonate conditions.   Obviously, then, the conditions necessary to pit the psychological against the pharmacological explanation of the effects of stress on smoking have been established.   Subjects in High Stress conditions are considerably more tense than are subjects in Low Stress conditions, whether they have taken a placebo or bicarbonate.   In the placebo conditions, however, where pH is uncontrolled, stress acidifies whereas in the bicarbonate conditions, it does not.

The effects of these manipulations on smoking are presented in Figure 17.3 which plots the mean number of puffs taken by subjects once the stress manipulation had begun.   It is clear that with placebo, there is considerably more smoking in high than in low stress conditions while with bicarbonate, stress has absolutely no effect on smoking (interaction $p < .01$).   It does appear, then, that smoking under stress has nothing to do with psychological, sensory or manipulative needs that are presumably activated by the state of stress but is explained by the effects of stress on the rate of excretion of nicotine.   The smoker under stress smokes to replenish nicotine supply, not to relieve anxiety.

Obviously, the research presented is an openly reductionist attempt to explain some

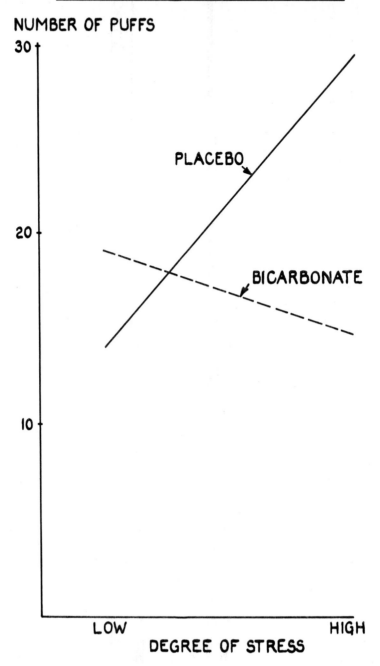

Fig. 17.3

of the effects of psychological variables without making use of the conceptual equipment of psychology. I believe that in the case of stress, the attempt has been successful for given the facts outlined, attempts to formulate the stress-smoking relationship in psychological terms (Ferster, 1970; Hunt, 1970; Marcovitz, 1969; Nesbitt, 1973; Schachter, 1973) seen unnecessary *ad hoc* constructions. In addition to stress, there is evidence suggesting that this may also be the case for the widely reported effects of party-going on smoking. In two studies, Silverstein, Kozlowski and Schachter (1977) have found that party-going does increase smoking and have also found that parties markedly increase urinary acidity. This is true for non-smokers as well as smokers – a finding which indicates that it is not smoking which is the cause of acidity and which makes somewhat more plausible the guess that the urinary pH mechanism may also be responsible for the party smoking relationship. I suspect that many of the presumed psychological and situational determinants of smoking behaviour may prove reducible to these elementary biochemical terms.

It must be admitted, however, that satisfactory though this mechanistic view of smoking may be for understanding the behaviour of many, perhaps most, smokers, the apparent exceptions to this model are maddeningly various. There are smokers (Schachter, 1973) who do not track nicotine content. Though it is known (Isaac and Rand, 1972) that plasma nicotine level is zero on awakening, there are smokers who find cigarettes distasteful in the morning and do not light up their first cigarette before lunchtime. Though withdrawal is a necessary component of virtually any model of addiction, some orthodox Jewish smokers, forbidden to smoke on the Sabbath, report that they can do so without a qualm. And so on.

Just how to cope with such blatant exceptions is problematic. Perhaps it is necessary to invent psychological typologies (McKennell, 1973; Russell, 1974b; Tomkins, 1968) to accommodate the distressing apparent variety of smokers, but I find this an unsatisfying scientific stratagem. As a working hypothesis, I propose instead that virtually all long-time smokers are addicted and suggest that many, perhaps all, exceptions to an addiction model can be understood in terms of such notions as self-control, concern with health, restraints etc. Certainly all smokers are aware of the dangers and expense of smoking. To the extent that such concerns are prominent, the smoker probably inhibits his smoking by such devices as imposing an upper limit on his daily consumption, scheduling his smoking, and so on – devices intended to lower consumption and which would tend to mask such behavioural manifestations of addiction as tracking nicotine content.

If this is correct, we should expect to find other, less obvious indications of addiction and, of these, I would suggest that withdrawal is the key. Obviously anyone can give up smoking, limit his daily intake or restrict smoking to particular times or occasions if he is willing and able to put up with the withdrawal syndrome. If it is correct that virtually all long time smokers are addicted, it should be anticipated that smokers who don't smoke in the morning will be more irritable at that time of day than in the afternoon; that smokers who restrain their smoking will be more volatile people than heavy smokers, and so on. To test such expectations, Perlick (1977) in the experiment described earlier, compared a group of heavy, unrestrained smokers to a matched group of highly restrained smokers, mostly former heavy smokers who on a variety of indices indicated that they were deliberately and successfully attempting to cut down, though not eliminate, smoking by a combination of devices such as smoking cigarettes only half way, smoking very low nicotine cigarettes, counting daily intake and the like. On the average these restrained smokers reported smoking at a rate less than half of their former level. As described earlier, all subjects rated how annoying they found the noise of each of a series of simulated aircraft over-flights while, depending on condition, they were either prevented from smoking or permitted *ad lib* smoking of high or of low nicotine cigarettes. It should be noted first that in the conditions where they were permitted to smoke, restrained former heavy smokers smoked only half as much as did current heavy smokers. They behaved in the laboratory, then, as they report they do in life. The effects of these manipulations on the two groups of smokers are presented in Figure 17.4.   As noted earlier, the extent to which heavy, unrestrained smokers were annoyed depends on the nicotine manipulation. When they did not smoke or smoked very low nicotine cigarettes they

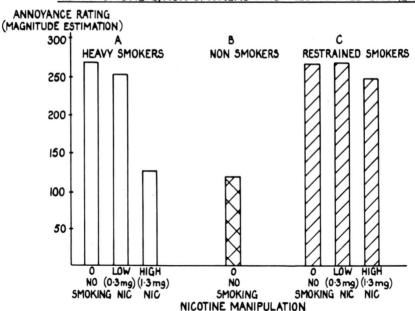

Fig. 17.4

were markedly more annoyed than when they smoked high nicotine cigarettes. The restrained, former heavy smokers stand in fascinating contrast for they were chronically annoyed — as they should be even in the high nicotine condition where they were still getting considerably less nicotine than in former days was their want. In other tests of the same hypothesis, Perlick (1977) demonstrates that such restrained smokers eat more than do heavy smokers when given free access to candy and also do worse at a proofreading task requiring concentration. Restrained smokers appear to be chronically more irascible, to nibble more and to have poorer concentration than

unrestrained smokers. It is possible to control and restrict smoking but at a price
– and the price appears to be a chronic state of withdrawal.* It does appear that one
of the exceptions to a purely addictive view of smoking is no exception. I suspect
that this shall be the case with most of these exceptions[†] and that by taking account
of withdrawal we can understand those studies (Finnegan et al, 1945) (Goldfarb
et al, 1970) which fail to demonstrate nicotine regulation.

Let us review our conclusions so far. For the confirmed smoker:

1. The psychological and probably the sensory and manipulative gratifications
of smoking are illusory. Serious smokers smoke to prevent withdrawal.

2. Smokers regulate nicotine intake.

3. Variations in smoking rate which customarily have been interpreted in
psychological terms seem better understood as an attempt to regulate nicotine.

4. Apparent exceptions to a regulatory model of smoking seem understandable
in terms of withdrawal. The smoker who fails to regulate suffers withdrawal.

Given this array of facts a formidable case can be made for a predominantly
pharmacological, addictive view of cigarette smoking and it would certainly seem
that the campaign for low nicotine cigarettes is misguided and rests on a set of
fallacious premises. It must be noted, however, that with the exception of the
Perlick (1977) study these conclusions are all based on studies in which the state
of nicotine deprivation or lowered nicotine intake is maintained from an hour or
so to, at most, a few days as in the Schachter (1977) study. Can we expect that,
in real life, shifting to a low nicotine cigarette will lead to a permanent increase in
amounts smoked or is there some sort of adaptation process so that eventually the
smoker returns to former levels of consumption? The question is crucial and
particularly so in light of (a) Hammond et al's (1976) demonstration that heavy smokers
of low nicotine cigarettes are in considerably more danger than light smokers of high
nicotine cigarettes even when tar and nicotine intake, by my calculation from their
data, are probably roughly equivalent and (b) Ross's (1976a, 1976b) evidence that
carbon monoxide, hydrogen cyanide and nitrogen oxide delivery is considerably
greater in most of the popular brands of low nicotine, filter cigarettes than in high
nicotine, non-filter cigarettes.

The only evidence I know of on the long-time effects of switching brands derives
from a major study conducted by the American Cancer Society (Hammond and
Garfinkel, 1964) and a considerably smaller scale version of the same study sponsored
by the Public Health Service (Waingrow and Horn, 1968). In both studies subjects
were interviewed about their smoking habits twice over a two-year period. Since

---

* One alternative interpretation of these data must be considered. It is conceivable that naturally
irascible people are most likely to restrain their smoking. If so, these results could be attributable
to self-selection rather than withdrawal. Acutely aware of this possibility, Perlick (1977) compared
these groups on numbers of personality and demographic variables and found no differences between
the two groups.

† With one exception - there are a small number of long-time, light smokers who give no evidence
of nicotine regulation Schachter (1977) and no indication of withdrawal when deprived of nicotine
Perlick (1977). What to make of such cases is, at this time, equivocal but by any of the standard
criteria of addiction they appear to be genuinely non-addicted smokers.

over this period many subjects switched brands of cigarettes, it is possible to evaluate the effects of changing brands on the number of cigarettes smoked. On the basis of such analysis, these investigators conclude that switching to a cigarette with lower nicotine content does not increase the amount smoked and on this basis Hammond *et al,* (1976) justify the campaign for low nicotine cigarettes.

It shall be my contention that the particular mode of analysis employed in these studies unfortunately obscures the relationship of shift in nicotine level to amount smoked and in fact what trends exist in these data suggest, for many smokers a conclusion that is opposite to that drawn by these authors. Though both studies are similar, I shall restrict my discussion to the Hammond and Garfinkel (1964) paper for in the Waingrow and Horn (1968) study the number of subjects who switch to lower nicotine brands is so small (N = 161) and the data are presented in such a way that it is impossible from the published material to make the kind of analysis required. Hammond and Garfinkel (1964) divide their group of 98,632 male smokers into four categories – those who in 1959-60 smoked less than ten cigarettes a day; 10-19 cigarettes a day; 20-39 cigarettes a day; and forty or more cigarettes a day. An interviewee is categorised as changing the amount smoked only if in 1961-62 his answer to the question 'how many cigarettes do you usually smoke a day?' moves him from one category to another. Thus if a 1959 pack-a-day smoker were in 1961 to report that he smoked 35 cigarettes a day, he would not be classified as increasing in smoking; only if in 1961 he reported smoking forty or more cigarettes a day would be be so classified.

To understand the problems created by this particular mode of categorisation it is necessary to examine a frequency distribution of smoking behaviour. Since Hammond & Garfinkel present only grouped data, I have plotted in Figure 17.5 the distribution of answers to a question about daily cigarette smoking included in some of my own surveys. It is immediately evident first, that most smokers answer such a question in round numbers, that is, they say they smoke twenty, thirty or forty cigarettes a day and second, that in each of the Hammond-Garfinkel categories by far the heaviest concentration of smokers fall at the lower end of the category. Thus in the 20-39 cigarettes a day category, 66% of the subjects report that they smoke twenty cigarettes and 77% report that they smoke fewer than thirty cigarettes a day. Given this distribution it can be simply calculated that if *every* subject in the 20-39 cigarette category were to increase smoking by 25%, the Hammond-Garfinkel criteria would permit us to classify only 3.5% of these subjects as increasing. Similarly, if *every* subject in this category were to increase his smoking by 50% only 24% of all of the subjects would be classified as increasers. Though not as extreme the same unfortunate circumstance obtains in each of these categories except the 40+ cigarettes category where, by definition, no one can increase smoking for 40+ is the maximum category. It can scarcely be considered surprising that these investigators find relatively few people who increase smoking with time and find that changing brands has no effect on the amount smoked.

Even more perversely a breakdown of the Hammon-Garfinkel data indicates in Table 17.5 a significant tendency for a shift to a lower nicotine cigarette to result in an increase in amount smoked in those categories (1-9) and (10-19) where, as indicated in Figure 17.5, because a larger proportion of subjects are at the upper end of the category, the distributions are such as to make it more likely that changes will

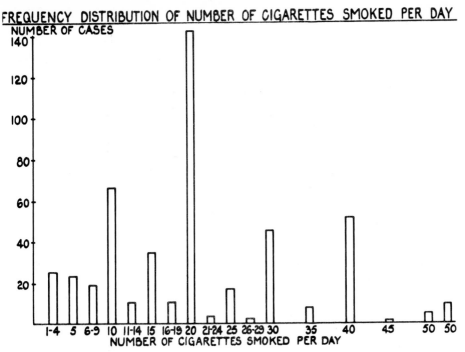

Fig. 17.5

be detected.   Though these differences are small, they are highly significant and do
at least suggest that an analysis based on a less stringent criterion of change might
very well reveal that switching to low nicotine cigarettes has a marked effect on
amounts smoked. Though the results of my own work obviously bias me to this
expectation, it is clear that this point is hardly yet proven within the context of a
large scale, long time field study. It is also clear, however, that the major body of
data that has been used to justify the campaign for low nicotine cigarettes does nothing
of the sort.

Table 17.5 Changes in number of cigarettes smoked per day in relation to decrease in
in nicotine content per cigarette (Adapted from Hammond and Garfinkel, 1964, Table 8)

	1961-62 cigarette smoking of men who smoked:					
	1 - 9 cigarettes a day in 1959-60		10-19 cigarettes a day in 1959-60		20-39 cigarettes a day in 1959-60	
Changes in nicotine content of cigarettes smoked in 1961-62 vs. 1959-60	Total N	% who increase to 10+	Total	% who increase to 20+	Total	% who increase to 40+
No change	5136	39.9	14047	42.4	51456	9.3
Decreased nicotine	532	47.4	1333	47.3	4648	9.1
x^2		11.17		12.12		0.2
p		.001		.001		n.s.

Acknowledgements

I am indebted to Dr. Jeremiah Barondess and Dr. David Rush for their critical reading of this paper.   The permission of the editor of Annals of Internal Medicine to reproduce this article is gratefully acknowledged.

References

Ashton, H. & Watson (1970) Puffing frequency and nicotine intake in cigarette smokers. *British Medical Journal,* **3**, 679-681.

Beckett, A.H., Rowland, M. & Triggs, E.G. (1965) Significance of smoking in investigations of urinary excretion rates of amines in man. *Nature, London,* **207**, 200-201.

Beckett, A.H. & Triggs, E.G. (1967) Enzyme induction in man caused by smoking. *Nature, London,* **216**, 587.

Domino, E.F. (1973) Neuropsychopharmacology of nicotine and tobacco smoking. In *Smoking Behaviour: Motives and Incentives,* ed. Dunn, W.L. pp.5–31, Washington: V.H. Winston & Sons.

Ferster, C.B. (1970) Comments on paper by Hunt and Matarazzo. In *Learning Mechanisms in Smoking,* ed. Hunt, W.A. Chicago: Aldine.

Finnegan, J.K., Larson, P.S. & Haag, H.B. (1945) The role of nicotine in the cigarette habit. *Science, N.Y.,* **102**, 94-96.

Frith, C.D. (1971) The effect of varying the nicotine content of cigarettes on human smoking behaviour. *Psychopharmacologia,* **19**, 188-192.

Goldfarb, T.L., Jarvik, M.F. & Glick, S.D. (1970) Cigarette nicotine content as a determinant of human smoking behaviour. *Psychopharmacologia,* **17**, 89-93.

Goodman, L.S. & Gilman, A. (1958) *The Pharmacological Basis of Therapeutics,* New York: MacMillan.

Hammond, E.C. & Garfinkel, L. (1964) Changes in cigarette smoking. *Journal of the National Cancer Institute,* **27**, 419-442.

Hammond, E.C., Garfinkel, L., Seidman, H. & Lew, E.A. (1976) Some recent findings concerning cigarette smoking.   Paper presented at a meeting on "The Origins of Human Cancer." at Cold Springs Harbor Laboratory on September, 14, 1976.

Heimstra, N. (1973) The effects of smoking on mood change. In *Smoking Behaviour: Motives and Incentives.* ed. Dunn, W.L., pp. 197-207. Washington: V.H. Winston & Sons.

Heimstra, N. W., Bancroft, N.P. & DeKock, A.R. (1967) Effects of smoking upon sustained performance in a simulated driving task. *Annals of the New York Academy of Sciences,* **142**, 295-307.

Herman, C.P. (1974) External and internal cues as determinants of the smoking behavior of light and heavy smokers. *Journal of Personality and Social Psychology,* **30**, 664-672.

Hunt, W.A. (1970) (ed) *Learning Mechanisms in Smoking.* Chicago: Aldine.

Isaac, P.F. & Rand, M.J. (1972) Cigarette smoking and plasma levels of nicotine. *Nature, London,* **236**, 308.

Jarvik, M.E., Glick, S.D. & Nakamura, R.K. (1970) Inhibition of cigarette smoking by orally administered nicotine. *Clinical Pharmacology and Therapeutics,* **11**, 574-576.

Kozlowski, L.T., Jarvik, M.E. & Gritz, E.R. (1975) Nicotine regulation and cigarette smoking. *Clinical Pharmacology and Therapeutics,* 17, 93-97.

Larson, P.S., Haag, H.B. & Silvette, H. (1961) *Tobacco. Experimental and Clinical Studies.* Baltimore: Williams & Wilkins.

Lucchesi, B.R., Schuster, C.R. & Emley, G.S. (1967) The role of nicotine as a determinant of cigarette smoking in man with observations of certain cardiovascular effects associated with the tobacco alkaloid. *Clinical Pharmacology and Therapeutics,* 8, 789-796.

Marcovitz, E. (1969) On the nature of addiction to cigarettes. *Journal of the American Psychoanalytic Association,* 17, 1074-1096.

McKennell, A.C. (1973) *A Comparison of Two Smoking Typologies.* Research Paper 12. London: Tobacco Research Council.

Nesbitt, P.D. (1973) Smoking, physiological arousal, and emotional response. *Journal of Personality and Social Psychology,* 25, 137-145.

Perlick, D. (1977) The withdrawal syndrome: Nicotine addiction and the effects of stopping smoking in heavy and light smokers. (Unpublished doctoral dissertation). Columbia University.

Ross, W.S. (1976a) Poison gases in your cigarettes, Part I: Carbon Monoxide. *Reader's Digest,* November, 1976.

Ross, W.S. (1976b) Poison gases in your cigarettes, Part II, Hydrogen Cyanide and Nitrogen Oxides. *Reader's Digest,* December, 1976.

Russell, M.A.H. (1974a) Realistic goals for smoking and health. *Lancet,* I, 254-258.

Russell, M.A.H. (1974b) The smoking habit and its classification. *Practitioner,* 212, 791-800.

Russell, M.A.H., Wilson, C., Patel, U.A., Cole, P.V. & Feyerabend, C. (1973) Comparison of effect on tobacco consumption and carbon monoxide absorption of changing to high and low nicotine cigarettes. *British Medical Journal,* 4, 512-516.

Schachter, S. (1973) Nesbitt's paradox. In *Smoking Behaviour: Motives and Incentives.* ed. Dunn, W.L. pp. 147-155. Washington: V.H. Winston & Sons.

Schachter, S. (1977) Nicotine regulation in heavy and light smokers. *Journal of Experimental Psychology: General,* 106, 5-12.

Schachter, S., Kozlowski, L.T. & Silverstein, B. (1977a) Effects of urinary pH on cigarette smoking. *Journal of Experimental Psychology: General,* 106, 13-19.

Schachter, S., Silverstein, B., Kozlowski, L., Herman, C.P. & Liebling, B. (1977b) Effects of stress on cigarette smoking and on urinary pH. *Journal of Experimental Psychology: General,* 106, 24-30.

Schachter, S., Silverstein, B. & Perlick, D. (1977c) Psychological and pharmacological explanations of smoking under stress. *Journal of Experimental Psychology: General,* 106, 31-40.

Silverstein, B. (1976) An addiction explanation of cigarette-induced relaxation. (Unpublished doctoral dissertation). Columbia University.

Silverstein, B., Kozlowski, L.T. & Schachter, S. (1977) Social life, cigarette smoking, and urinary pH. *Journal of Experimental Psychology: General,* 106, 20-23.

Smith, G.M. (1970) Personality and smoking: A review of the empirical literature. In *Learning Mechanisms in Smoking,* ed. Hunt, W.A. Chicago: Aldine.

Surgeon General's Report (1972) *The Health Consequences of Smoking,* U.S. Department of Health, Education and Welfare.

Tomkins, S. (1968) A modified model of smoking behaviour. In *Smoking, Health and Behavior.* ed. Borgatta, E.F. & Evans, P.R. Chicago: Aldine.

Waingrow, S. & Horn, D. (1968) Relationship of number of cigarettes smoked to "tar" rating. *National Cancer Institute Monograph,* **28**, 29-33.

18. The role of nicotine in the tobacco smoking habit

A K ARMITAGE

Tobacco smoking, particularly when the smoke is inhaled, has been recognised for many years as an efficient way for the self-administration of nicotine (Armitage, Hall and Morrison, 1968).

The importance of nicotine to the tobacco smoker. The evidence that one of the reasons why many people smoke cigarettes is to dose themselves with nicotine is substantial (Russell, 1976) but the crucial experiment to show that cigarettes are unacceptable if they are nicotine-free but otherwise identical in every way, has not been performed. One of the earliest experiments that provided evidence, albeit somewhat anecdotal, that nicotine is of importance to the cigarette smoker dates back to 1942 when Johnston showed that injected nicotine was an acceptable alternative to a cigarette for an unspecified number of the 35 subjects. Johnston gave himself three or four injections of nicotine a day with some smoking; after this course he preferred an injection of 1.3 mg of nicotine to inhaling cigarette smoke and feelings of deprivation were experienced when the injections were discontinued. In another early study Finnegan, Larson and Haag, (1945) examined the acceptability to 24 habitual cigarette smokers (all stated to be inhalers) of cigarettes made from tobacco naturally low in nicotine and of cigarettes made from tobacco to which sufficient nicotine had been added to give a final content of about 2%. Throughout the experiment each subject kept a daily record of the number of cigarettes smoked. For the first month, subjects smoked their accustomed brand in order that a record of their normal smoking habits might be obtained. The number of cigarettes smoked in the experimental period did not differ significantly from the number smoked in the control period. Six of the 24 subjects experienced no change in physical and mental tranquillity during their period on low nicotine cigarettes; six experienced an initial vague lack of the satisfaction that they normally derived from smoking; three definitely missed the nicotine but became adapted to the change in one to two weeks; nine definitely missed the nicotine and continued to do so throughout the experimental period. The authors concluded from these results that with some individuals nicotine was a major factor in their cigarette habit, but equally so, with some individuals, it was not. The obvious weakness of this experiment was the inherently different taste and aroma of the low nicotine tobacco, although some attempt was made to allow for this factor in the experimental design. Another pioneer experiment to which reference must be made, was that of Lucchesi, Schuster and Emley (1967) who studied the effect of intravenously administered nicotine on smoking behaviour in smokers who were unaware of the nature of the administered drug and the true purpose of the study. Smoking behaviour was not significantly altered when nicotine was administered at a dose of 1 mg per hour for six hours. A significant decrease in smoking frequency was obtained, however, when nicotine was administered at the rate of 2 to 4 mg/hour and in addition, the butt lengths of the cigarette smoked were longer than in the control experiments. This was a well designed experiment of Lucchesi *et al* but the dose of nicotine was inappropriate as the data to be presented will show.

The amount of nicotine available to a cigarette smoker. The human smoker is able to control the dose of nicotine he takes into his mouth very subtly by adjusting either the size of the puffs (puff volume) or the rate at which he puffs on a cigarette. This is clearly illustrated in Table 18.1 which shows data, quoted by Wakeham (1972) relating to how smokers puff cigarettes.

Table 18.1 How smokers puff cigarettes.

Puff	Lowest	Standard		Highest
Volume (V ML)	17.0	35.0	Nicotine	73.0
Duration (D Sec)	0.9	2.0	Yield	3.2
Interval (I Sec)	22.0	60.0	100%	72.0

With variable puff volume (D & I Standard), nicotine yields in range 55% to 150%*
With variable interval (V & D Standard), nicotine yields in range 75% to 133%*
With extreme parameters (V_{Low}, I_{High}) or (V_{High}, I_{Low}) nicotine yields perhaps range from 30% to 200%?

*Based on data of Bush *et al* (1972) and hitherto unpublished data (Hazelton Laboratories, Europe).

Puff volumes ranged from 17 to 73 ml and puff interval from 22 to 72 sec. The nicotine yields were determined by machine smoking. With standard parameters, most cigarette smokers will take into their mouths anything from 0.5 to 3 mg of nicotine while they smoke a cigarette. The table shows how nicotine yields can change considerably by manipulation of one or more parameters, particularly if the whole cigarette is smoked in an extreme way. The larger the puff volume, the quicker will the cigarette be smoked, with more nicotine appearing in the smoke each puff.

The nicotine in acidic cigarette smoke or alkaline cigar smoke, taken by the smoker into his mouth, can be inhaled into the lungs (very deeply, moderately deeply, slightly or not at all); it can be absorbed through the mucous membranes of the mouth and nose; it can be swallowed and absorbed from the gastrointestinal tract or it can be exhaled. These are the only possibilities, the first two of which will be discussed in some detail. It is therefore hardly surprising that the correlation between incidence of tobacco smoking related diseases and number of cigarettes or cigars smoked is poor in some epidemiological studies; it is not the number of cigarettes smoked that is important but the manner in which they are smoked.

Animal experiments

The amount of nicotine absorbed from tobacco smoke taken into the mouth and lungs must be central to any discussion of the role of nicotine in the tobacco smoking habit. In order to measure this quantitatively, Armitage *et al* (1974) designed a smoking machine that would smoke cigarettes to standard parameters and which was capable of introducing a portion of a puff into the lung of an anaesthetised cat in a way which was believed to imitate the smoking behaviour of an inhaling cigarette smoker. The machine took a 25 ml puff of smoke into a chamber, 20 or 22.5 ml of the smoke was allowed to escape and the 5 ml or 2.5 ml sample was held in the chamber for the cat to draw into its lungs when it next inspired.

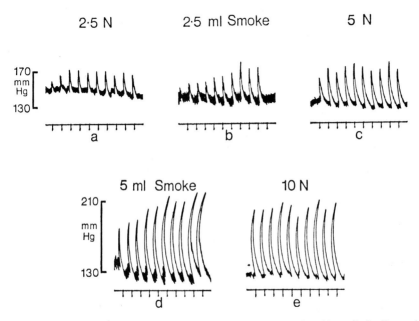

Fig. 18.1 Cat, 3.1 kg, chloralose anaesthesia, given atropine (1 mg/kg). Records of femoral blood pressure. b and d, effects of tobacco smoke (2.5 and 5 ml). a, c and e, effects of nicotine (N) administered intravenously, the dose being indicated in μg/kg. Time marker: 60 sec.

Fig. 18.1 shows the effects on blood pressure of successive puffs of smoke (2.5 ml in b, 5 ml in d), taken at one minute intervals. There was a rise in blood pressure within seconds of the smoke reaching the lungs, and these effects of smoke could be matched by injecting a small amount of nicotine into a vein. The response is clearly dose related and the effects are reproducible for many hours. The 2.5 ml samples of smoke were shown to contain 4 g of nicotine and the 5 ml samples about 11 g of nicotine. Absorption of nicotine through the lungs and into the pulmonary veins is therefore a highly efficient and exceedingly rapid process. Other experiments showed that the effect of an intravenous dose of nicotine could be matched by roughly half that dose injected into the left atrium. The results of these experiments on cats indicated that each time a cigarette smoker inhales a puff of tobacco smoke, the dose of nicotine he is likely to receive can be mimicked reasonably accurately by a suitable intravenous injection of nicotine of the order of 1 - 2 μg/kg.

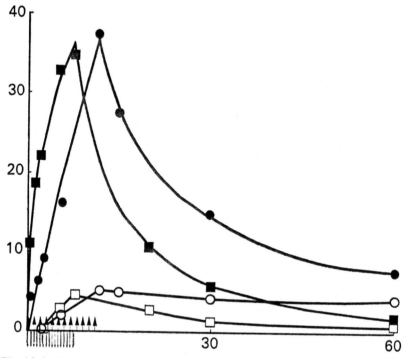

Fig. 18.2 Carotid blood levels in ng/ml of nicotine (● and ■) and cotinine (○ and □) following the administration of tobacco smoke containing $1 - (2' - {}^{14}C)$ nicotine to the lungs of anaesthetised cats. In one experiment twelve 5 ml puffs of smoke were administered every 60 sec and in the other sixteen 2.5 ml puffs were administered every 30 sec, as shown by the arrows. Abscissa: time in minutes.

Fig. 18.2 illustrates an experiment using the same machine in which the amount of nicotine that appeared in the cat's blood following the administration of tobacco smoke containing $1 - (2' - {}^{14}C)$ nicotine was measured. In one experiment 2.5 ml of smoke was administered at thirty second intervals and in another, 5 ml puffs of smoke at one minute intervals. In both experiments the peak concentration of nicotine in the blood stream was between 30 and 40 ng/ml. As a result of smoking a single cigarette in this way, nicotine appears rapidly in the arterial blood and when the cigarette is finished the nicotine disappears rapidly. The concentration of cotinine, one of the better known metabolites of nicotine, is shown at the bottom of Figure 18.2. It should be emphasised that the smoking in the animal experiments illustrated in Figs. 18.1 and 18.2 corresponds with the deepest possible inhalation in man.

In another series of similar experiments, tobacco smoke was introduced into the mouth of anaesthetised cats. The smoke was excluded from the lungs and the stomach so that nicotine could be absorbed only from the mouth. Changes in blood pressure and movements of the cat's ears, caused by tobacco smoke or by solutions of nicotine introduced into the mouth, were recorded. Twitching of the ears is an action which is highly specific for nicotine and compounds with nicotine-like actions and is an indication that nicotine has reached the brain. It was necessary to administer between twenty and thirty whole puffs of tobacco smoke in order to elicit a measurable pharmacological response. A typical experiment is shown in Fig. 18.3. Cigar smoke caused a slow rise in blood pressure (b) whereas a similar quantity of cigarette smoke had very little, if any, effect on (a). Cigar smoke, but not cigarette smoke, usually caused the cat's ears to twitch towards the end of the smoke administration period and the twitching persisted for approximately ten minutes. These observations indicated that there was a gradual accumulation of nicotine in the brain followed by a gradual decline but it should be noted how relatively inefficient was the absorption of nicotine through the mouth. Thirty 25 ml puffs of cigar smoke in the mouth had a smaller and quite different effect to 5 ml of smoke taken into the lungs. Considering that the contact time in the mouth was 10 sec compared with probably no more than 2 sec in the lungs, the efficiency with which nicotine is absorbed via these two routes differs by a factor of hundreds rather than tens. It is to be expected that slight inhalation (allowing absorption from the upper airways) will be a more effective way of obtaining nicotine than non-inhalation and moderate inhalation will be still more effective.

Fig. 18.3 also shows an experiment in which solutions of nicotine in 0.1 M phosphate buffer in a concentration range of 0.2 to 1.2 mg/ml were put in the mouth for ten minutes. The concentration of nicotine at pH 7 required to produce a given rise of blood pressure was about six times the concentration required at pH 8. The concentration of nicotine as free base, however, was similar at pH 7 and pH 8. In cigar smoke (pH8) the nicotine is predominantly present as the uncharged free base which diffuses through the membranes lining the mouth more readily than the positively charged nicotinium ion which predominates in cigarette smoke (pH 5).

When these data were published (Armitage and Turner, 1970) the paper concluded with a statement that 'the present evidence indicates that cigarette smokers who do not inhale may not obtain a stimulant dose of nicotine from relatively acidic cigarette smoke. It may, however, be possible for a cigar smoker to obtain such a dose without inhaling'. The findings of this paper have been misquoted on many occasions. Some nicotine can undoubtedly be absorbed from cigar smoke without inhaling, provided a large enough dose is given, but no one has yet shown conclusively that realistic smoking doses exert any effects on the brain in either human or animal experiments. So much for these fairly old but nevertheless relevant animal experiments.

Human experiments

Effects of smoking on heart rate. Studies of the effect of cigarette and cigar smoke on the heart rate of human subjects suggested that these observations in cats did have some relevance to the human smoking situation. The upper trace in Fig. 18.4 shows the effect on heart rate of a relaxed female subject, sitting in a chair, reading a book, when she smoked her first cigarette of the day.

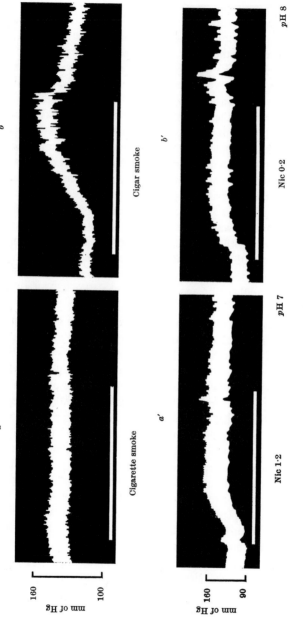

Fig. 18.3 Records of femoral blood pressure. Thirty puffs of cigar smoke introduced into the mouth of an anaesthetised cat during 14.5 min caused a slow rise in blood pressure (b) whereas a similar quantity of cigarette smoke had very little effect (a). In another experiment, a' and b' show the effects of buffered solutions of nicotine containing 1.2 mg/ml nicotine base at pH 7 and 0.2 mg/ml at pH 8, when put into the mouth and left there for ten minutes.

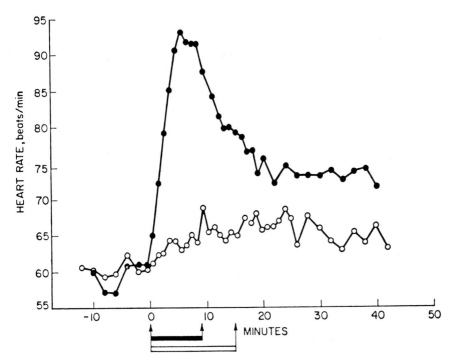

Fig. 18.4 Effects on the heart rate of two human subjects smoking a cigarette
(●—●) or a cigar (O—O) during the period shown by the arrows on the abscissa.

Ten puffs were taken at exactly one minute intervals. There was a very rapid
increase in heart rate, which reached a peak after the sixth puff. Of ten subjects
studied, there was a rapid effect similar to this in six of them, presumed to be
inhalers, there was a doubtful effect in three, presumed to be non-inhalers and
there was an intermediate effect in one subject. The lower trace showed the effect
on heart rate of a male subject smoking his first cigar of the day during which 16
puffs were taken at one minute intervals. The increase in heart rate was less than
ten beats per minute and the peak effect occurred about twenty minutes after
starting to smoke. This type of response was observed in several subjects who
smoked only cigars and had never smoked cigarettes.

The amount of nicotine absorbed during the smoking of a cigarette or cigar.
Experiments with cigarette and cigar smokers, in which subjects smoked a single
cigarette or cigar spiked with $1 - (2' - {}^{14}C)$ nicotine bis-(di-P-toluoyl-D-tartrate) have
recently provided the human counterpart of the cat experiments (Armitage *et al*,
1975; Armitage *et al*, 1978). The cigarette or cigar was mounted in a smoking
cartridge, which consisted of a vertically mounted glass cylinder with a port in
one side. The burning tip projected into the cylinder and the butt protruded
out of the port. A stream of air was drawn through the cartridge at a constant
rate to support combustion of the cigarette and to collect for analysis particulate
and vapour phase sidestream smoke (that is the smoke emanating from the lit

cigarette between puffs). Exhaled smoke was collected into an anaesthetic face mask applied over the subject's nose and mouth for the two exhalations immediately after puffing on the cigarette. The exhaled smoke was collected into a polythene bag which was emptied continuously by a pump, the smoke being drawn on to a filter disc and vapour phase absorption system identical with that used for the collection of the sidestream smoke. Radioactivity in sidestream smoke, exhaled smoke and the unsmoked butt was measured and knowing the amount of radioactivity with which the cigarette was spiked, the dose of nicotine taken into the smoker's mouth could be calculated.

The heart rate of the subject was continuously recorded and a T cannula was inserted in the brachial artery so that blood samples could be taken as required. This cannula was connected to a transducer so that a continuous record of arterial blood pressure was also obtained.

Cigarettes. The subjects did not smoke after midnight in the evening before the experiment. After preparing the subjects for the experiment, heart rate and blood pressure were monitored until these parameters were steady. The radiolabelled cigarette was then smoked, at the rate of one puff per minute until the cigarette was smoked down to a standard butt length. Apart from this constraint each subject was asked to smoke in his usual manner.

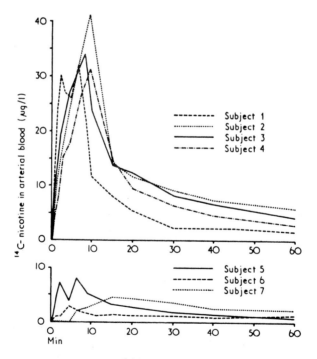

Fig. 18.5 Arterial blood levels of ^{14}C-nicotine in habitual smokers, presumed to inhale (subjects 1 - 4), in an inhabitual smoker presumed to inhale less deeply (subject 5) and in non-smokers (subjects 6 & 7) after smoking one cigarette labelled with ^{14}C-nicotine.

Fig. 18.5 shows the arterial blood concentration profiles of nicotine in the seven subjects for which measurements were made. Subjects 1 to 4 absorbed most of the nicotine they took into their mouths and the maximum arterial concentration attained ranged from 31.3 to 41.0 ng/ml. The remaining three subjects (numbers 5 to 7) achieved much lower concentrations ranging from 2.5 to 8 ng/ml and these smokers were presumed to be no more than modest inhalers.

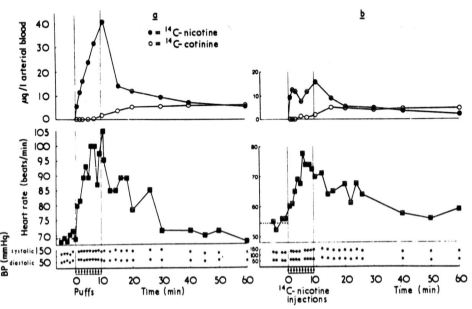

Fig. 18.6 Subject 2 of Fig. 18.5. Arterial blood levels of ^{14}C-nicotine (●) and ^{14}C-cotinine (O) heart rate (■), and blood pressure (*) during and after smoking a cigarette labelled with ^{14}C-nicotine (a) and during and after intravenous administration of 1 mg ^{14}C-nicotine given in ten divided doses, each of 0.1 mg (b).

Fig. 18.6 shows the result of two experiments on subject 2, who smoked a cigarette (a) and received intravenous injections of nicotine (b) on different occasions. In the first experiment, his resting heart rate was around seventy beats per minute. While smoking a cigarette, which lasted ten minutes, heart rate increased to 105 beats per minute which coincided with the peak arterial nicotine concentration of 40 ng/ml. Heart rate returned to resting level after about thirty minutes. The effect of smoking on blood pressure was negligible. After sixty minutes the nicotine blood level was about 5 ng/ml and still falling,   By this time the concentration of cotinine in the blood was greater than the concentration of nicotine. The dose of nicotine taken by the subject was calculated to be 1.9 mg.   On the right hand side of this figure are shown the effects of ten intravenous injections of nicotine, each of 100 μg given at one minute intervals. The dose of nicotine was thus about half that received during the smoking of the cigarette. The effect on heart rate was less (25 beats per minute increase) and the peak arterial nicotine concentration was only 16 ng/ml. If larger intravenous doses of nicotine had been given to this subject it is likely that the effects of smoking would have been very closely matched.

The results of these human experiments were remarkably similar to the earlier results obtained with cats. They amply confirm that each time a cigarette smoker inhales a puff of tobacco smoke the dose of nicotine he receives can be mimicked reasonably accurately by a suitable intravenous injection of nicotine. That dose is perhaps closer to 2 - 3 μg/kg rather than the 1 - 2 μg/kg originally predicted. It depends very much on the inhaling pattern of the subject.

Cigars. The results of the cigar experiments performed on five subjects are shown in Fig. 18.7

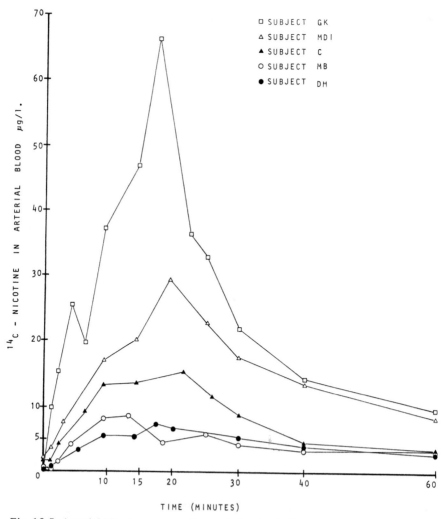

Fig. 18.7 Arterial blood concentrations of nicotine in five subjects during and following the smoking of a single small cigar labelled with ^{14}C-nicotine. (From Armitage, Alan, Dollery, Colin, Houseman, Terry, Kohner, Eva, Lewis, Peter J., and Turner, David: Absorption of nicotine from small cigars, Clin. Pharmacol. Ther. 23: 143 - 151, 1978).

The cigars used for these experiments were 83 mm long and experiments were conducted in an identical way to the cigarette experiments, that is to say puffs were taken every minute and the cigar was smoked down to a butt length of 20 mm. It took about twice as long to smoke a cigar as to smoke a cigarette and in subjects 1 and 2 the calculated dose of nicotine retained was very much greater (4.5 mg and 3.3 mg) than for any of the cigarette smoking subjects. The five subjects of these experiments were mixed smokers; they all smoked cigarettes and cigars and because of this it is likely that there were similarities in the way they smoked the two products. Subject 1 almost certainly inhaled fairly deeply in view of the fact that the blood nicotine profile was similar to that of the cigarette smokers who inhaled. The rate at which the concentration of nicotine in the blood rose in the other subjects was less, due either to modest inhalation, and/or perhaps some contribution due to the relatively slow absorption of nicotine from the alkaline smoke through the buccal membranes.

Table 18.2 Differences in the biological effects observed on smoking the first cigarette or cigar of the day.

Presumed smoking habit	Cigarette Smoker		Cigar Smoker	
	Inhaler	Slight inhalers & non-smokers	Inhaler	Slight inhalers
Estimated dose of nicotine (mg)	$2.11^+_-0.2$ (4)	$0.83^+_-0.2$ (4)	$3.12^+_-0.8$ (3)	$1.29^+_-0.2$ (4)
Peak plasma nicotine level (ng/ml)	$34.5^+_-2.2$ (4)	$5.1^+_-1.5$ (3)	$36.9^+_-15.3$ (3)	$5.4^+_-2.7$ (3)
Estimated plasma half-life (min)	$33.3^+_-3.7$ (4)	$32.5^+_-4.5$ (2)	$35.8^+_-7.2$ (3)	$48.9^+_-14.6$ (2)
Increase in heart rate (beats/min)	$17.0^+_-2.3$ (4)	$4.0^+_-3.0$ (3)	$9.0^+_-2.6$ (3)	$3.0^+_-1.5$ (3)
Increase in percentage COHb	$2.0^+_-0.6$ (4)	No data	$2.24^+_-0.6$ (3)	$0.3^+_-0.2$ (3)

The figures in parenthesis refer to the number of subjects.
Data are expressed as means $^+_-$ SEM.

Table 18.2 highlights the main differences between the observations of these cigarette and cigar smoking experiments. Firstly, carbon monoxide can be absorbed only from the alveoli so that the increase in COHb after smoking is another index of inhalation. Cigars of the type used in this study, however, yield approximately 9% (v/v) CO per puff in contrast to the 'medium tar' cigarette yield of 4% (v/v). The mean increase in COHb in the comparable cigar and cigarette groups was very similar suggesting that some inhalation of smoke had occurred with the cigar smokers but to a lesser extent than with the cigarette smokers. This would also explain why **the heart rate** changes observed during cigar smoking were less than after cigarette smoking. Secondly, the data on the elimination half life of nicotine suggests that the decline in blood nicotine levels is slower in the poor or non-inhaling group of cigar smokers than in the inhaling cigarette or cigar smokers. This may be due to a late absorption of nicotine occurring after smoking had stopped indicative of a slow buccal absorption from the cigar smoke. Such an occurrence would explain why the heart rate of the cigar smoking subject in Fig. 18.4 continued to rise after stopping smoking. These cigarette and cigar experiments by their very nature were somewhat artificial and the number of subjects was small. Nevertheless they are considered to provide valid data.

Arterial nicotine levels in human smokers. What are the consequences likely to be so far as blood nicotine levels are concerned, of inhaling tobacco smoke deeply, moderately, slightly or not at all? The nicotine blood profile illustrated in Fig. 18.2 was misleading because blood samples were taken halfway between puffs and the levels when plotted were joined together in a smooth curve. The sorts of profile that might theoretically be obtained if it was technically possible to take very frequent or ideally continuous blood samples are illustrated in Fig. 18.8. The rate at which nicotine appears in the bloodstream on deep inhalation of tobacco smoke or administration of intravenous shots must be near instantaneous and the curve is steep and very spikey (1). At the other extreme (non-inhalation - (3)) the rate at which nicotine appears in the bloodstream is very slow and steady; the curve is shallow with no spikes. In between these two extremes (that is slight to moderate inhalation) there are numerous possibilities. The rate of rise will be intermediate and peaks and troughs will be much less prominent as shown in the middle curve (2). To exert pronounced pharmacological effects, it is necessary for a threshold level of nicotine to be achieved quickly and intermittent intravenous injections of nicotine have been shown to be more efficient than a continuous infusion at the same "dose/ min". Rate of change of nicotine blood levels may be more important than absolute blood levels. Thus a type (3) smoker with a nicotine blood level of X ng/ml may not be experiencing the same pharmacological effects as a type (1) smoker with the same measured levels.

Nicotine thresholds and sensitivity. The number of experiments in which human subjects have been given nicotine intravenously is naturally few. It is impossible to predict how similar would be the response of the smoking population to a fixed intravenous dose of nicotine or indeed what variation there would be in the threshold dose necessary to produce a particular pharmacological response. The threshold dose of nicotine, however, required to release adrenaline from the adrenal glands of anaesthetised cats has been determined. The upper trace of Fig. 18.9 shows contractions of the denervated nictitating membrane which is supersensitive to adrenaline. The threshold dose of nicotine to contract the membrane in this experiment was >2.5 and <5.0 μg/kg. The mean value in a series of experiments was 8 $\pm$ 2 μg/kg, the lowest threshold being 2.5 and the highest 17.5 μg/kg, that is a sevenfold difference between lowest and highest. It is doubtful whether there is such a large difference in sensitivity among chronic cigarette smokers; it is also not known whether sensitivity can change over the years in an individual smoker.

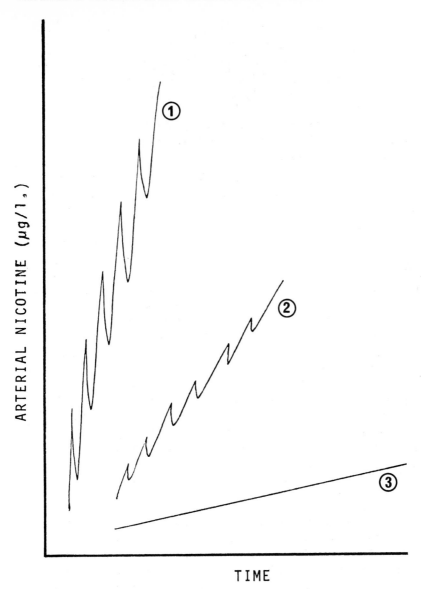

Fig. 18.8 Theoretical arterial nicotine profiles for different types of smoker. (1). Deep inhalation or intermittent intravenous injections. (2). Moderate inhalation. (3). Buccal absorption or slow intravenous infusion.

The nicotine content of cigarettes   So how much nicotine does a smoker require from a cigarette? In 1975 the sales weighted average of all brands in the UK was 1.37 mg nicotine/cigarette, (classified 'middle tar'), compared with 2.08 mg/cigarette in 1965, which would be currently classified as 'middle to high tar' (Lee, 1976). Currently 70% of the smoking population voluntarily choose to smoke cigarettes in the middle tar range. In Germany the corresponding figure has recently been quoted as 0.66 mg/cigarette, though it must be stressed that the figures are not

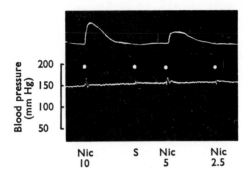

Fig. 18.9 Cat, 3.2 kg, chloralose anaesthesia, right superior cervical ganglion removed 18 days earlier. Top trace: contractions of denervated nictitating membrane. Bottom trace: femoral blood pressure. Nic = nicotine, S = saline; doses are expressed as μg/kg of base injected into the femoral vein.

strictly comparable because of differences in machine smoking. One cannot escape from the possibility that Germans are apparently currently satisfied with cigarettes containing substantially less nicotine than UK smokers. But are their blood nicotine levels during and after cigarette smoking any different? And are the blood nicotine levels of UK smokers in 1975 any different from the levels in 1965? Clearly any one, or a combination of the factors already discussed could almost certainly account for this apparent anomaly. Nicotine and cigarette smoke have been shown to have such pronounced and variable CNS effects that it is difficult to believe that these are coincidental and unconnected with the reasons why people smoke. One does begin to wonder whether the population of cigarette smokers smoke for different pharmacological effects: deep inhalers smoke for one effect, moderate inhalers for another and perhaps buccal smokers and slight inhalers for another. The picture is far from clear!

Nicotine in relation to smoking and health problem Numerous studies over the last 25 years have shown that tobacco smoking is associated with an increased incidence of certain diseases compared with their incidence in non-smokers. The major reason why smoking and health problems exist is that cigarette smokers inhale smoke into their lungs and they adopt this habit to obtain a 'pharmacologically satisfying' dose of nicotine. Smokers who inhale deeply are probably dependent on nicotine. Such smokers find the habit very difficult to give up and will find that nicotine taken in other ways (e.g. chewing-gum) is most unlikely to be a satisfactory substitute. Nicotine dependence of itself, however, may be no more detrimental to health than caffeine dependence. There is no evidence to suggest that the central effects of nicotine are harmful; indeed in the brain nicotine appears to modulate normal physiological mechanisms and to initiate responses which can occur without intervention of a drug. There is some circumstantial evidence to suggest that some of the peripheral pharmacological effects of tobacco smoking, and by inference therefore of nicotine, may be harmful but this is certainly not yet proven. During the absorption of nicotine by inhalation, however, the lung is exposed to hundreds of other components of tobacco smoke, many of which are not absorbed, but are deposited in the airways. Provided the normal mechanisms for clearing substances from the lungs and respiratory tract are functioning efficiently, there would probably be no great harm. Unfortunately, these mechanisms are adversely affected by the chronic administration of any tobacco smoke, but not by nicotine, and it is regrettable that research in this general area seems to have been rather overlooked in the quest for 'the safer cigarette'.

Acknowledgements

The permission of the editors of the following journals to reproduce Figs 18.1 and 18.2 (Quarterly Journal of Experimental Physiology), Fig. 18.3 (Nature), Figs. 18.5 and 18.6 (British Medical Journal) and Fig. 18.7 (Clinical Pharmacology and Therapeutics) is gratefully acknowledged.

References

Armitage, A.K., Hall, G.H., & Morrison, C.F.(1968) Pharmacological basis for the tobacco smoking habit. *Nature, London,* **217**, 331-334.

Armitage, A.K. & Turner, D.M. (1970) Absorption of nicotine in cigarette and cigar smoke through the oral mucosa. *Nature, London,* **226**, 1231-1232.

Armitage, A.K., Houseman, T.H., Turner, D.M. & Wilson, D.A. (1974) The evaluation of a machine for introducing tobacco smoke into the lungs of anaesthetised animals during spontaneous respiration. *Quarterly Journal of Experimental Physiology,* **59**, 43-54.

Armitage, A.K., Dollery, C.T., George, C.F., Houseman, T.H., Lewis, P.J. & Turner, D.M. (1975) Absorption and metabolism of nicotine from cigarettes. *British Medical Journal,* **4**, 313-316.

Armitage, A.K., Dollery, C.T., Houseman, T.H., Kohner, E.M., Lewis, P.J. & Turner, D.M. (1978) The absorption and metabolism of nicotine from cigars. *Clinical Pharmacology and Therapeutics.* (accepted for publication).

Bush, L.P., Grunwald, C. & Davis, D.L. (1972) Influence of puff frequency and puff volume on the alkaloid content of smoke. *Journal of Agricultural and Food Chemistry,* **20**, 676-678.

Finnegan, K.J., Larson, P.S. & Haag, H.B. (1945) The role of nicotine in the cigarette habit. *Science, N.Y.,* **102**, 94-96.

Johnston, L.M. (1942) Tobacco smoking and nicotine. *Lancet,* **2**, 742.

Lee, P.N. (1976) *Statistics of Smoking in the United Kingdom.* Tobacco Research Council Research Paper, 1, 7th edition.

Lucchesi, B.R., Schuster, C.R. & Emley, G.S. (1967) The role of nicotine as a determinant of cigarette smoking frequency in man with observations of certain cardiovascular effects associated with the tobacco alkaloid. *Clinical Pharmacology and Therapeutics,* **8**, 789-796.

Russell, M.A.H. (1976) Tobacco smoking and nicotine dependence. In *Research Advances in Alcohol and Drug Problems,* Vol. III, ed. Gibbins, R.J. *et al*; pp. 1-47. New York: Wiley & Sons.

Wakeham, H. (1972) Recent trends in tobacco and tobacco smoke research. In *The Chemistry of Tobacco and Tobacco Smoke,* ed. Schmeltz, I., pp. 1-20. New York-London: Plenum Press.

19. Is tobacco smoking a form of nicotine dependence?

R KUMAR, E C COOKE, M H LADER AND M A H RUSSELL

Introduction

The pharmacological basis of the tobacco-smoking habit remains surprisingly obscure, although it is generally assumed that nicotine plays some part in this bizarre and widespread compulsion to burn dried leaves. An average-strength cigarette delivers slightly over 1 mg of nicotine in its mainstream smoke, most of which can be rapidly absorbed into the blood-stream following inhalation (Armitage *et al*, 1975). Such 'smoking doses' of the alkaloid produce many effects in the brain and peripherally (Agué, 1974; Brown, 1973; Coffman, 1969; Friedman, Horvath and Meares, 1974; Russell, 1976), but the psychological actions of nicotine are variable and there is only circumstantial evidence that tobacco-smoking is a form of nicotine dependence.

Smokers can partially regulate their intakes of nicotine when offered cigarettes of varying strengths (Ashton and Watson, 1970; Finnegan, Larson and Haag, 1945; Frith, 1971; Turner, Sillett and Ball, 1974), but other constituents of tobacco smoke such as tar, covary in amount with nicotine (Russell *et al*, 1973), and factors such as the taste and 'quality' of the smoke can markedly influence the amounts of smoking (Goldfarb, Jarvik and Glick, 1970). Recent tests (Goldfarb *et al*, 1976) in which tar and nicotine yields of cigarettes were independently varied do, however, implicate nicotine as a reinforcer of smoking. This view is also supported by the observation (Stolerman *et al*, 1973) that smoking increases when subjects are given mecamylamine, which is, among other things, a central antagonist of nicotine. Other evidence for the nicotine hypothesis comes from studies of the effects of nicotine-containing chewing-gum upon smoking (Brantmark, Ohlin and Westling, 1973; Kozlowski, Jarvik and Gritz, 1975), but the most direct tests have been done with injected doses of the drug.

In 1942 Johnston commented that when habitual smokers were given hypodermic injections of nicotine they 'almost invariably thought the sensation pleasant, and, given an adequate dose, were disinclined to smoke for some time thereafter'. The same author also injected himself repeatedly with nicotine and came to prefer the injections to inhaling cigarette smoke; he later experienced feelings of deprivation when the injections were discontinued. These are all hallmarks of a dependence disorder and it can be argued that habitual smokers are physiologically dependent upon nicotine and that they repeatedly self-administer this drug in order to ward off the onset of withdrawal symptoms. There is some evidence for a nicotine-abstinence syndrome comprising psychological responses such as craving, tension, irritability, restlessness, impaired attention and performance, as well as a number of minor cardiovascular and neurophysiological changes (Finnegan *et al*, 1945; Hall *et al*, 1973; Knapp, Bliss and Wells, 1963; Ulett and Itil, 1970).

There seems to have been only one study of the effects of intravenous doses of nicotine upon smoking behaviour. This is one of the most direct ways of examining the possible reinforcing actions of the drug and the experiments were done by Lucchesi, Schuster and Emley (1967) who demonstrated small, but significant, reductions in the numbers of cigarettes smoked following continuous slow intravenous infusions of nicotine bitartrate. In order to try and confirm these findings and extend the assessment of the role of nicotine in smoking, we devised a laboratory test which permitted the continuous and automated recording of puffing and also of several physiological measures. The units of measurement were thus obtained from individual puffs rather than from counts of cigarettes that were smoked. Because nicotine has a relatively short half-life (Beckett, Gorrod and Jenner, 1971; Isaac and Rand, 1972), it was possible to examine the effects upon smoking of different doses of this drug during a single session. An important feature of the design of the study was that it covertly reduced the possibly over-riding influences of the habits and rituals of cigarette smoking. Somewhat unexpectedly, our results do not support the hypothesis that smokers are dependent upon and hence need regular doses of nicotine.

Methods

Subjects

The subjects were 12 paid volunteers, seven male and five female, aged between 24 and 38 years; their weights ranged between 44 and 83 kg. They were all screened as fit on the basis of a medical history and physical check, including an electrocardiogram. All the subjects were moderate/heavy cigarette-smokers; they reported smoking between 25 and 60 cigarettes daily for at least two years previously. Counts of smoking during three days before one of the tests confirmed these estimates.

Procedure

Each subject was required to attend the laboratory three times. The first occasion was for familiarisation with the apparatus and procedure and with the 'aims' of the study. The actual purpose of the experiments that were to be done was concealed and the subjects were told that 'habituation' of several important physiological measures differed in smokers and non-smokers. It was explained that these measures had never been recorded while subjects smoked 'normally', nor had the effects of intravenous nicotine on habituation been studied in this way. They were told that, in order to obtain adequate recordings from the various electrodes, they would not be able to move about freely, nor to light nor handle cigarettes. In order to circumvent this problem a shielded holder, containing a permanently lit and regularly replaced cigarette, would be placed very near their mouths while they sat in a comfortable chair for the duration of each experiment (approximately three-and-a-half hours) in a small semi-isolated test room. They could thus take a puff whenever they wanted. All subjects were asked to bring their own reading matter. A glass of orange drink would be available throughout. Excessive hand movements would be discouraged as well as conversation.

It was explained that during the first experiment they would be asked at intervals to take a number of deep puffs, so that their 'habituation' responses to these could be compared with the results of the second test a few weeks later when, instead of puffs, they would receive pulsed injections of comparable doses of nicotine through an intravenous infusion which would be running into an arm vein throughout the session. The final requirement was that they should take a total of nine grammes of enteric-coated tablets of ammonium chloride at set intervals during the 24 hours preceeding each of the two tests. The importance was stressed of acidifying the urine to reduce variations in the urinary excretion of nicotine, a weak base (Beckett *et al,* 1971). There were no restrictions upon the subjects' smoking or diet prior to the tests.

Drugs

The plan of the two experiments is outlined in Figure 19.1. In the first experiment the doses of nicotine were given by inhalation of tobacco smoke and in the second experiment, about a month later, roughly comparable doses of nicotine were given to the same subjects by intravenous injection. Two doses of the drug and a control were tested in each experiment; the order in which they were given to individual subjects was counterbalanced according to a Latin square design (Cochran and Cox, 1957).

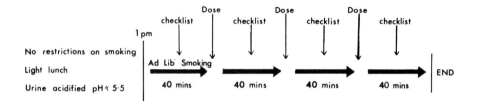

Measurements

Smoking:	Frequency of puffing
	Intervals between puffs
	Amplitude of puffs

Physiological:	Skin conductance
	Skin temperature
	Heart rate (ECG)
	EEG : 4 wave bands

| Psychological: | Checklists of mood and bodily symptoms |

Figure 19.1 Summary of the procedure adopted for both experiments

Experiment 1   The independent variable was inhaled smoked containing three 'doses' of nicotine. Each dose consisted of 12 deep puffs that were inhaled and held for 3-5 seconds; the puffs were spaced at one-minute intervals. Dose 'O' consisted of 12 puffs at a nicotine-free, herbal cigarette, and dose '2' was 12 puffs at the equivalent of a strong cigarette (six puffs from each of two small cigarettes with a machine smoked delivery of 1.3 mg of nicotine - the total intake was thus about 2.6 mg). The intermediate dose '1' was obtained by alternating puffs at the herbal and the strong cigarette. In all cases, immediately after the last puff of each dose had been taken, a medium-strength cigarette was placed in the holder and the subject was told he could resume puffing whenever he wanted.

Experiment 2   The procedure for *ad libitum* puffing remained the same, but here the doses were administered by intravenous injections through a saline infusion which ran continuously into an arm vein. Each dose was made up in distilled water to a volume of 50 ml, and was given in ten five-second pulses (5 ml) at one-minute intervals. The injections into the infusion were made via a two-way tap situated behind the subject and each "bolus' was flushed in by the infusion, thus overcoming possible errors due to the dead space. Dose '0' consisted of distilled water alone, dose '1' contained 0.035 mg /kg of nicotine bitartrate in distilled water, and dose '2' contained 0.07 mg./kg. of nicotine bitartrate. Thus, dose '2' for a 70 kg. man comprised an absolute amount of nearly 5 mg of the bitartrate, which is equivalent to about 1.7 mg of the alkaloid. The subjects were allowed to puff whenever they wanted during the ten-minute periods of intravenous dosing.

Measures of smoking behaviour
The dependent variable in both experiments was the amount and rate of *ad libitum* puffing at medium-strength, filter-tipped cigarettes (nicotine yield 1.3 mg - normally extracted by about ten puffs) during the three forty-minute sessions which followed each dose. These cigarettes were regularly replaced and thus a lit cigarette was continuously available to the subjects. Smoking behaviour was monitored by a pressure transducer connected to the cigarette holder which gave a continuous record of the number of puffs taken and of the inter-puff intervals. In addition, the duration and depth of each puff gave an estimate of the volume of smoke sucked through the holder. Calibration tests with known volumes (range 10-50 ml) confirmed the validity of the volumetric estimates. The amounts of smoke actually inhaled could not be measured.

Physiological measures
The following measures were recorded continuously.
   Heart rate: wrist and ankle electrodes were used.
   Skin temperature: a thermistor was strapped to the middle finger of the dominant hand.
   Skin conductance: the recording and earth electrodes were attached to the thumb and forearm of the non-dominant hand and measures of basal conductance and its variance (an estimate of the fluctuations) were obtained.
   EEG: two scalp leads (vertex and left parieto-temporal) were used and the output was analysed via broad wave-band filters. The mean rectified, integrated voltage of the EEG in the δ, θ , α and β wave-bands was recorded continuously (i.e. 2.3-4.0 Hz; 4.0-7.5 Hz; 7.5-13.5 Hz; 13.5-26.0 Hz respectively).
   The physiological measures were averaged over one-second periods and then further processed by computer (PDP12) and stored on tape together with the smoking scores. Polygraph recordings of the ECG, skin conductance and puffs were also taken.

Psychological measures
Linear analogue scales (Bond and Lader, 1974) covering a range of items corresponding

to mood and to somatic symptoms of anxiety were administered twenty minutes after the start of the experiment and twenty minutes after the end of each dose of the drug; these were completed by the subjects within two to five minutes.

Analysis of results

The scores for puffing and for the physiological measures were first averaged over ten-minute blocks and this gave four consecutive scores for each measure after every dose. Multivariate analyses showed that the scores for the first ten minutes after the inhaled doses (Experiment 1) were significantly different from the scores over subsequent ten-minute blocks and it appeared that the main effects due to doses had occurred during the first ten-minute block. Further analyses of variance were then done on the data for the first ten minutes after the doses in both experiments and also for selected measures that were taken during the times that the doses were being given (12 minutes in Experiment 1 and ten minutes in Experiment 2).

Results and discussion

Figure 19.2 illustrates segments of the polygraph records for two of the subjects; it shows how, once they had settled down, these subjects tended to puff in a regular way. Subjects differed considerably between themselves in their rates of puffing, but individual rates tended to remain broadly stable during the test session. Furthermore, there was a relatively good correlation between the overall rates of puffing by individual subjects across the two experiments which were about a month apart ($r = 0.66$ df 10 $p < 0.02$).

These puff-by-puff recordings are reminiscent of behavioural research into drug dependence in animals where drugs may be self-administered according to simple schedules of reinforcement. In this study the schedule can be described as fixed ratio - 1, i.e. one response (sucking at holder) producing one reinforcement (dose of smoke). It was not possible to measure the amounts of smoke actually inhaled and we elected in this experiment not to disturb the smoking behaviour of our subjects by taking repeated blood samples for nicotine and carbon monoxide estimations. Puffing and inhalation seem closely related, but our conclusions must remain tentative until the method is further developed to incorporate estimates of smoke inhaled. This technique does, however, improve on studies in which either numbers of cigarettes smoked or numbers of puffs are counted. Estimates of the volume puffed add greatly to the sensitivity of the measures and the validity of these scores was checked by correlating them with estimates of nicotine remaining in the filter-tips. The filters from Experiment 2 were pooled in batches of four corresponding to each forty-minute period; two batches were lost and there were therefore 46 possible comparisons ($r = 0.88$ df 44 $p < 0.001$). The filter nicotine measures give a good indication of the smoke that has passed through the filter-tip and this result confirms the validity of the puff volume scores.

Effects of inhaled and intravenous doses of nicotine upon smoking

Figure 19.3 shows the average rates of puffing by the subjects after each of three doses of inhaled or intravenous nicotine. After the inhaled doses (Experiment 1) there were no overall differences during the full forty-minute periods ($F < 1$), but comparisons of puffing scores over the successive ten-minute blocks showed that

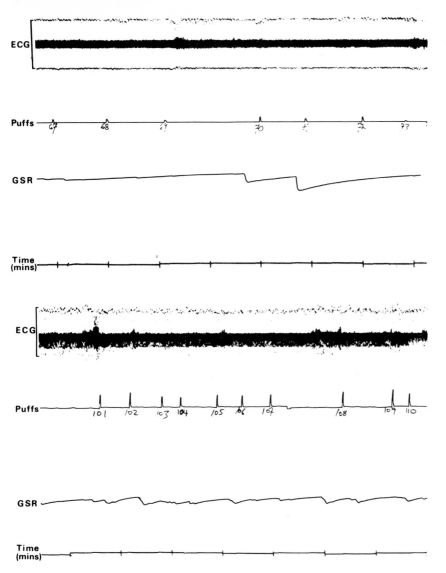

Figure 19.2. Sections of polygraph records of two subjects, The measures in each case are of the heart-rate, puffing, skin conductance and a time-marker indicating one-minute intervals. Individual puffs have been numbered on the tracings.

the rates at which puffing changed were a linear function of the doses which had previously been inhaled (F = 13.01 df 1,20 p<0.002). For example, there was a marked initial reduction after the large inhaled dose which was then followed by a gradual recovery. Roughly comparable doses of nicotine were given intravenously in Experiment 2 and it can be seen in Figure 19.3 that puffing rates remain unaffected over the forty minutes (F<1). The subjects did, however, tend to puff more frequently irrespective of the dose which had been injected.

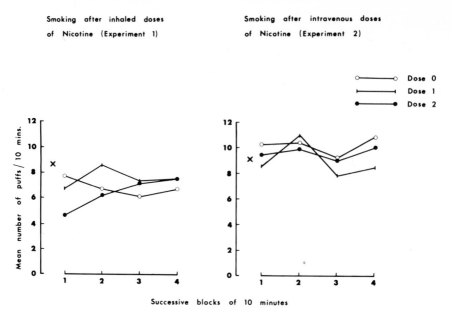

Figure 19.3. Inhaled tobacco smoke depresses the subsequent rate of puffing in a dose-related way (Experiment 1) and the biggest effect is seen during the first ten minutes. Comparable intravenous doses of nicotine (Experiment 2) do not alter subsequent rates of puffing. The crosses indicate the average number of puffs taken by the subjects during the last ten minutes of the initial settling-down period, i.e. just before any doses were given.

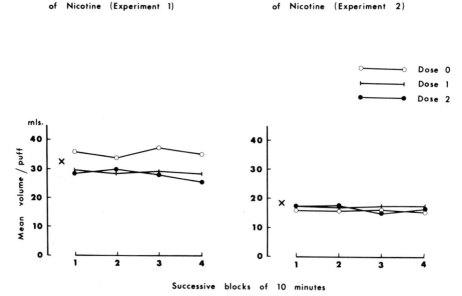

Figure 19.4. The average size of each puff is reduced by both inhaled doses of tobacco smoke to a similar extent and this effect persists throughout the forty minutes after the doses. Intravenous doses of nicotine do not change the size of puffs, but in Experiment 2 the subjects take much smaller puffs throughout, even before any doses are given (as illustrated by the two crosses).

The average volumes per puff are shown in Figure 19.4.   After both the inhaled doses of tobacco smoke the subjects took smaller puffs and this effect persisted throughout the forty minutes (F = 4.54 df 2,20 p<0.05). The sizes of the puffs that were taken after the intravenous doses did not differ significantly from each other (F < 1), but there was a striking general reduction in the volumes per puff even before any doses were injected.

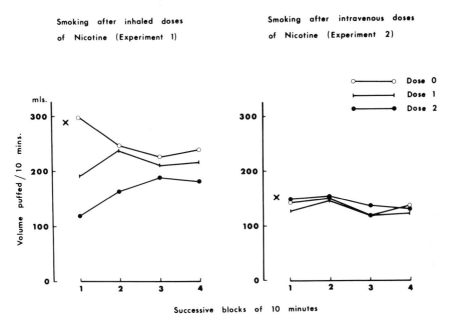

Figure 19.5. Inahled doses of tobacco smoke reduce the amount of smoke that is subsequently puffed in a dose-related way (Experiment 1) and this effect is greatest during the first ten minutes after the doses. Comparable intravenous doses of nicotine have no effect upon the volumes that are puffed in Experiment 2. Although the subjects are puffing more often (see Fig. 19.3), the fact that they take smaller puffs (see Fig. 19.4) results in a general fall in the volumes puffed in Experiment 2; this difference between the two experiments, which is evident before any doses are given, is also shown by the crosses indicating the volumes puffed during the last ten minutes of the settling-down period.

The average volumes of smoke puffed in successive ten-minute blocks are plotted in Figure 19.5; these scores are, in effect, the product of the two previous measures (numbers of puffs and volumes per puff). The inhaled doses reduced the volumes subsequently puffed in an orderly manner (F = 8.78 df 1,20 p<0.01) and the clearest effect was seen in the first ten minutes after the doses. As might be expected (see Figures 19.3 and 19.4) the intravenous doses did not modify the amounts of smoke subsequently puffed (F <1).

The total volumes puffed were smaller in Experiment 2 in spite of the increased rates of puffing; perhaps this was a response to the more stressful conditions produced by the intravenous infusions, but a number of observations fail to support this interpretation. In Experiment 2 the subjects' check-list scores showed that they were not feeling more tense or anxious or experiencing somatic symptoms of anxiety to any greater degree than in the test with the inhaled doses. The physiological measures (see below) were consistent with the self-reports. Finally, if the altered patterns of smoking in the intravenous test had been caused by increased anxiety, the scores might have shown signs of habituation as the experiment progressed over successive sessions of forty minutes; this was not the case (F = $<$1, F = 1.90 and F = 1.43 df 2,20, for numbers of puffs, volume per puff and volume puffed respectively). Thus, while there is no satisfactory explanation for the differences in patterns of puffing between the two experiments, an effect of intravenous nicotine should, in principle, have been possible either through a reduction in the numbers of puffs taken or by a further depression of the volumes puffed.

Puffing during the first ten minutes after doses
Since the main effects seemed to be confined to the first ten minutes of each period the analyses of variance were restricted to this initial block and tested for dose-response relationships in the form of linear trends. The two experiments were analysed separately, but the results obtained from *within* each experiment are, however, presented and discussed side by side.   Figure 19.6 summarises the scores for four measures of puffing which are plotted against increasing doses.

    In Experiment 1 there was clear evidence that doses of inhaled tobacco smoke reduced subsequent puffing in a dose-related manner: there were significant linear dose trends for the volumes puffed (F = 15.24 df 1,20 p $<$0.001), the numbers of puffs (F = 6.22 df 1,20 p$<$0.025) and the volume per puff (F = 7.20 df 1,20 p$<$0.02). In Experiment 2, the doses of intravenous nicotine failed to affect the volumes puffed (F$<$1), the numbers of puffs (F$<$1) and the volume per puff (F = 1.3), df 1,20 in each case.

    In order to check for possible short-lived effects of intravenous nicotine the latencies to the first puff after the end of each dose period were compared by the Friedman two-way analysis of variance; this non-parametric test (Siegel, 1956) was used because of the non-normal nature of the scores.   Inhaled doses of smoke significantly altered the latencies (x r^2 = 13.50 df 2 p 0.01) while intravenous doses were without effect ($x$$r^2$= 1.17 df 2). However, since this was the only measure which suggested that intravenous doses might be affecting smoking (see Figure 19.4), the scores were further checked by tests for linear trends following reciprocal transformations. While inhaled doses systematically reduced the speed to the first puff (F = 13.19 df 1,20 p$<$0.002) intravenous nicotine did not (F$<$1).

Puffing during the periods of dose administration
The average volumes of smoke that were puffed for doses 0, 1 and 2 were 473 ml., 491 ml. and 478 ml. respectively and, as these values did not differ significantly (F$<$1), it seems reasonable to assume that any subsequent effects on smoking were due to the content of the doses.

    In Experiment 2 the subjects were allowed to puff *ad libitum* during the ten-minute periods of infusion. This procedure was adopted because of the greater likelihood of detecting very short-lasting effects of intravenous nicotine upon smoking.   As it happened there were no differences due to the doses in any of the smoking measures, i.e. number of puffs (F$<$1), volume per puff (F $<$1) and in their

Smoking during the first ten minutes after each of three doses of nicotine

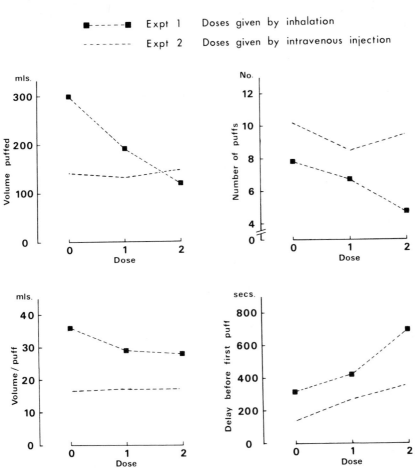

Figure 19.6. Dose-response effects of inhaled smoke and intravenous nicotine are compared. The three doses of smoke were roughly matched in terms of potency with the doses of intravenous nicotine and both are expressed on the arbitrary interval scale — 0, 1 and 2. Four smoking measures show that inhaled doses of tobacco smoke depress subsequent *ad libitum* smoking whereas comparable intravenous doses of nicotine are without effect. Three of the measures, volume puffed, the number of puffs, and the volume per puff, are presented as average scores over the first ten minutes after each dose. The fourth variable is the average delay before taking the first puff and after the end of each dose.

product, total volume puffed during the ten minutes ($F < 1$); the scores are shown in Figure 19.7. Had any such differences been detected, they would, of course, have had to be taken into account in comparisons of the periods *after* the doses.

Measures of smoking during the intravenous infusion of three doses of Nicotine (Expt. 2)

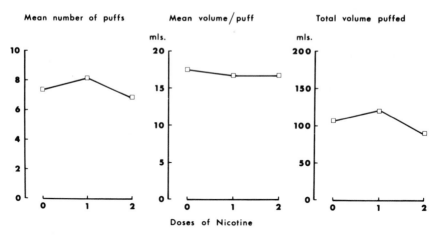

Figure 19.7. The subjects were allowed to puff *ad libitum* during the ten minute periods in Experiment 2 when the intravenous doses of nicotine were being infused. This diagram shows that there are no very short-lasting effects due to nicotine. The rates of puffing, the volumes per puff and the total volumes puffed during the ten minutes when each dose was infused are very similar.

Physiological measures.   Heart rate: In both experiments the heart rate was systematically altered by doses of the drug.   The average rates in the ten minutes after the inhaled doses were 75.9, 77.2 and 79.3 beats per minute for dose 0, dose 1 and dose 2 respectively (F = 10.22 df 1,20 p$<$0.005). Intravenous nicotine produced very similar effects; the corresponding average rates were 73.5, 76.0 and 78.2 beats per minute (F = 23.85 df 1,20 p$<$0.0001).   These results are consistent with previous tests of the effects of inhaled and intravenous nicotine (Agué, 1974; Coffman, 1969).

Skin conductance: No dose-related effects of nicotine upon this measure were found in either experiment.

Skin temperature: As a result of apparatus failure several measures were lost and the remaining data were not analysed.

EEG mean rectified, integrated voltage: Inhaled doses of nicotine were without a clear effect on any of the bands although there was a tendency for β activity to be systematically increased by the drug both during (F = 2.91 df 1,20 p$<$0.10) and in the ten minutes after the dose (F = 3.37 df 1,20 p$<$0.08). A similar and significant effect was seen during (F = 5.37 df 1,20 p$<$0.03) and after the intravenous doses of nicotine (F = 21.0 df 1,20 p$<$0.0002). The mean scores for β activity after the inhaled doses were 1.92, 1.94 and 2.07 μV and in the ten minutes after the intravenous dose the corresponding scores were 1.57, 1.70 and 1.80 μV. The mean β values during the last ten minutes of the settling-down periods, i.e. before any doses were given, were 1.87 μV and 1.56 μV in Experiments 1 and 2 respectively.

Psychological measures Analyses of the self-ratings made in both the mood check list and the anxiety symptom scale failed to show any consistent effects after doses of inhaled smoke or intravenous nicotine. This may well have been due to the fact that these ratings were not made until twenty minutes had elapsed after each dose. The ratings were not done sooner as they took two to five minutes to complete and this would have disrupted the principal measure, i.e. smoking. There was, however, a significant trend in the infusion study for subjects to rate themselves as more drowsy and more relaxed as the experiment progressed. Paradoxically, they also reported feeling more energetic and this somewhat complicates interpretation of the data.

Conclusions

The real aim of the experiment was successfully concealed and this meant that subjects puffed freely and as naturally as possible. Intervals between lighting-up the manner of lighting, handling, puffing and extinguishing cigarettes all tend to follow firmly ingrained patterns. By allowing only the terminal response of puffing it was hoped to obtain measures of *ad libitum* smoking which were as free as possible from such habits and were thus more sensitive to pharmacological manipulations. The physiological measures provided parallel assays of the potency of nicotine in the two experiments. Acidifying the urine reduces variations in excretion of nicotine and thus improving control over circulating levels of the drug. Another important element was the use of dose-response analyses without which it is extremely difficult to draw meaningful conclusions about the effect of drugs on biological systems.

Experiment 1 showed that inhaled 'doses' of smoke systematically postponed and reduced subsequent puffing and that this was a function of the content of the smoked doses. The second experiment took the analysis a stage further by directly examining the role of nicotine as the putative reinforcer. Contrary to expectation, the intravenous doses were without effect on smoking behaviour. The physiological tests showed that the doses of nicotine clearly modified the heart-rate and also the EEG (β activity) and very comparable effects were seen in the two experiments. Thus, the lack of effect of intravenous nicotine on smoking cannot be ascribed either to inadequate dosage or to a failure of the drug to enter the blood and the brain. Some of the subjects did complain of some aching and pain in their arms at the time the doses were injected into the infusion, but neither they, nor the experimenters, were able to guess which doses were active and which were not, at levels better than chance. Finally, the failure of intravenous nicotine to modify smoking cannot be ascribed to an insensitive method (cf. Experiment 1).

Our negative findings, therefore, re-open the question whether physiological dependence upon nicotine really is the basis for the tobacco smoking habit. Is it possible that there is some other rewarding constituent of tobacco smoke? Alternatively, if relief or avoidance of nicotine-abstinence is unimportant, could the drug be acting as a primary positive reinforcer rather in the way that amphetamine and other stimulant drugs are thought to sustain self-administration behaviour? (Pickens and Thompson, 1971). If this were so, one might expect that, *within limits,* increasing the nicotine content of cigarettes would result in increased reinforcement and more smoking; if anything, the opposite seems to be the case (Goldfarb *et al*, 1976). Although there is now an immense literature on intravenous self-administration behaviour in animals relating to drugs of dependence (Kumar and Stolerman, 1977), there seems to be only two brief reports (Deneau and Inoki, 1967; Lang *et al*, 1977) that nicotine can serve as a reinforcer in this way.

Much money and effort are being spent on attempts to reduce tobacco smoking and to make the habit less damaging to health. Some recent suggestions and developments include nicotine-containing chewing-gum, cigarettes made from tobacco substitutes, cigarettes with low nicotine and tar yields, or cigarettes with high nicotine and low tar yields. The rationale for such measures is lacking since the role of nicotine and the mechanisms of pharmacological reinforcement in tobacco smoking remain virtually unexplored.

Acknowledgements

We thank Dr. M.V. Driver for screening the electrocardiograms of our subjects, Mr. B. Aschkenasy for preparing the nicotine solutions for injection and Dr. Griffith Edwards for his advice and support.

This is an expanded version of a paper entitled 'Is nicotine important in tobacco smoking?' reproduced with permission from *Clinical Pharmacology and Therapeutics,* **21**, 520-529 (1977); copyright The C.V. Mosby Company, St. Louis, Missouri, U.S.A.

References

Agué, C. (1974) Cardiovascular variables, skin conductance and time estimation; changes after the administration of small doses of nicotine. *Psychopharmacologia,* **37**, 109-125.

Armitage, A.K., Dollery, C.T., George, C.F., Houseman, T.H., Lewis, P.J. & Turner, D.M. (1975) The absorption and metabolism of nicotine from cigarettes. *British Medical Journal,* **4**, 313-316.

Ashton, H. & Watson, D.W. (1970) Puffing frequency and nicotine intake in cigarette smokers. *British Medical Journal,* **3**, 679-681.

Beckett, A.H., Gorrod, J.W. & Jenner, P. (1971) The analysis of nicotine-1'-N-oxide in urine, in the presence of nicotine and cotinine, and its application to the study of *in vivo* nicotine metabolism in man. *Journal of Pharmacy and Pharmacology,* **23 Suppl.** , 55S-61S.

Bond, A. & Lader, M. (1974) The use of analogue scales in rating subjective feelings. *British Journal of Medical Psychology,* **47**, 211-218.

Brantmark, B., Ohlin, P. & Westling, H. (1973) Nicotine-containing chewing-gum as an anti-smoking aid. *Psychopharmacologia,* **31**, 191-200.

Brown, B.B. (1973) Additional characteristic EEG differences between smokers and non-smokers. In *Smoking Behavior: Motives and Incentives,* ed. Dunn, W.L. pp. 67-81. Washington: V.H. Winston & Sons.

Cochran, W.G. & Cox, G.M. (1957) *Experimental Designs,* 2nd Edition. New York: Wiley.

Coffman, J.D. (1969) Effect of propranolol on blood pressure and skin blood flow during cigarette smoking. *Journal of Clinical Pharmacology,* **9**, 39-44.

Deneau, G.A. & Inoki, R. (1967) Nicotine self-administration in monkeys. *Annals of the New York Academy of Sciences*, **142**, 277-279.

Finnegan, J.K., Larson, P.S. & Haag, H.B. (1945) The role of nicotine in the cigarette habit. *Science, N.Y.*, **102**, 94-96.

Friedman, J., Horvath, T. & Meares, R. (1974) Tobacco smoking and a 'stimulus barrier'. *Nature, London*, **248**, 455-456.

Frith, C.D. (1971) The effect of varying the nicotine content of cigarettes on human smoking behaviour. *Psychopharmacologia*, **19**, 188-192.

Goldfarb, T., Gritz, E.R., Jarvik, M.E. & Stolerman, I.P. (1976) Reactions to cigarettes as a function of nicotine and "tar". *Clinical Pharmacology and Therapeutics*, **19**, 767-772.

Goldfarb, T.L., Jarvik, M.E. & Glick, S.D. (1970) Cigarette nicotine content as a determinant of human smoking behavior. *Psychopharmacologia*, **17**, 89-93.

Hall, R.A., Rappaport, M., Hopkins, H.K. & Griffin, R. (1973) Tobacco smoking and evoked potential. *Science, N.Y.*, **180**, 212-214.

Isaac, P.F. & Rand, M.J. (1972) Cigarette smoking and plasma levels of nicotine. *Nature, London*, **236**, 308-310.

Johnston, L.M. (1942) Tobacco smoking and nicotine. *Lancet*, **2**, 742.

Knapp, P.H., Bliss, C.M. & Wells, H. (1963) Addictive aspects of heavy cigarette smoking. *American Journal of Psychiatry*, **119**, 966-972.

Kozlowski, L.T., Jarvik, M.E. & Gritz, E.R. (1975) Nicotine regulation and cigarette smoking. *Clinical Pharmacology and Therapeutics*, **17**, 93-97.

Kumar, R. & Stolerman, I.P. (1977) Experimental and clinical aspects of drug dependance. In *Handbook of Psychopharmacology*, Volume 7, ed. Iversen, L.L., Iversen, S.D. & Snyder, S.H. pp. 321-367. New York: Plenum Press.

Lang, W.J., Latiff, A.A., McQueen, A. & Singer, G. (1977) Self administration of nicotine with and without a food delivery schedule. *Pharmacology, Biochemistry and Behaviour*, **7**, 65-70.

Lucchesi, B.R., Schuster, C.R. & Emley, C.S. (1967) The role of nicotine as a determinant of cigarette smoking frequency in man with observations of certain cardiovascular effects associated with the tobacco alkaloid. *Clinical Pharmacology and Therapeutics*, **8**, 789-796.

Pickens, R. & Thompson, T. (1971) Characteristics of stimulant drug reinforcement. In *Stimulus Properties of Drugs*, ed. Thompson, T. & Pickens, R. pp. 177-192. New York: Appleton-Century-Crofts.

Russell, M.A.H. (1976) Smoking and nicotine dependence. In *Recent Advances in Alcohol and Drug Problems*, Volume III, ed. Gibbins, R.J. *et al*, New York: Wiley & Sons.

Russell, M.A.H., Wilson, C., Patel, U.A., Cole, P.V. & Feyerabend, C. (1973) Comparison of effect on tobacco consumption and carbon monoxide absorption of changing to high and low nicotine cigarettes. *British Medical Journal*, **4**, 512-516.

Siegel, S. (1956) *Non-parametric Statistics for the Behavioral Sciences*, New York: McGraw-Hill.

Stolerman, I.P., Goldfarb, T., Fink, R. & Jarvik, M.E. (1973) Influencing cigarette smoking with nicotine antagonists. *Psychopharmacologia*, **28**, 247-259.

Turner, J.A.McM., Sillett, R.W. & Ball, K.P. (1974) Some effects of changing to low-tar and low-nicotine cigarettes. *Lancet,* **2,** 737-739.

Ulett, J.A. & Itil, T.M. (1970) Quantitative electroencephalogram in smoking and smoking deprivation. *Science, N.Y.,* **164,** 969-970.

20. Smoking behaviour in Germany—the analysis of cigarette butts (KIPA)

W SCHULZ AND F SEEHOFER

Smoking behaviour in Germany 1968-1977

When we started our work concerned with smoking behaviour, in 1968, we had ventured into new territory. The only known factors were some results from observations and puff profile recordings of smokers (Keith and Hackney, 1962) which may have influenced machine smoking conditions.

At about the same time measurements and observations were made to determine differences in smoke deliveries between 'free smoking' or natural smoking, and 'restricted smoking' or machine smoking. Additionally ideas were put forward to estimate smoke intake by analysing the amount of smoke retained in the tobacco butt and on the filter tip.

There were also first thoughts and proposals for the reproduction of human smoking by means of a 'slave-smoker' or 'puff duplicator',

Our ideas stemmed from the observation that the range of human smoking behaviour is very wide and we would have to study many subjects. Experimental methods should be chosen or developed which would allow us to draw conclusions about the behaviour of the average smoker.

Of all methods available, we thought that the examination of cigarette butts discarded by smokers would be most successful. This was the only totally non-invasive way to estimate the amounts of smoke taken by human smokers, and such cigarette butts are available in large enough samples to answer many questions. The butt analysis 'KIPA' (from Kippen, a slang term for cigarette end) is limited to filter cigarettes, which formed approximately 85% of the cigarette consumption in Germany.

The basis of KIPA is the correlation of the amount of smoke retained in the filter with the actual amount of smoke taken in by the smoker. Under constant smoking conditions (puff volume and puff duration, which is equivalent to constant flow rate) the ratio between the amount of smoke retained in the filter and the actual intake of smoke is constant. One can therefore calculate the amount of smoke taken by the smoker from the amount of smoke retained by the filter. Unfortunately, this is not the case in natural smoking. Smoking conditions are not constant, and the ratio of the smoke retained by the filter and the amount of smoke taken by the smoker is not necessarily constant.

Additional information about smoking behaviour and knowledge about the dependance of filtration coefficients (for individual smoke components) on smoking conditions are therefore necessary. Only then can the actual intake of smoke be calculated.

A simple approach would be to examine the ratios of various smoke components in the filter (e.g. condensate, nicotine and phenols) with respect to puff volume, puff duration, puff frequency and butt length (for single cigarettes) and to check that these ratios remain constant for cigarettes smoked naturally. By use of the appropriate retention value the actual amount of the smoke component taken could be calculated. The values obtained by this method would be hypothetical and would need to be checked by machine smoking, using the calculated conditions. It is also possible to assume initially that some smoking parameters, e.g. puff duration, puff interval, puff number and butt length, are fixed values which may be obtained from sufficient observations. An average puff volume can be calculated from a sufficient number of flow profile recordings which would be exact enough to check the assumed values. The first tests in the years 1968-71 showed that such simplified test models are not sufficiently accurate to describe natural smoking. The lack of consistency in smoking conditions whilst the cigarette was smoked proved to be the biggest problem.

Butt length

In butt analysis it is assumed that there is a relationship between the amount of tobacco smoked and the amount of smoke retained in the filter tip. It is known from machine smoking that per puff smoke deliveries increase as the cigarette is smoked. It can be assumed that the last few puffs are very important for the smoker and that small differences in butt length can have considerable effects on smoke deliveries. How do these presumptions agree with reality?

Butt lengths of 22 mm for filter cigarettes and 19 mm for cigarettes without filters, were found in West Germany by von Bethmann (1959). Ten years later we noted a butt length of 30.6 mm for filter cigarettes and 25.6 mm for cigarettes without filters (Schulz and Seehofer, 1970), although average smoke deliveries, especially in filter cigarettes, were lowered dramatically in the meantime. Butt lengths increased until 1972 (Schulz, 1974) but have since decreased, probably for economic reasons such as an increase in tax and a recession (Schulz, 1974; Schulz and Seehofer, 1976).

Table 20.1 Butt lengths in West Germany

Time of collection	Filter Cigarettes		Cigarettes without filter	
	Number sampled	Butt Length (mm)	Number sampled	Butt Length (mm)
1959 (1)		22.1		19.3
1968 (2)	19543	30.6	935	25.6
1972 (3) (Aug.)	26965	33.8	4364	28.2
1972 (2) (Oct.)	36411	33.2	3623	28.0
1974 (4)	31203	32.8	7099	26.5

These tests show that the range for single butt lengths for different brands was considerable. However, it was possible to calculate very exact average values as large numbers of butts were collected. There are significant differences in butt length for different sections of the population, e.g. sex, place, occupation, geographic location, and economic conditions, brand etc. (Schulz and Seehofer, 1970; Schulz, 1972; Schulz and Seehofer, 1976). The question arises as to the importance of these differences with respect to the amounts of smoke drawn.

An analysis of the amount of smoke retained in filters with respect to butt lengths can give very variable results for some smokers, ranging from a disproportionate increase during the last few millimeters of the cigarette smoked, to a level which was too low to be detected during the last third of the cigarette smoked. For this reason it is necessary to proceed with different types of smokers typical of the different smoking classes. The average of all smokers or large groups of smokers shows a uniform picture - the increase of smoke retained in the filter is only very small during the last few puffs. The average smoker puffs only a little during the last part of the cigarette and the amount of smoke taken from these puffs is small (Figures 20.1 and 20.2).

Observed smoking parameters

Puff number, puff interval and total time alight can be measured relatively easily by observing smokers with timing devices (stopclocks, cassette recorders with constant run speed etc.). It is considerably more difficult to measure puff duration as the actual drawing of the puff does not have to be identical with the time the cigarette is held in the mouth or with a visible onset of glow. Puff volume cannot be determined by observation.

In two experiments carried out in 1971 and 1974 in Hamburg a large number of smokers (two groups of 100 and 218) were observed surreptitiously and puff number, puff duration and puff interval were measured. Puff duration was defined as the time for which the cigarette was held in the mouth. In most of these surreptitious tests it was impossible to determine the brand name or butt length. Observations were made in public houses, railway stations, on the road or at work, which means in nearly all situations possible. Table 20.2 shows the average values for puff number, puff duration, puff interval and total of the puff durations. Some of these values show a remarkably high consistency in smoking behaviour over a long time period, especially the value for total puff duration which, of all the values shown in Table 20.2, is most relevant to smoke deliveries.

Table 20.2 Smoking parameters of smokers observed in Hamburg 1971 and 1974

	Puff Number		Puff Duration (sec)		Puff Interval (sec)		Total Puff Duration (sec)	
	1971	1974	1971	1974	1971	1974	1971	1974
Men	10.2	10.9	1.47	1.47	52.9	42.1	15.0	16.0
Women	10.9	13.3	1.31	1.17	46.0	40.7	14.3	15.5
All	10.5	11.8	1.41	1.34	50.3	41.5	14.8	15.8

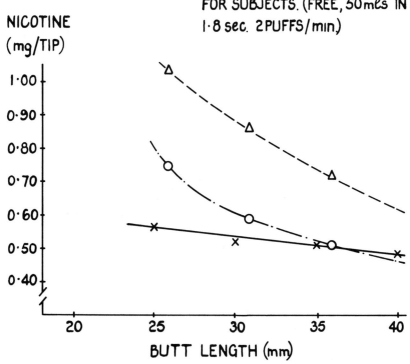

AMOUNT OF NICOTINE RETAINED IN THE FILTER WITH RESPECT TO BUTT LENGTH

× AVERAGE VALUES FOR ALL SUBJECTS (SERIES I)

O STANDARD MACHINE SMOKING CONDITIONS (FREE, 35mℓs. IN 2·0 sec. 1 PUFF/ min.)

Δ MACHINE SMOKED CIGARETTES. UNDER CONDITIONS DETERMINED FOR SUBJECTS. (FREE, 50mℓs IN 1·8 sec. 2 PUFFS/min.)

NICOTINE (mg/TIP)

BUTT LENGTH (mm)

Fig. 20.1

AMOUNT OF TPM RETAINED IN THE FILTER
WITH RESPECT TO BUTT LENGTH

X AVERAGE VALUES FOR ALL
   SUBJECTS (SERIES I)

O STANDARD MACHINE SMOKING
   CONDITIONS (FREE, 35mℓs IN 2·0sec
   I PUFF/min)

Δ MACHINE SMOKED CIGARETTES
   UNDER CONDITIONS DETERMINED
   FOR SUBJECTS. (FREE, 50mℓs IN
   1·8 SEC, 2 PUFFS/min)

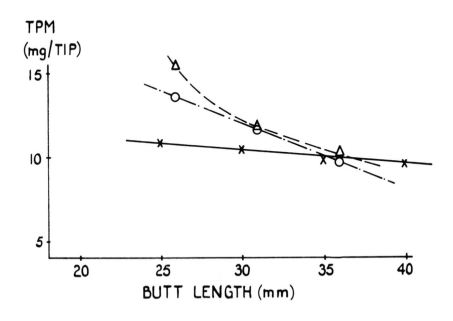

Fig. 20.2

There are some significant differences in observed smoking behaviour between men and women. Women leave a longer butt (on average approximately 2 mm longer) and have a shorter puff duration than men; they seem to compensate for this with a higher number of puffs and have therefore the same total puff duration (puff duration x puff number). There seems to be a trend for a shortening of puff duration with increasing age in men. In women however there is no such difference in smoking behaviour (Table 20.3).

Table 20.3 Smoking parameters with respect to age (1974)
(average number of all subjects 16-36)

Age	Puff Number		Puff Duration (sec)		Puff Interval (sec)	
	Men	Women	Men	Women	Men	Women
15-25	10.7	13.2	1.57	1.17	39.5	39.5
25-35	11.2	14.6	1.49	1.15	39.6	39.6
35-45	10.7	13.6	1.42	1.21	42.8	40.5
45-55	10.7	13.0	1.40	1.16	41.3	38.6
55-75	11.4	--	1.37	--	48.0	--

No differences were observed between cigarette brands or different types of cigarettes as far as smoking behaviour was concerned with the exception that puff durations were clearly longer when cigarettes manufactured from air-cured tobaccos were smoked (1.8 instead of 1.4 sec).

It was observed that smoking in situations that caused physical stress (e.g. when waiting) resulting in a shortening of puff interval (35 instead of 43 sec). In men the puff duration was shortened as well (puff duration 1.25 instead of 1.38 sec).

All the values discussed above are averages of how a whole cigarette was smoked. The distribution of the values for single puffs (puff duration and puff interval) shows a definite trend with respect to puff number (Figures 20.3 - 20.5).

Men and women show a trend for a shorter puff duration with increasing puff number (Figure 20.3). The frequency with which long duration puffs occur decreases from the first to the last puff, the frequency of occurrence of the shortest puff is equally low during the first five puffs but increases from then on until the last puff (Figure 20.4).

Puff interval increases with increasing puff number (Figure 20.5). In summary one can deduce from a decreasing puff duration and an increasing puff interval a decreasing smoking intensity dependent on puff number. These results agree with the small increase of smoke retained in the filter during the last few puffs.

Smoking parameters from puff profile recordings

When puff profiles are recorded with a differential pressure transducer (e.g. Lorenz and Seehofer, 1971) data are obtained about the intensity of puffs and the distribution of the intensity during puffs in addition to puff numbers, puff durations and puff

PUFF DURATION WITH RESPECT TO PUFF NUMBER

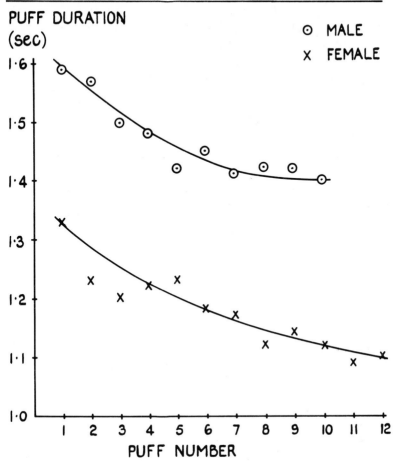

Fig. 20.3

intervals. Important data can be deduced from a knowledge of the puff profile. The puff volume may be obtained by integration of the profile area, the peak flow rate can be obtained from the height of the profiles and the time in which the volume was drawn can also be obtained.

Such profiles were recorded from a large number of smokers in 1970, 1971 and 1977. The values obtained from these experiments agree with some of the observations made but disagree with others (Table 20.4).

15 to 19 puffs were recorded as average values for larger groups (about fifty smokers) when puff profile recordings were made compared with 11 puffs in other recording situations or when observed surreptitiously. This shows that the survey procedure and the recording situation have an influence on smoking behaviour which can be quite considerable. The puff interval, which reduced from 42-50 sec to 30-35 sec. is compatible with the increased number of puffs. It is difficult to estimate values obtained for puff volume as comparative values could not be obtained from surreptitious observation. Three experiments in 1970-77 showed between

FREQUENCIES OF THE LONGEST(A) & SHORTEST (B) PUFFS MALE AND FEMALE

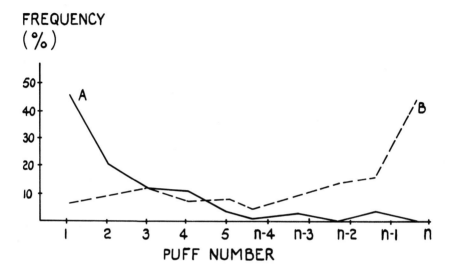

Fig. 20.4

Table 20.4 Smoking parameters from observations and profile recordings (Mean values for groups of 30-218 subjects)

Parameter	Observations		Profile Recordings		
	1971	1974	1970	1971	1977
Puff number	10.5	11.8	15-19	14	11
Puff duration (sec)	1.41	1.34	1.8	1.7	--
Puff interval (sec)	50.3	41.5	30	35	--
Puff volume (ml)	--	--	50	60	55

50 and 60 ml per puff (Table 20.4). Most smokers seem to reduce their puff volume after the first three to four.puffs.   This reduction could not be found in our profile recordings which suggests that the measurement and recording procedure influences not only puff number but also puff duration and puff volume.

PUFF INTERVAL WITH RESPECT TO THE NUMBER OF INTERVALS BETWEEN PUFFS

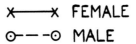

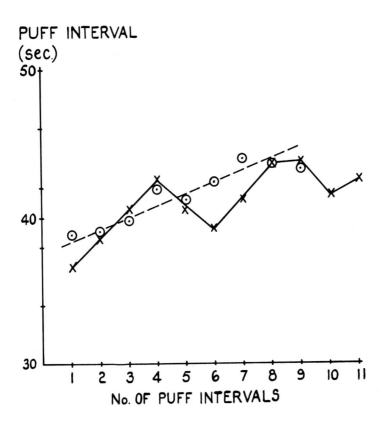

Fig. 20.5

Smoking parameters, as deduced from the amount of smoke retained in the butt

Assumptions about the smoking behaviour, especially the average puff volume, can be made from the amount of smoke retained in the butt. It is, however, necessary to know, from comparable tests, the dependence of the amount retained in the cigarette butt at various flow rates for several smoke components. For this reason we determined this relationship for nicotine, condensate and phenol retained in the butt of one test cigarette (German blend with usual cellulose acetate filter). It can be seen in Figures 20.6 - 20.8 that for this cigarette the amount of phenol and condensate retained, with respect to puff volume (constant puff duration and frequency) was similar, apart from a slightly different gradient. With decreasing butt length and increasing puff volume the amount of phenol and condensate retained increases disproportionately. This disproportionate increase was not seen in the amount of nicotine retained. It was examined under conditions similar to human smoking and the ratios of nicotine:condensate:phenol found were 0.5:12:0.13. The results showed that these values coincide with a puff volume of more than 65 ml and a butt length of at least 43 mm (Figures 20.6 - 20.8). The smokers in this test group must have taken a very large volume of, on average, approximately 65-75 ml during the first few puffs. During the last few puffs (at least from a butt length of 43 mm onwards) they could have hardly drawn any smoke at all. The true average volume for the whole cigarette smoked in these tests does not seem to have greatly exceeded the standard volume of 35 ml.

To confirm this hypothesis, special smoking engines (puff duplicator, slave smoker and others) are necessary which are able to smoke to such programs.

Amounts of smoke drawn from the cigarette

Retention coefficients were obtained for the filter tips using the smoking parameters already mentioned. The amount of actual smoke taken from one test cigarette (Figures 20.6 - 20.8) was then calculated (Tables 20.5 (a) and 20.5 (b)).

Table 20.5 (a) Average smoking parameters of test smokers (see Table 20.4, 1970).

Puff duration	(sec)	1.8
Puff interval	(sec)	30
Puff volume	(ml)	50
Butt length	(mm)	31

Table 20.5 (b) Actual amount of smoke taken by test smokers (from KIPA values) (120 subjects)

Smoke components	Amount of smoke retained in the butt (KIPA values) (mg)	Retention Coefficients from Table 20.5 (a) %	Actual amount o smoke intake (mg/cig)
Nicotine	0.51	40	0.77
Condensate (dry)	10.8	34	21.0
Total phenols	0.131	63	0.077

AMOUNT OF NICOTINE RETAINED IN THE BUTT
WITH RESPECT TO BUTT LENGTH AND PUFF VOLUME

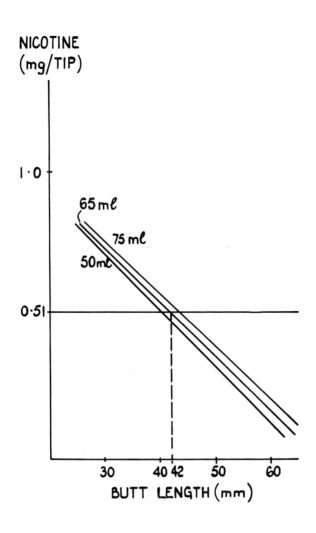

KIPA VALUES FOR ALL
TEST SMOKERS 1970

Fig. 20.6

AMOUNT OF CONDENSATE RETAINED IN THE BUTT
WITH RESPECT TO BUTT LENGTH AND PUFF VOLUME

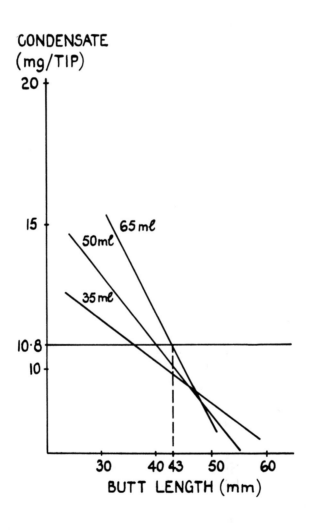

Fig. 20.7

AMOUNT OF PHENOL RETAINED IN THE BUTT WITH RESPECT TO BUTT LENGTH AND PUFF VOLUME

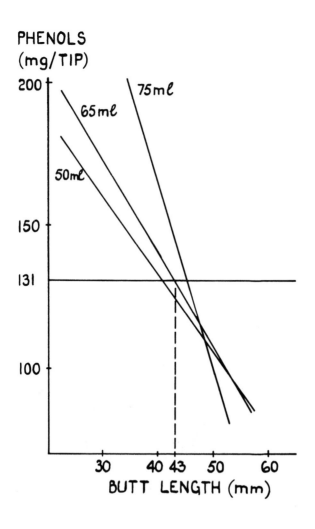

Fig. 20.8

The actual amount of nicotine taken was calculated in the same way for various cigarette brands. The amount of smoke retained in collected butts was measured to determine how values obtained from natural smoking relate to standard analysis values. For comparison the same brands were smoked according to standard smoking conditions DIN 10240 (CORESTA - standard method) i.e. free smoking with a butt length of 33 mm (compare with Table 20.1 1972-74). The nicotine values for these brands (A–I) for natural compared with standard smoking are shown in Table 20.6. In column 6 of Table 20.6 the percentage differences for nicotine intake, comparing natural smoking and standard smoking are shown.

Table 20.6 Nicotine values according to natural smoking (collection 1974; Table 20.1) and according to standard smoking for various brands.

Cigarette Brand	Amount of Nicotine retained in butts (KIPA) (mg/tip)		Amount of actual nicotine intake (mg/cig)		Difference (%) natural smoking - standard smoking
	Natural smoking	Standard smoking	Natural smoking	Standard smoking	
A	0.51	0.61	0.82	0.98	-16
B	0.52	0.53	0.60	0.61	-2
C	0.52	0.58	0.81	0.90	-10
D	0.56	0.48	0.66	0.56	18
E	0.58	0.64	0.74	0.81	-9
F	0.61	0.62	0.73	0.74	-1
G	0.61	0.87	0.76	1.09	-30
H	0.91	0.71	1.04	0.81	28
I	0.96	0.70	0.84	0.61	38

For brands with equivalent standard values, such as B and I with 0.61 mg nicotine/cigarette of E and H with 0.81 mg nicotine (Table 20.6, column 5) very variable results were obtained between natural and standard smoking (-2 and 38% or -9 and 28% respectively). This shows that smokers do not have a uniform smoking pattern for all types of cigarettes. Because of these smoking behaviour differences, it is necessary to proceed with various groups of smokers who prefer certain types of cigarettes. In Table 20.6 for example the following 3 types could be differentiated:

Type I, brand A, C, E, F, G	No* or negative deviation from standard values in medium amounts of smoke taken. (0.73-0.82 mg nicotine/cig)
Type II, brands B and D	No* or slightly positive deviation from standard values in low amounts of smoke taken. (0.60-0.66 mg nicotine/cig)

*Differences for brands B and F considered to show no deviations.

Type III, brands H and I   Strong positive deviation from standard
values in high amounts of smoke taken.
(0.84-1.04 mg/cig)

All the smoke values mentioned so far (Figures 20.6 - 20.8, Tables 20.5 (a) and 20.6) are average values from fairly large test groups or from representative numbers of butts collected.

But how much do these values mean? Are such values reproducible? What deviation is there between smokers, or within a smoker but on different days?

In Table 20.7 all KIPA mean values obtained since 1968 for the amount of nicotine retained in the filter of some brands were assembled to illustrate the reproducibility (for the corresponding values of the amount of nicotine in the smoke from these brands compare Table 20.6, column 4). The brands C and D showed in 4 out of 5 tests a coefficient of variance of only 4.0 to 6.7%.

Table 20.7 Average amounts of nicotine retained in butts of natural smoked cigarettes of different brands in KIPA tests from 1968-77.

| Brand | Nicotine /Filter (mg) | | | | | | | $\bar{x}$ | CV |
	1968*	1970**	1971**	1972*	1974*	1976**	1977**		(%)
A				0.51	0.59				
B	0.41			0.52	0.50				
C	0.49			0.52	0.54		0.52 0.52		4.0
D		0.51	0.48	0.56	0.51	0.56	0.52		6.7
E				0.58	0.58				
F	0.63			0.61	0.62				
G				0.63	0.63				
H	0.72			0.91	0.89				
I				0.96	0.84				

*   Butts from general collection in West Germany.
**   Butts obtained from test smokers (number of subjects 30-120).

The variation in average values is shown to be small for brands, but the average variation for days (average values of all cigarettes smoked in one day) in individual smokers, is twice as high, with a coefficient of variance of 10% and for various smokers of the same brand a coefficient of variance of 25% was obtained. These variations are not constant for all brands, for example in an extremely low delivery brand a coefficient of 66.5% was found (Table 20.8).

Reaction of the smoker to changed products

Apart from the tests carried out to determine the average smoking behaviour, the behaviour of individuals towards various products was examined. Questions were asked about the physiological effect of certain smoke components from brands with

Table 20.8 Variation of KIPA values in natural smoking. (Tests on one brand at a time).

	Coefficient of variance (%)		
	Nicotine	Condensate	Phenols
Average variation in days measured on single smokers	10	10	10
Measured in various smokers	25*	25	30

*In very low delivery brands values up to 66.5%.

variable deliveries (Schievelbein, 1978). It was also expected to get some objective results or at least indications that smokers who change to a low delivery product would react to it by increasing their consumption of cigarettes or smoking individual cigarettes more intensely.

For this purpose two experiments were carried out in 1976 and 1977 in which thirty subjects smoked cigarettes of a different brand for one to two weeks. The actual amount of smoke intake was calculated from the butt analyses. The range in nicotine intake is less than in nicotine deliveries measured under standard conditions (Table 20.9) in the first test (1976) and this tendency to 'levelling out' the difference between brands increases in the following test in 1977.

Table 20.9 Amount of nicotine taken from various cigarettes during smoke tests.

Test Cigarette	Amount of Nicotine in smoke under standard conditions (mg/cig)	Nicotine Intake in test smokers (mg/cig)	
		1976 (n=30)	1977 (n=30)
K	1.05	1.10	0.80
L	0.54	0.70	--
M	0.40	0.63	0.70
N	0.64	0.59	--
O	0.75	--	0.69

On average the high delivery cigarettes K, N and O were smoked less intensively and the low delivery cigarettes were smoked more intensively than under standard smoking conditions. From puff profile recordings it can be assumed that 'levelling out' of the smoking values was carried out mainly by increasing or decreasing the puff volume (e.g. cigarette K: 50 ml/puff, cigarette M: 60 ml/puff).

There were no significant differences between cigarettes for butt length and number of cigarettes smoked per day.

The results of these tests (Table 20.10) in which heavy smokers (average consumption 20-25 cig/day) had to smoke for a short time (one to two weeks) brands with very different deliveries show significant differences in smoking behaviour compared to 'normal' smokers.   The test smokers (heavy smokers from the medium delivery class) tried to smoke both groups of cigarettes (medium and low delivery class) according to their smoking habit, which is to take similar amounts of smoke and to smoke the same number of cigarettes per day (Table 20.9).

Normal test smokers from the medium delivery class distinguish themselves clearly from smokers in the low delivery class. The amounts of smoke taken from these classes are similar to the standard yields of these classes (Table 20.10). The daily cigarette consumption is significantly higher in the strong to medium delivery class than in the low delivery class.

Table 20.10 Smoke and cigarette consumption in various cigarettes with respect to cigarette strength (Collection in West Germany, 1974, 440-4350 butts).

Class	Standard Values (mg/cig)		Natural Smoke Values (mg/cig)		Cigarette Consumption (period/day)
	Nicotine	Condensate	Nicotine	Condensate	
	1.09	15.2	0.76	16.1	16.3
Medium	0.90	15.3	0.81	15.3	16.8
Del.	0.81	13.6	1.04	13.1	16.6
Class	0.81	13.2	0.74	13.4	17.5
	0.74	12.6	0.73	13.3	16.7
$\tilde{x}$	0.87	14.0	0.82	14.2	16.8
Low	0.61	11.8	0.84*	12.1	15.3*
Del.	0.61	11.3	0.60	11.9	13.6
Class	0.56	12.6	0.66	12.4	13.6
$\tilde{x}$	0.59	11.9	(Without 0.63*) 0.70	12.1	(Without 13.6*) 14.2

* This cigarette has a delivery level which makes its classification into medium or low arbitrary.

Acknowledgement

Translated by Mrs. U.C. Hopkins, British-American Tobacco Co. Ltd., Southampton, U.K.

References

Bethmann, M.von. (1959) Personal communication.
Keith, C.H. & Hackney, E.J. (1962) Human smoking characteristics, *16th Tobacco Chemists Research Conference,* Richmond, Virginia.
Lorenz, H.W. & Seehofer, F. (1971) Zur messung von abrauchparametern mit hilfe von messgroessenumformern. *Beiträge zur Tabakforschung,* **6**, 1-6.

Schievelbein, H. (1978) Metabolic aspects of smoking behaviour. *This volume.*

Schulz, W. (1974) Die auswirkung der tabaksteuererhohung vom 1.9.1972 auf die lange der cigarettenstummel in der Bundesrepublik Deutschland. *Beiträge zur Tabakforschung,* 7, 203-205.

Schulz, W. & Seehofer, F. (1970) Uber die lange von cigarettenstummeln in der Bundesrepublik Deutschland im jahre 1968. *Beiträge zur Tabakforschung,* 5, 198-200.

Schulz, W. & Seehofer, F. (1976) Die auswirkung der wirtschaftlichen rezession auf die lange der cigarettenstummel in der Bundesrepublic Deutschland. *Beiträge zur Tabakforschung,* 7, 455-458.

21. Instruments to measure, record and duplicate human smoking patterns

D E CREIGHTON, M J NOBLE, AND R T WHEWELL

Introduction

For the purposes of comparing the delivery of different cigarette brands standard smoking conditions have been introduced in many countries and the information resulting from standard smoking has formed the basis for the construction of league tables of 'tar' and nicotine deliveries.

There is, however, an interaction between cigarette smoke and the smoker. It is possible, by varying the size of the puffs and the rate of puffing, for a smoker to take more or less smoke from a cigarette than is delivered when standard machine smoking conditions are used, i.e. the smoker may receive different deliveries of smoke components than is indicated by league tables.

In order to measure the way in which cigarettes are smoked various techniques, reviewed by Hausermann (1972), have been used. A further method has been published by Guillerm and Radziszewski (1975) but Adams (1966, 1972) deserves special attention as his work in the fields of puff profile recording and duplication has formed the starting point for our own developments. Most techniques rely on the subject smoking a cigarette through a holder. The holder is pneumatically connected to a device that converts pressure to a proportional voltage which may be recorded on a moving chart. The analysis of such data relies on the manual measurement of the traces, which is both tedious and inherently inaccurate.

An important requirement of smoking behaviour studies is to be able to measure the amount of 'tar', nicotine and gas phase components taken from the cigarette by the smoker. Filter tip analysis can provide an estimate of some smoke deliveries but makes the assumption that the filtration efficiency of the brand is constant under all smoking regimes and conditions. It is known that the filtration efficiency of a filter is dependent on the velocity of smoke passing through the filter especially with filters such as cellulose acetate (Overton, 1973). Our observations show that human smokers use a range of flow rates (typically up to 60 cm^3 s^{-1}) which frequently exceed those used for standard machine smoking. It is, therefore, to be expected that inaccuracies may result from filter tip analysis.

A better estimate of the amount of material presented to a smoker may be made by smoking similar cigarettes by a machine to the same smoking pattern as that used by the smoker. Before the smoking pattern can be duplicated it is necessary to measure and record the pattern accurately. Alternatively the human smoking measurement system might be made to control a 'Slave'machine so that both cigarettes were smoked simultaneously. The advantages of recording the smoking pattern are that it may be used to control a duplicator repetitively **so that several** cigarettes may be smoked by the machine for each one smoked by the subject. Recorded data may also be analysed to show if and how smoking patterns have been modified by smokers in response to changes in cigarette design.

This paper describes the structure, functions and operation of a smoking analyser and data logger designed to monitor the way human subjects smoke cigarettes and a puff duplicator which smokes cigarettes to the recorded smoking patterns. The equipment has been designed and developed in the B.A.T. Services Ltd., Group R. & D. Centre, Southampton in association with Projects CGC Ltd., of Cheltenham.

The smoking analyser and recorder

The cigarette to be smoked by the subject is held in a cigarette holder which is connected by light plastic tubes to a small wooden case. The case contains a pair of transducers and their power supplies and is connected by a long lead to the main analyser and data logger so that a subject may smoke a cigarette in a room adjacent to the equipment. The arrangement of the analogue measurement system is shown in Fig. 21.1.

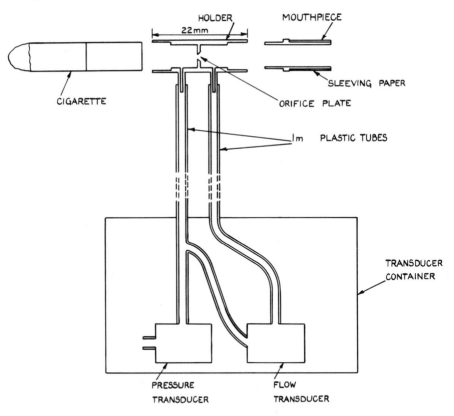

Fig. 21.1 Pressure and flow measurement apparatus.

The cigarette holder is moulded in a hard plastic material with a central orifice plate that contains a hole slightly less than 1 mm in diameter. The hole in the orifice plate is made to have a sharp edge by dishing the lower pressure side. A mouthpiece, usually sleeved with cork-tipping paper, is fitted into the low pressure side. The draw resistance of a typical holder is 6.5 cm W.G. (1 cm W.G. = 98 N m^{-2}) at a flow rate of 17.5 cm^3 s^{-1}.

Light plastic tubes about 1 m long and 2.5 mm internal diameter are attached to side-arms either side of the orifice plate. The tube in front of the orifice plate is connected to a National Semiconductor Inc. transducer (LX 1701D) which has a range $\pm$5 p.s.i. (1 p.s.i. = 6890 N m^{-2}). The other inlet to this transducer is open to atmosphere, so the transducer measures the pressure used to draw smoke from the cigarette, relative to atmosphere. The second transducer, which is of the same type as the pressure transducer, measures the difference in pressure across the orifice plate, which is related to the flow through the holder.

The output voltage from the pressure transducer is linearly related to the pressure applied to its diaphragm. Signal conditioning consists of a ranging amplifier with a zero control and a gain control which are adjusted to calibrate the measurements over the desired range (0.1-100 cm W.G.) and in the appropriate units. A water manometer is used as the standard for calibration.

The conditioning of the flow transducer signal is more complex as the relationship between the difference in pressure across an orifice plate in a tube and the flow through the tube is approximately square root (Prandtl, 1957). A lineariser is used to convert the flow signal to a voltage directly proportional to the flow. The lineariser consists of a series of linear and logarithmic amplifiers with potentiometric controls that allow the output characteristics to be bent or straightened and to set zero and gain. The flow signal is calibrated against a rotameter so that it is linear over the range 1-100 cm^3 s^{-1}.

After signal conditioning, the outputs of both the pressure and flow channels are voltages proportional to the pressure and flow in the cigarette holder. These voltages may be displayed directly on an oscilloscope or pen recorder to trace the pressure and flow profiles of puffs. The voltages are also converted (by voltage to frequency converters) into frequencies proportional to the voltages. The frequencies are sampled and counted at the rate of fifty flow readings and fifty pressure readings per second. The outputs of the count registers are used to drive digital displays of the instantaneous pressure and flow. The instantaneous pressure and flow signals are both integrated and displayed as the integrated pressure used to draw the puff and as the volume of the puff respectively. A digitiser is then employed to convert the samples of the frequency signals into Binary Coded Decimals (BCD). The timing of these operations is synchronised by a crystal controlled clock. The BCD outputs are further arranged into a form suitable to be stored on magnetic tape. This requires the insertion of fixed characters, punctuation and a code change to ASCII (American Standard Code for Information Interchange). An output from the crystal clock is used to display the duration of each puff and in a separate register the interval between puffs. These data are also recorded on magnetic tape. A functional block diagram of the smoking analyser and data logger is shown as Figure 21.2.

K*

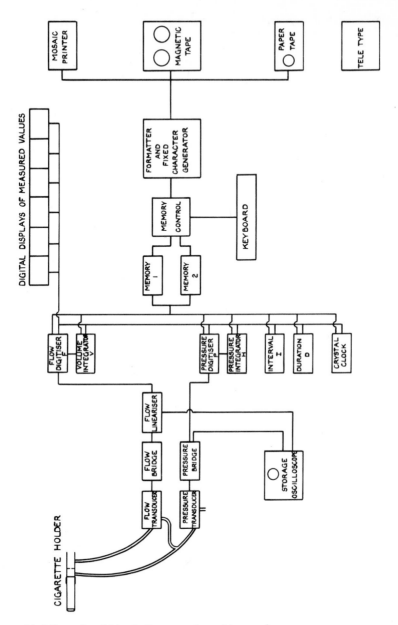

Fig. 21.2 Functional block diagram of smoking analyser

The system has been constructed so that a puff is said to have started when the pressure in the cigarette holder rises above 0.1 cm W.G.   When this occurs the volume, duration and total pressure registers and displays are reset to zero and start counting.   The instantaneous pressure and flow are displayed and recorded for the duration of the puff.   When the pressure falls below 0.1 cm W.G. the **puff** is defined as terminated.   The displays of volume, total pressure and puff duration remain at the last reading, the instantaneous pressure and flow displays read zero but the interval display resets and starts counting the interval between puffs.

The output from the formatting module is stored temporarily in a split buffer memory store. Each half of the store has a capacity of 256 characters. When half of the memory is full it automatically switches in the other half of the memory and empties itself onto the magnetic tape. When the second half of the memory is full it switches in the first half which is again empty and discharges its 256 characters to tape. In this way a memory store of modest capacity can handle the data from long duration puffs. The alternative would be to use a memory store with capacity of at least 7,000 characters. The tape recorder used is an R.D.L. 10500 which is of the incremental, nine track, NRZ, 800 BPI type with both read and write capabilities.

Data recording

A keyboard which has a full set of upper case letters and numbers is provided with the instrument. A row of 18 indicator and control function keys is also set into the keyboard.

To record a smoking pattern, the end of the last test on the tape is located and the data highways to the tape recorder are opened. Header data, to identify the subject, date, cigarette brand, replicate number, test number etc. are typed into the memory store directly from the keyboard and then transferred to magnetic tape. Tape marker gaps are usually inserted to separate keyboard data from puffing data. The instrument is then ready to receive and record the puffing data. The transfer of puffing data to the tape recorder is fully automatic.

When the smoker has finished the cigarette, the clock is stopped manually and the last puff data transferred to magnetic tape by pressing a button. A further tape marker gap is inserted followed by 'trailer' data from the keyboard which includes information such as the length of the cigarette butt. The instrument is then reset to close the data highways to the tape recorder, but can still be used for display only.

Data retrieval

The magnetic tape is rewound and stopped. The data for a particular test may then be located by searching the header records for any or all of the first 26 characters in the header. The header data are typed in via the keyboard and a 'search' key pressed. The tape moves forward until the data are located. The data may be read from the magnetic tape in several different forms:

(a) Mosaic printer A Mullard 60SR mosaic printer operates when a 'tape to print' key is pressed. Twenty characters per line are written on a paper strip 58 mm wide. Blocks of data are read singly so 'tape to print' has to be pressed at the start of each block of data.

The mosaic printer is used mainly for checking and fault finding as it reads directly from the magnetic tape. The data are not formatted in columns so do not provide the most convenient record or display of the stored data.

(b) Paper tape punch Data may be read from the magnetic tape onto a paper tape punch in three formats.

(i) *Full format* Two blanking zeros are introduced after each pressure and each flow reading. Carriage return and line feed signals are inserted after every 32 characters. Decimal points are introduced where appropriate. Two pressure and two flow readings are printed on each line so that the data form columns as successive rows are printed, when the tape is read by teletype.

All the data on the magnetic tape are transferred to the paper tape. From such print-outs the pressure and flow profiles may be reconstructed. Peak values of pressure and flow and the times taken to reach the peak values can be read from the print-out. The interval, volume, duration and integrated pressure readings are printed at the end of each puff after the final flow reading.

(ii) Reduced format Only the interval, duration, volume and integrated pressure readings are punched. The formatting board introduces spaces, carriage return and line feed characters so that when printed, the results are written in columns with spaces between the columns. Print-outs in this form may be scanned to identify the smoking pattern characteristics of an individual. It is also a convenient format for totalling and averaging the data manually as the format is clear and unambiguous.

(iii) Duplication format In this form the paper tape is punched with only the interval, pressure and flow data. Blanking zeros, carriage return, line feed and decimal point characters are omitted or suppressed. The puff volume, integrated pressure and puff duration are not punched as these data are derived from the pressure and flow readings. This tape format is used to control the machine which smokes cigarettes to the same pattern as that used by a human smoker.

(c) Direct to computer The magnetic tape may be read directly through a translator (code changer) into a disc store in a computer configuration. The data may then be manipulated into different forms and combinations for statistical analysis.

The puff duplicator
The puff duplicator, of which a general view is shown as Figure 21.3, is of modular construction. The digital functions are housed to the right of the smoking control module and the analogue functions to the left. The analogue valve is located on top of the smoking control module, in a vacuum chamber covered by a removable glass dome and safety screen. A balloon to collect the gas phase may be placed under the dome. The box on the front of the instrument is to catch the paper tape as it is read by the tape reader.

A functional block diagram of the duplicator is shown as Figure 21.4. Paper tapes, made in the duplication format, (i.e. pressure, flow and interval data only) are read by an Elliott T10 200 optical tape reader. The paper tape is passed through the reader at 1000 c.p.s. (characters per second) to read the pressure from the tape into a memory store. This store may be updated by a higher reading so that only the peak pressure is retained. The paper tape is then repositioned in the tape reader on the first character of the first puff.

The peak pressure held in the store is used to set the vacuum level in the analogue valve housing to be sufficient to draw the highest puff pressure on the tape. The pressure within the valve housing is measured against atmospheric pressure by a transducer. The voltage output of the transducer is compared across a bridge with a voltage reconstruction of the value held in the peak pressure memory store.

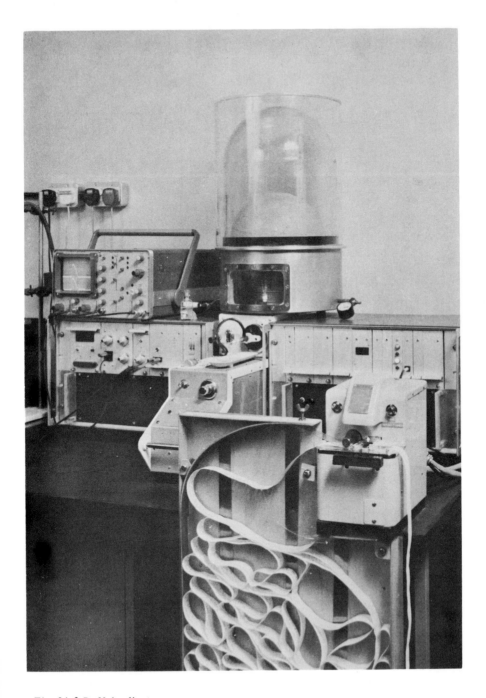

Fig. 21.3 Puff duplicator

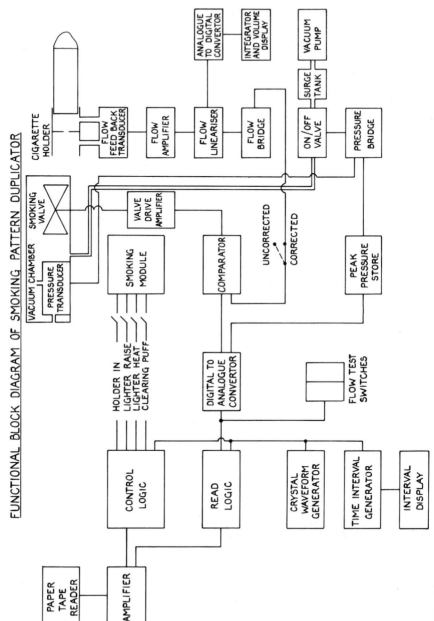

FUNCTIONAL BLOCK DIAGRAM OF SMOKING PATTERN DUPLICATOR

Fig. 21.4

If the difference in pressure between that called for by the memory store and that measured by the transducer exceeds 1 cm W.G. a valve is opened to reduce the pressure in the valve housing. The volume of the valve housing is about 35 litres.

The analogue valve, within the low pressure housing, consists of a 75 watt loud-speaker motor about 300 mm in diameter. The cone has been removed and an adjustable linkage attached to the centre of the diaphragm. The linkage is connected to a pair of pinch rollers which open against a light spring when power is applied to the speech coil. A pair of latex tubes pass through the pinch rollers. The upper ends are connected by a 'Y' piece to a latex balloon which rests on a shelf above the valve and within the glass dome. The lower ends of the latex tubes are connected by a 'Y' piece which passes through a seal in the low pressure valve housing and is further sealed into the smoke path.

The cigarette to be smoked is held in a similar cigarette holder to that used by the subject to smoke the original cigarette. The cigarette holder is held by a rubber seal in an arm which can be driven in and out by a pneumatic piston. The end of the cigarette holder is held 40 mm away from a Cambridge filter holder during the intervals between puffs (free smoking) but is drawn in to seal against the Cambridge filter holder three seconds before a puff is drawn (restricted smoking). When the cigarette holder is sealed to the Cambridge filter holder the analogue valve opens in a controlled way, so that the appropriate volume of smoke is drawn from the cigarette into the Cambridge filter holder. The particulate matter and nicotine alkaloids are trapped on the Cambridge filter pad and the gas phase of the smoke passes through the latex tubes in the analogue valve to the collecting balloon above. At the end of a puff, the cigarette holder is driven out from the Cambridge filter holder and a clearing puff of 20 cm^3 volume drawn through the Cambridge filter holder. The clearing puff draws the smoke in front of the filter pad onto the filter and clears the gas phase past the pinch rollers in the analogue valve. The clearing puff sequence is initiated by a microswitch on the free/restricted drive rod but is electronically timed so that the clearing puff is not drawn until the cigarette holder is 10 mm clear of the Cambridge filter holder.

The duplicator is designed to copy the flow pattern recorded on the paper tape. The flow readings are read from the tape at the rate of fifty readings per second, the same as the recording rate. The digital values read from the tape are converted to analogue voltages and applied to a comparator bridge which controls the analogue valve through a power amplifier. The side-arms of the cigarette holder are connected to a National Semiconductor Inc. LX 1701D transducer by light plastic tubes. The output of this transducer is linearised and calibrated in a similar way to the flow measurement circuit of the smoking analyser, except the rotameter readings are set against digital values injected by a pair of edge switches so that they mimic digital values read from the paper tape. The output of the flow lineariser is in the same calibration units (1 volt/10 cm^3s^{-1}) as the voltage reconstruction of the flow signal read from the paper tape. This signal is a measure of what is happening in the cigarette holder which may be compared, across the comparator bridge, with what should be happening according to the flow signal derived from the paper tape. If there is a discrepancy, the difference between the flow feedback signal and the analogue reconstruction voltage is used to open or close the analogue valve so that there is no difference between the 'slave' and 'master' profiles.

The interval between puffs is located at the end of each flow profile on the paper tape. This reading is used to set a count-down timer, with digital display in seconds, that indicates the length of the interval before the next puff. The count-down timer is operated from a crystal controlled clock that supervises all the timed functions of the equipment.

Voltage outputs may be taken from the lineariser and analogue to digital converter in the flow circuits to display the 'slave' and 'master' flow profiles on an oscilloscope. These profiles are superimposable when the equipment is calibrated, except the 'slave' profile lags behind the 'master' profile by about 8 ms. The voltage output from the lineariser is also converted into a proportional frequency, then counted and integrated to drive a digital display of the 'slave' volumes. During operation the volumes displayed on the integrator should be the same as read from a reduced format printout of the original data.

Discussion

It was realised at the outset that smokers do not normally smoke through a cigarette holder to which a pair of tubes are attached. As far as we are aware it is, however, the only practical way to measure the pressure and flow profiles with a sufficient degree of accuracy. We have made surreptitious observations of smokers where puff duration, puff number, butt length and intervals between puffs were noted and found that the results from these observations were comparable with measurements made using the smoking analyser and data logger.

In order to measure the flow through a cigarette holder it is necessary to build a restriction into the holder. We have chosen to use an orifice plate because it removes very little material from the smoke stream.

The orifice, which is about 0.9 mm in diameter, contributes very little to the overall draw resistance experienced by the smoker at low flow rates. It is not until the flow rate reaches about 30 ml/sec that the draw resistance of the holder equals that of a typical lit U.K. cigarette. The cigarette holder may therefore place some restriction on the peak flow rates a smoker might take as he has to overcome the combined draw resistance of the holder and the cigarette. In practice we have found some smokers who have drawn peak flow rates of 60-70 $cm^3 s^{-1}$ but few smokers comment on any difficulties experienced in drawing smoke.

An inherent source of error exists in the measurement system in that the cigarette holders are calibrated in air but are used with cigarette smoke. The viscosity and density of smoke are different from air. The composition of smoke may vary, however, according to tobacco type, degree of filtration and ventilation and other factors associated with the combustion of the tobacco, so there is no simple way to correct for these errors. We have determined the error in volume measurement for a typical U.K. flue-cured tobacco cigarette smoked at a representative range of volumes and found the average error to be +2.7 (+2.3 to +3.2)%. The volumes quoted are therefore slightly over-estimated. When a smoking pattern is duplicated, the duplicator is similarly calibrated in air but measures in smoke. Any errors in absolute measurements of puff volume should therefore cancel out and not affect the deliveries determined after duplication.

The delivery of a cigarette is related to the volume of smoke drawn from it and therefore we have chosen to duplicate the flow signal. The pressure used to draw a puff is related to the flow when the draw resistance is constant. Previous studies (Baker, 1975) indicate that the draw resistance of a lit cigarette is not constant and is not predictable from a measurement of the unlit draw resistance. It was therefore necessary to include a flow feedback loop to make continuous corrections to the flow profile to overcome the varying draw resistance of a lit cigarette. The flow feedback circuit on our instrument is able to correct the valve position by about ±30% which means that we can achieve very good matching of slave and master profiles (Figure 21.5).

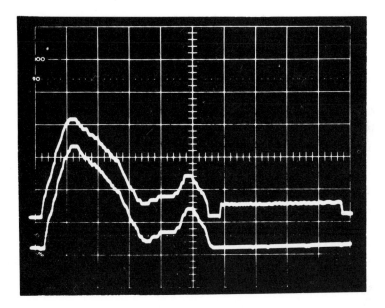

Fig. 21.5 Master profile with clearing puff shown above slave profile. Photographed by oscilloscope camera.

The pressure signals recorded on the paper tape are those measured by the analyser between the orifice plate and the end of the cigarette. The pressure used to draw the puff must, however, be equal to the mouth pressure used by the smoker to overcome the draw resistance of the orifice plate and the cigarette. By ratioing the pressure measured behind and in front of the orifice at a represent-ative range of flow rates (10-100 cm^3 s^{-1}) we found a factor of 1.2-1.7. We therefore multiply the pressure from the pressure memory stores by 1.8, which converts the pressure in front of the orifice plate to slightly more than the mouth pressure. The excess pressure is a safety margin to overcome the additional draw resistance of the Cambridge filter pad and of the smoke path through the instrument, and to act as spare capacity during flow correction by the feedback circuit.

The use of a specific pressure setting for each tape allows for greater calibration accuracy. The maximum peak flow rates seen have been 60-70 cm^3 s^{-1}; whereas average peak flow rates are 25-35 cm^3 s^{-1}. If a pressure suitable to draw 70 cm^3 s^{-1}, when the analogue valve was fully open, was used for a 25 cm^3 s^{-1} flow rate then the valve would be less than half-way open. By using the measured pressure from each tape to set the vacuum level, the flow feedback circuit can be calibrated over the range used by that specific smoker. The peak flow rate in a particular smoking pattern is therefore reproduced when the analogue valve is close to its maximum opening.

We have used this instrument to duplicate the smoking patterns of a number of subjects who participated in a test to study the effects of changing brands. We have found that the accuracy of volume duplication is generally within 1.0% and the timing of both puff durations and intervals between puffs to be within 0.02 seconds.

Summary

Apparatus has been constructed which records the smoking patterns of smokers. The data may be displayed in numeric form and stored in digital form on magnetic tape. The magnetic tape may be read in several forms so that print-outs of the pressures, flows, volumes, durations and intervals between the puffs may be made in a number of ways. Paper tapes are made to control the functions of a puff duplicator which smokes cigarettes to the same pattern as the human smoker, enabling the 'tar', nicotine and gas phase components to be collected for analysis.

References

Adams, P.I. (1966) Measurements on puffs taken by human smokers. *20th Tobacco Chemists' Research Conference.* Winston-Salem, N.C.

Adams, P.I. (1972) Cigar smoking: Measurement of the human smoking regime and its relationship to smoking machines. *26th Tobacco Chemists' Research Conference.* Williamsburg.

Baker, R.R. (1975) Contributions to the draw resistance of a burning cigarette. *Beiträge zur Tabakforschung,* 8, 124-131.

Guillerm, R. & Radziszewski, E. (1975) Une nouvelle méthode d'analyse de l'acte du fumeur. *Annales du Tabac,* 1, 101-110. Paris: SEITA.

Hausermann, M. (1972) Report and literature survey presented to the meeting of the CORESTA Smoke Study Group, Williamsburg Va. U.S.A. October 26-27 1972.

Overton, J.R. (1973) Filtration of cigarette smoke: Relative contributions of inertial impaction, diffusional deposition, and direct interception. *Beiträge zur Tabakforschung,* 7, 117-120.

Prandtl, L. (1957) *Essentials of Fluid Dynamics,* Blackie & Sons, p. 170.

22. The effect of different cigarettes on human smoking patterns

D E CREIGHTON AND P H LEWIS

Introduction

In most parts of the world the design of cigarettes is being modified and the deliveries of tar (or TPM) and nicotine, as determined by machine smoking, have been declining. TPM is the total particulate matter trapped on a Cambridge filter and is determined by direct weighing. Tar usually refers to the total particulate matter less the weights of nicotine and water. Although this trend has been particularly noticeable in recent years with the introduction of 'league' tables of cigarettes ranked by deliveries, the reduction in deliveries has been going on for some time; e.g. in a survey of U.K. smoking patterns records, the 1973 deliveries of nicotine and tar were 47% and 57% respectively of the deliveries obtained in 1935 (Todd, 1975).

It is often assumed by smokers and implied by others that it is preferable to change to a brand which offers lower deliveries of tar and nicotine, and to an increasing extent such advice is becoming more explicit, e.g. 'Smoke a brand of cigarettes in a lower 'tar' group than the brand you smoke at present and aim progressively to reduce still further' (D.H.S.S., 1976). However, there is a considerable body of evidence (Ashton and Watson, 1970; Frith, 1971; Adams, 1976; Gritz, Baer-Weiss and Jarvik, 1976) that shows that smokers alter their smoking patterns when they change to a brand of cigarettes with different delivery characteristics. If a smoker of relatively high delivery cigarettes changes to a brand with substantially lower deliveries, he may actually increase his intake of tar and carbon monoxide in his attempts to compensate for the reduced delivery of nicotine (Russell, 1974). Compensation is a subconscious control of the intake of one or more smoke components by a change in the smoking pattern so that similar intakes are achieved from cigarettes with dissimilar machine smoked deliveries.

Much of the evidence for compensation has been obtained under laboratory conditions and has involved comparisons of single cigarette smoking measurements. It is, however, possible that a smoker can change his behaviour with time and become accustomed to a brand offering higher or lower deliveries, especially if he smokes the 'new' brand exclusively.

It was therefore decided to carry out an experiment in which the cigarettes of interest would be smoked *ad libitum* for a reasonably long period of time, smoking behaviour being measured, in the laboratory, on a number of occasions throughout this period. A panel of smokers of a medium delivery cigarette (about 1.4 mg nicotine) would be monitored for a period of about one month and then asked to smoke, for a similar period, a brand with a substantially different nicotine delivery (about 1.0 mg for half of the panel and about 1.8 mg for the other half of the panel). For the final period the smokers would revert to smoking the brand delivering 1.4 mg nicotine.

Methods

The panel

The subjects selected for this test were eight male and eight female smokers recruited from the laboratory staff employed at the B.A.T. Group R. & D. Centre, Southampton, England. All of the subjects had participated in previous experiments in which smoking patterns were recorded and were thus familiar with the apparatus, procedures and environment that we use for such measurements. They were regular smokers who normally smoked king size filter tipped cigarettes with a delivery of about 1.4 mg nicotine.

Data recording

Smoking pattern data were recorded on a smoking analyser and data logger (Creighton, Noble, Whewell, 1978) developed at Southampton. This instrument measures and records the pressures and flows in an orifice plate cigarette holder connected to a pair of transducers. Both the pressure and flow signals are conditioned, digitised and stored on magnetic tape in a computer compatible form together with the volume and duration of each puff, the pressure used to draw each puff and the interval between puffs.

The data stored on magnetic tape can be copied directly onto a paper tape that can be read by a standard teletype machine to obtain a printed record of the data. An alternative form of the paper tape can be used to control a machine known as a puff duplicator (Creighton *et al,* 1978) that smokes a cigarette to the same pattern as used by the human smoker.

Cigarettes

Three king sized cigarettes designated A, B and C, were used in this study. The physical dimensions and analytical data when smoked under standard conditions are shown in Table 22.1. Throughout this paper the terms 'control' or 'medium delivery cigarette' refer to cigarette A, 'high delivery' to cigarette B and 'low delivery' to cigarette C. These cigarettes were slected as being typical of the range of cigarettes available on the U.K. market at the time of the experiment, and all three were variants of the same brand.

All cigarettes smoked by the subjects in the laboratory were selected to be within the draw resistance range 12-14 cm W.G., when measured at a flow rate of 17.5 cm^3 sec^{-1}. The cigarettes were not weight selected. The cigarettes issued to the subjects to smoke outside the smoking behaviour laboratory were in sealed packs of twenty.

Cigarettes smoked in the laboratory

When a subject reported to the laboratory, he was allowed to settle in an armchair in an air-conditioned room. The room is sound-attenuated to prevent the intrusion of extraneous noise. Throughout the test the subject listened to tape recorded music of his choice. During the settling down period, information to identify the

Table 22.1 Physical dimensions and analytical data for the cigarettes when smoked under standard conditions.

		A	B	C
Overall length	(mm)	83	82	83
Tobacco rod length	(mm)	65	68	64
Circumference	(mm)	24.5	24.5	25
Filter mouth section (length and type)	(mm)	6 Cellulose acetate	14 Cellulose acetate	6 Cellulose acetate
Filter tobacco section (length and type)	(mm)	12 Myria	--	13 Myria*
Printed tipping paper length	(mm)	21	23	24
Draw resistance at 17.5 cm^3 sec^{-1} (cm W.G.) **		12-14	12-14	12-14
Total particulate matter (TPM)	(mg)	23.3	35.7	16.1
Total nicotine alkaloids (TNA)	(mg)	1.4	1.8	1.0
Carbon monoxide	(% v/v)	4.5	5.4	3.0
Carbon monoxide	(mg)	18.6	21.6	12.9
TPM/Nicotine ratio		16.6	19.8	16.1

* Ventilated filter.
** 1 cm Water Gauge = 98 Nm^{-2}.

smoker, cigarette replicate etc. was recorded on the smoking analyser and data logger via a keyboard. When the subject was ready he picked up the cigarette in its holder, lit it and smoked the cigarette completely at will. When a smoker had finished smoking, the cigarette was extinguished by placing it in a tray containing granulated solid carbon dioxide. The smoker was watched during the test through a one way mirror as a safety measure and to observe when the cigarette had been extinguished.

The number of cigarettes issued to the subject was recorded and at the end of a phase any unsmoked cigarettes were returned and their number noted. In this way it was possible to have some measure of the cigarette consumption throughout the three phases of the experiment. The length of the cigarette butt left by the smoker was measured and recorded on the magnetic tape.

Experimental design

Phase 1   All subjects were given the medium delivery cigarette (A) to smoke exclusively for four weeks. Cigarettes were issued *ad libitum*. During this time each subject was monitored on ten occasions. The spacing of recordings was as even as possible throughout the period; half of the recordings were taken during the morning and half in the afternoon to minimise any effects due to time of day.

Phase 11   Half of the subjects changed to the high delivery brand (B) and half changed to the low delivery brand (C). A further ten smoking pattern measurements were recorded from all the panel members evenly spaced throughout the next four weeks.   The changeover was arranged so that the first example of the replacement brand was smoked in the laboratory and recorded. Cigarettes of the replacement brand were also issued to the subjects *ad libitum.*

Phase 111   All the smokers returned to the medium delivery brand (A). A further ten measurements were taken over the four weeks with, as far as possible, equal spacing between records. The first cigarette smoked by each subject in this final phase was recorded and, as before, subjects smoked the brand exclusively.

Analysis of data
480 cigarettes were smoked by the panel in our laboratory. The data collected by the smoking analyser and data logger were read into a computer using a program which validates the data, processes the data and produces a file suitable for analysis by statistical programs. The results of the primary data reduction are shown in Table 22.2.   These data were analysed by a univariate analysis of variance technique to show the significance of the changes.   Table 22.3 shows the results of the statistical analysis.

Table 22.2 Effect of changed delivery on smoking pattern.

Parameter		Delivery in Phase II	Phase I	Phase II	Phase III
Total puff volume	(cm^3)	Higher	546	433	534
		Lower	571	625	522
Average puff volume	(cm^3)	Higher	43.8	39.6	44.5
		Lower	46.1	53.4	46.1
Average puff duration	(sec)	Higher	2.27	2.14	2.34
		Lower	2.44	2.77	2.41
Average interval between puffs	(sec)	Higher	38.5	36.5	39.2
		Lower	36.5	37.2	40.9
Average lit draw resistance*	(cm W.G.)	Higher	18.9	19.4	18.6
		Lower	18.6	16.6	19.2
Average number of puffs		Higher	13.0	11.5	12.6
		Lower	12.6	12.0	11.4
Average butt length	(mm)	Higher	31.4	33.9	30.7
		Lower	31.2	32.8	31.5
Total time alight	(sec)	Higher	468	395	452
		Lower	467	451	458
Estimated number of cigarettes smoked per day		Higher	33.2	29.9	33.3
		Lower	31.1	32.5	32.8

*Average lit draw resistance is the total of the pressures used to draw the puffs divided by the total duration of the puffs.

Table 22.3 Summary of significant differences in smoking pattern between delivery levels and between sex groups (level of significance 0.10)

Parameter	GROUP 1		GROUP 2	
	Those who smoked the high delivery cigarette in phase II		Those who smoked the low delivery cigarette in phase II	
	High delivery relative to control cigarette	Women relative to men	Low delivery relative to control cigarette	Women relative to men
Total puff volume	Lower	No change	Higher	No change
Average puff volume	Lower	Lower	Higher	Lower
Average puff duration	Shorter	No change	Longer	No change
Average interval between puffs	No change	No change	Phase I to II: No change; Shorter in II than III	No change
Average lit draw resistance	Higher	Lower	Lower	No change
Average number of puffs	Lower	No change	Phase I to II: No change; Higher in II than III	Higher
Average butt length	Longer	No change	Longer	No change
Total time alight	Shorter	No change	No change	No change
Estimated number of cigarettes smoked per day	No change	No change	No change	No change

Duplication of human smoking patterns

In the past, filter tip analysis was the only practical method to estimate the intake of smoke components by smokers. This method assumed that the filtration efficiency of a filter is independent of the way in which the cigarette is smoked. It has, however, been shown that the filtration efficiency of a filter depends, for example, on the velocity of smoke passing through it (Overton, 1973). To obtain a better estimate of the deliveries of smoke components from a cigarette it is necessary to smoke an identical cigarette in the same way that a subject smoked it and to collect the mainstream smoke. The puff duplicator developed in Southampton (Creighton *et al,* 1978) is programmed by a paper tape made from the smoking analyser and data logger. The instrument will smoke a 'slave' cigarette to the same flow profiles (hence puff volumes and shape) and with the same intervals between puffs as those taken by a subject to smoke the original cigarette. Unfortunately, cigarettes taken from the same packet are not identical; even if cigarettes are selected to be within a close weight and draw resistance range, the deliveries of individual cigarettes may differ by $\pm$ 15% of the mean when smoked under standard conditions. Due to these differences it is desirable to smoke many cigarettes by the puff duplicator for each of the recorded human smoking patterns. It was not practical to smoke replicate (perhaps twenty) cigarettes to each of the 480 smoking patterns recorded in this test. It was, therefore, decided to select one tape from each phase of the experiment for each subject which was close to the mean smoking pattern for that subject and phase. The criteria used for this selection were the total volume of smoke drawn and the number of puffs used to draw it. Five cigarettes were smoked by the puff duplicator for each of the 48 selected tapes.

In addition to these results, which have provided panel average figures for the deliveries of the cigarettes when smoked by human subjects, the results from two male and two female subjects were selected at random and all thirty records of the smoking pattern obtained from each of these subjects were used to smoke a single cigarette on the puff duplicator. This showed that the coefficient of variation for nicotine delivery measurements from the replicate smokings of a single brand for an individual was on average about 14% (range 8% to 24%). This is considerably lower than the coefficient of variation between nicotine deliveries for different people smoking the same brand which was about 30% (range 24% to 38%).

Success in choosing typical tapes to represent these individuals was confirmed since the nicotine delivery of the selected replicate was always within 15% of the means of the ten replicates.

The particulate matter in the smoke drawn from the cigarettes smoked by the puff duplicator was collected on a Cambridge filter pad. The gas phase of the smoke, which passes through a Cambridge filter, was collected in a latex balloon. The TPM delivery was measured by direct weighing and the nicotine estimated as total nicotine alkaloids by a cyanogen bromide auto-analyser method. The carbon monoxide content of the gas phase was measured by an infra-red gas analyser. No corrections have been made for atmospheric temperature and pressure as the instrument was calibrated daily with standard gas mixtures under ambient conditions.

The results obtained by duplicating the smoking patterns are shown in Table 22.4.

Table 22.4 Deliveries measured from duplication of human smoking patterns

		Sex	Delivery in Phase II	Phase I	Phase II	Phase III
Nicotine on Cambridge Filter pad	(mg)	M	Higher	2.2	2.1	2.2
		F	Higher	2.0	2.2	1.9
		M	Lower	2.3	1.7	2.3
		F	Lower	1.9	1.0	1.6
Nicotine in filter tip	(mg)	M	Higher	1.8	0.9	1.9
		F	Higher	1.7	1.0	1.8
		M	Lower	1.9	2.6	2.0
		F	Lower	1.7	1.9	1.5
TPM on Cambridge filter pad	(mg)	M	Higher	32.3	30.0	34.9
		F	Higher	25.0	23.2	22.5
		M	Lower	34.6	22.1	34.8
		F	Lower	23.5	10.8	19.0
Carbon monoxide delivery	(% v/v)	M	Higher	4.2	4.8	4.6
		F	Higher	3.9	4.6	4.3
		M	Lower	4.1	2.9	4.8
		F	Lower	3.5	2.2	3.8
Carbon monoxide delivery	(mg)	M	Higher	30.4	28.7	33.1
		F	Higher	24.4	22.4	27.7
		M	Lower	31.6	25.0	36.5
		F	Lower	21.3	15.2	21.6
TPM:Nicotine ratio		M	Higher	14.4	13.5	15.1
		F	Higher	12.2	10.6	11.6
		M	Lower	15.2	13.0	14.3
		F	Lower	12.5	11.1	11.7

Effect of time on smoking pattern

It has been implied that it is preferable for a smoker to change to a brand offering lower deliveries (D.H.S.S., 1976). Although he may smoke a lower delivery brand more intensively to begin with, it is assumed that he will soon become used to it and revert to his former smoking pattern and be satisfied with the lower deliveries.

In order to test for a significant carry over from one phase to the next or an acclimatisation process on switching to a different delivery, the replicates for individuals in each of the three phases were divided into three sub-phases, the first containing replicates 1 to 3, the second, replicates 4 to 6 and the third, replicates 7 to 9. Replicate 10 was dropped. These first and last sub-phase averages in each phase are shown as Table 22.5. The nine-sub-phases were then regarded as 9 levels of a phase factor in a separate set of analyses of variance. The analysis of the new phase factor and the results of a comparison of means are shown in Table 22.6.

Table 22.5 Effect of time on smoking cigarettes with changed delivery

Parameter		Delivery in Phase II	Phase I		Phase II		Phase III	
			Sub-phase 1	Sub-phase 3	Sub-phase 4	Sub-phase 6	Sub-phase 7	Sub-phase 9
Total puff volume	(cm³)	Higher	533	566	453	425	572	504
		Lower	555	558	651	607	547	518
Average puff volume	(cm³)	Higher	40.4	46.2	40.4	39.3	44.8	43.8
		Lower	44.9	46.0	54.5	53.1	48.6	46.6
Average puff duration	(sec)	Higher	2.11	2.38	2.17	2.11	2.32	2.36
		Lower	2.49	2.35	2.84	2.70	2.62	2.38
Average interval between puffs	(sec)	Higher	36.3	39.9	37.4	36.8	37.3	41.6
		Lower	35.8	38.0	35.8	37.5	40.9	42.0
Average lit draw resistance	(cm W.G.)	Higher	19.5	18.8	19.8	19.4	18.5	18.3
		Lower	18.1	19.5	16.5	16.6	18.2	19.2
Average number of puffs		Higher	13.5	12.9	11.7	11.4	13.3	12.1
		Lower	12.5	12.3	12.3	11.8	11.4	11.2
Average butt length	(mm)	Higher	31.7	31.5	34.6	33.2	31.0	30.2
		Lower	31.3	31.0	33.8	32.5	32.3	30.8
Total time alight	(sec)	Higher	473	465	411	390	451	457
		Lower	462	469	448	443	458	458

NOTE: No estimate of the number of cigarettes smoked per day has been included in this table as the system of measurement used was not sufficiently accurate to provide reliable data.

Table 22.6 Significant differences between sub-phases

Parameter	Delivery in Phase II	Sub-Phase Difference				
		1-3	4-3	4-6	6-7	7-9
Total puff volume	Higher		*		*	*
	Lower		*			
Average puff volume	Higher	*	*		*	
	Lower		*		*	
Average puff duration	Higher	*	*		*	
	Lower		*			
Average interval between puffs	Higher					
	Lower					
Average lit draw resistance	Higher					
	Lower		*		*	
Average number of puffs	Higher				*	
	Lower					
Average butt length	Higher		*		*	
	Lower		*			
Total time alight	Higher		*		*	
	Lower					

* Indicates significance at 0.05. The direction of the changes can be obtained from Table 22.5.

Discussion

The results in Tables 22.2 and 22.3 show that smokers have altered their smoking patterns in response to both increased delivery by decreasing the intensity of smoking, and for reduced delivery by increasing the intensity of smoking. These alterations have involved almost every method that can be used on a single cigarette and, with the exception of butt length, significant changes were always in the direction which tended to equalise deliveries in the three phases. The butt length anomaly may be due to the smokers using the length of white paper between the cigarette coal and the tipping paper as a cue to the termination of smoking. It can be seen in Table 22.1 that the tipping paper lengths of the three brands are different.

Table 22.3 indicates that few significant differences in smoking pattern were detected between men and women. This was possibly due to the small number of subjects from which to estimate the variation between people.

Tables 22.2 and 22.3 also show that the lower total volumes of smoke taken from the higher delivery cigarettes were achieved, not only by a reduction in the number of puffs taken but also by shorter individual puff durations, smaller individual puff volumes and a shorter total time alight.

The higher total volumes taken from the low delivery cigarettes were achieved by longer individual puff durations and larger puff volumes.

Since the low delivery brand had a ventilated filter the smoke drawn is diluted with air and it is easier to draw a given volume. This is reflected in the lower average lit draw resistance for the low delivery cigarette.

One of the mechanisms by which a smoker might be expected to compensate for changes in delivery is by smoking different numbers of cigarettes per day. The evidence collected during this study suggests that the number of cigarettes smoked per day is reasonably constant, irrespective of the delivery of the cigarette. Similar results have been reported (Adams, 1976; Goldfarb et al, 1976) where only small differences in the number of cigarettes smoked per day were noted when subjects smoked cigarettes with different nicotine deliveries. It should be made clear, however, that the cigarette consumption figures quoted are approximate. Cigarettes were issued to the subjects on demand, and the figures quoted will include those given away.

Examination of the data for each individual (although not given) showed that all subjects made compensating changes in the way in which they smoked individual cigarettes. Although the individual changes for some of the parameters did not always reach statistical significance their collective effects on delivery were assessed by using the puff duplicator.

The results of smoking pattern duplication (Table 22.4) indicate that subjects almost equalised nicotine and TPM deliveries when changing between the medium and the high delivery brands. However, the subjects did not equalise nicotine or TPM deliveries when changing between the control and low delivery cigarettes, in spite of the increase in smoking intensity shown by these subjects. This may be due to a combination of effects. Ventilation of the filter dilutes the smoke drawn by the smoker in such a way that higher velocity puffs contain a larger proportion of air than low velocity puffs. Additionally the tipping paper length was longer on the low delivery brand so that the smokers were inhibited from taking the puffs closest to the filter which have the highest deliveries.

The ratios of the deliveries obtained when human subjects smoked the cigarettes, as well as the actual deliveries of TPM, nicotine and carbon monoxide, differ widely from those obtained by standard machine smoking conditions and published in the league tables. Our results show that most smokers obtained lower TPM to nicotine ratios than the standard smoking machines and that generally female smokers obtained lower TPM to nicotine ratios than the male smokers. These results and conclusions may, however, only apply to the panel of smokers studied in these experiments.

Nevertheless, we believe that the results indicate the complexity of the changes in smoking behaviour which occur when smokers change brands and the results emphasise the need for considering the possibility of such changes when assessing the intake of smoke components by smokers. The approach we have adopted, comparing the deliveries of cigarettes smoked by a puff duplicator, also gives realistic information as to how a particular type of cigarette has been smoked.

The data in Tables 22.5 and 22.6 were produced in an attempt to establish whether smoking patterns changed during the course of each one month phase of the experiment.

It can be seen from Table 22.6 that most of the significant differences are between sub-phases 3 and 4 and between sub-phases 6 and 7. These changes coincide with the changes in cigarette type from the medium delivery brand to the high or low delivery brand and back again. Only a few significant differences were detected in the way the first and the last groups of three cigarettes were smoked in phase I and phase III and no significant differences were detected between the first and last group of three cigarettes smoked in phase II. These observations indicate that although the subjects modified their smoking patterns in a consistent way when they changed from one brand to another with different delivery, no consistent modification with time was detected.

The observation that smokers have not changed their smoking patterns after one month of smoking a brand with changed deliveries suggests that any modifications to the physiological and psychological mechanisms which govern the intake of smoke by a smoker are longer term. This should be borne in mind if a smoker makes the decision to change to a brand offering substantially different deliveries to his usual brand.

Summary

Frequent measurements of the smoking patterns were recorded for 16 subjects who were changed from a control brand of cigarettes to either a higher or lower delivery brand. Each cigarette brand was smoked exclusively for about four weeks. Representative smoking patterns of each subject were duplicated by machine to measure deliveries of TPM, nicotine and carbon monoxide.

Analyses of these data showed that on average smokers increased the intensity with which they smoked the lower delivery brand and decreased the intensity of smoking the higher delivery brand when compared with the control brand. The number of cigarettes smoked per day did not alter significantly. The amounts of TPM, nicotine and carbon monoxide taken from the medium and high delivery brands by the smokers were similar, although the deliveries of these two brands differ considerably when smoked by machine under standard conditions. Although they smoked the low delivery brand more intensely, the smokers did not equalise the deliveries taken from the low and medium delivery brands.

A further analysis showed that the modified smoking patterns adopted to smoke the brands with changed deliveries were maintained for the period of smoking those brands. The smokers reverted to their former smoking patterns during the last phase of the experiment when they again smoked the control brand.

Acknowledgements

The authors gratefully acknowledge the technical assistance of Mrs. U.C. Hopkins, Mrs. J.R. Lavier, Mr. M.J. Derrick and Mr. S. Basevi.

References

Adams, P.I. (1976) Changes in personal smoking habits brought about by changes in cigarette smoke yield. *Proceedings of the 6th International Tobacco Science Congress.* Tokyo. 102-108.

Ashton, H. & Watson, D.W. (1970) Puffing frequency and nicotine intake in cigarette smokers. *British Medical Journal,* 3, 679-681.

Creighton, D.E., Noble, M.J. & Whewell, R.T. (1978) Instruments to measure, record and duplicate human smoking patterns. *This volume.*

Health Departments of the United Kingdom (1976) *Tar and Nicotine Yields of Cigarettes,* London, D.H.S.S., January 1976.

Frith, C.D. (1971) The effect of varying the nicotine content of cigarettes on human smoking behaviour. *Psychopharmacologia,* **19**, 188,192.

Goldfarb, T., Gritz, E.R., Jarvik, M.E. & Stolerman, I.P. (1976) Reactions to cigarettes as a function of nicotine and tar. *Clinical Pharmacology and Therapeutics,* **19**, 767-772.

Gritz, E.R., Baer-Weiss, V. & Jarvik, M.E. (1976) Titration of nicotine intake with full-length and half-length cigarettes. *Clinical Pharmacology and Therapeutics,* **20**, 552-556.

Overton, J.R. (1973) Filtration of cigarette smoke: Relative contributions of inertial impaction, difference deposition and direct interception. *Beiträge zur Takakforschung,* **7**, 117-120.

Russell, M.A.H. (1974) Realistic goals for smoking and health: A case for safer smoking. *Lancet,* **1**, 254-258.

Todd, G.F. (1975) *Changes in the Smoking Patterns in the U.K.* Tobacco Research Council, London.

23. The effect of smoking pattern on smoke deliveries

D E CREIGHTON AND P H LEWIS

Introduction

When the human smoking patterns recorded in a previous experiment (Creighton and Lewis, 1978) were duplicated it was shown that the TPM to nicotine ratios achieved by the panel were generally lower than when the same cigarettes were smoked by a standard smoking machine to the standard smoking conditions. This difference has been attributed to the way in which the human subjects smoked the cigarettes. From the results of the same experiment it was observed that female smokers tended to have lower TPM to nicotine ratios than male subjects and that generally there are differences between the way in which male and female subjects smoke cigarettes. The female smokers tended to take more puffs of smaller volume per puff at more frequent intervals than male smokers. The peak flow rates of the individual puffs taken by female smokers tended to be lower and the rising edge of the puff profile sharper than those taken by male smokers.

Evidence has been published (Frisch and Spivey, 1968; Seehofer and Wennberg, 1971) that the puff profile (shape) influences the deliveries of a cigarette. Early peaked profiles tended to increase the delivery of nicotine relative to the TPM components, whereas late peaked profiles tended to increase the delivery of TPM components relative to nicotine. The deliveries for other profiles examined were intermediate.

This report describes an experiment to investigate the main and interaction effects of puff shape, puff volume and interval between puffs on deliveries of TPM, nicotine and carbon monoxide, the ratios of the deliveries of these components and the filtration efficiencies for TPM and nicotine.

Method

The experiment made use of the puff duplicator developed in Southampton (Creighton, Noble and Whewell, 1978) which normally smokes cigarettes to human smoking patterns recorded on paper tape by the smoking analyser and data logger. However, it can be programmed to work as a versatile research smoking engine and in this experiment special paper tapes were prepared representing the specific smoking patterns to be studied.

A range of puff volumes and intervals between puffs were chosen to cover the range typically observed when human smokers have been studied. The puff volumes used were 23, 35, 52.5 and 78.8 cm^3 sec^{-1} and the intervals between puffs were 19, 33, 58 and 102 seconds. Human smoking patterns outside this range have been measured but such patterns may be considered as exceptional.

The puff profiles (shapes) selected for this study were not actual human profiles. Four shapes, early triangle, late triangle, sine curve (bell) and square were constructed mathematically to represent the main characteristics of human profiles. The puff duration was fixed at two seconds and a smoking pattern tape was constructed for each of the 64 combinations of the above factors (four shapes, four volumes, four intervals). Each tape consisted of a long series of identical puffs and intervals used to control the smoking of the test cigarettes on the duplicator.

The cigarette brand chosen for this study was typical of the king size filter tipped cigarettes at present available on the U.K.market. The dimensions and deliveries of this cigarette when smoked under standard conditions are shown in Table 23.1.

Table 23.1 Dimensions and analytical data for the cigarette (when smoked under standard conditions).

Tobacco Rod Length	(mm)	64
Tobacco Type		Flue-cured Blend
Filter Material		Cellulose Acetate
Filter Length	(mm)	20
Tipping Paper Length	(mm)	25
Draw Resistance ($17.5cc^3/sec^{-1}$)(cm W.G.)*		12-14
TPM Delivery	(mg)	31
Nicotine (TNA) Delivery	(mg)	1.6
Carbon Monoxide Delivery	(mg)	22
Puff Number		9.4

* 1 cm W.G. = 98 Nm^{-2}. The cigarette filter is not ventilated.

The duplicator was calibrated and operated as previously described (Creighton et al, 1978) except each cigarette was marked by pencil at 28 mm (tipping paper length + 3 mm). When the burn reached the mark the duplicator was stopped and the cigarette extinguished.

The delivery of TPM was measured by direct weighing of the Cambridge filter pad in its holder. The filter tip was cut from the cigarette, when it had been smoked, and weighed. Tips were also cut from forty unsmoked cigarettes, and an average weight found for comparison with the tips containing particulate matter. In this way an estimate could be made of the filtration efficiency of the filter to TPM. Both the filtration efficiency for TPM and nicotine were estimated by:

$$F.E. = \frac{\text{weight on tip x 100}}{\text{weight on tip + weight on pad}}$$

The nicotine contained in the filter tip and on the Cambridge filter pad were measured as total nicotine alkaloids by a standard autoanalyser method. The carbon monoxide content of the gas phase was measured as percentage by volume by an ·

infrared gas analyser. The number of puffs drawn from the cigarette, and hence the number of clearing puffs, were noted so that the percentage and weight of carbon monoxide in the whole smoke could be calculated.

Five replicates were smoked for each of the 64 tapes. The data from the five replicates were averaged and are shown in Tables 23.2 - 23.5. The data for the four volumes and four intervals are shown for each of the four puff shapes.

Table 23.2 Sine shaped puff profile

Puff Volume (cm^3)	Puff Interval (sec)	Number of Puffs	Butt Length (mm)	Butt TPM (mg)	Butt Nicotine (mg)	Cambridge Filter TPM (mg)	Cambridge Filter Nicotine (mg)	Carbon Monoxide (mg)
23	19	20.6	28.2	24.3	0.96	28.3	2.18	31.3
23	33	14.2	28.8	15.6	0.59	19.2	1.43	18.4
23	58	9.4	27.8	11.0	0.63	13.4	1.29	14.0
23	102	6.6	27.4	10.5	0.24	7.3	0.64	8.9
35	19	18.2	28.1	29.5	1.03	40.5	2.81	32.8
35	33	12.6	28.4	23.1	0.87	31.1	2.29	31.5
35	58	8.8	28.0	13.6	0.59	18.0	1.54	24.5
35	102	6.0	28.2	10.9	0.50	11.8	1.00	14.5
52.5	19	14.6	28.0	28.6	1.26	49.5	3.73	47.3
52.5	33	11.2	28.0	25.4	0.97	36.4	2.93	46.3
52.5	58	8.0	28.0	17.6	0.77	25.5	2.32	30.3
52.5	102	5.0	28.2	10.7	0.41	13.9	1.31	17.3
78.8	19	13.6	28.0	30.6	1.16	65.8	3.57	68.6
78.8	33	11.0	29.2	24.5	0.99	48.2	2.81	48.4
78.8	58	8.4	28.4	20.0	0.80	31.5	2.03	36.8
78.8	102	5.4	27.4	15.1	0.36	21.6	1.28	28.2

Analysis of data

The data from this experiment were coded, punched onto cards and read into a computer. They were analysed by a univariate analysis of variance technique.

The deliveries per unit volume were estimated using the total volume of smoke taken and the delivery ratios also calculated. The filtration efficiencies for TPM and nicotine were calculated, giving the following eight responses to be studied in this analysis.
1. TPM delivery (μg/cm^3)
2. TNA delivery (μg/cm^3)
3. Carbon monoxide delivery (μg/cm^3)
4. TPM/TNA delivery ratio
5. CO/TNA delivery ratio.

6. TPM/CO delivery ratio.
7. Filtration efficiency for TPM (%).
8. Filtration efficiency for nicotine (%).

A univariate analysis of variance was performed for each of the above responses using the following model for the observations:

$$Y_{ijkl} = \mu + V_i + I_j + S_k + VI_{ij} + VS_{ik} + IS_{jk} + VIS_{ijk} + \varepsilon_{ijkl}$$

where Y_{ijkl} represents the measured response.

Table 23.3 Early peak triangle puff profile

Puff Volume (cm³)	Puff Interval (sec)	Number of Puffs	Butt Length (mm)	Butt TPM (mg)	Butt Nicotine (mg)	Cambridge Filter TPM (mg)	Cambridge Filter Nicotine (mg)	Carbon Monoxide (mg)
23	19	19.8	29.0	18.8	0.92	25.8	2.09	21.6
23	33	14.6	27.8	16.9	0.81	10.8	1.84	18.0
23	58	10.0	27.8	13.1	0.56	13.9	1.32	13.0
23	102	6.4	27.5	10.1	0.41	6.4	0.77	6.4
35	19	18.2	27.8	30.1	0.93	38.6	2.51	32.0
35	33	13.0	28.6	20.5	0.65	27.3	1.89	23.3
35	58	9.0	27.6	12.8	0.58	19.5	1.65	19.4
35	102	6.0	27.6	14.9	0.40	12.2	0.96	11.4
52.5	19	16.2	28.4	29.7	1.06	49.3	3.10	47.2
52.5	33	12.0	28.4	25.6	0.85	36.0	2.53	39.8
52.5	58	8.0	27.1	19.9	0.90	27.4	2.29	28.4
52.5	102	5.8	27.6	17.1	0.51	16.3	1.41	22.3
78.8	19	13.0	27.4	30.8	1.01	60.0	3.19	53.8
78.8	33	11.2	28.0	29.2	0.93	45.4	3.04	46.8
78.8	58	8.4	28.3	19.4	0.60	30.5	2.06	31.5
78.8	102	6.0	27.6	17.2	0.42	21.1	1.39	22.6

μ represents the general mean
V_i (i = 1,4) represents the effect of volume i (fixed)
I_j (j=1,4) represents the effect of interval j (fixed)
S_k (k=1,4) represents the effect of shape k (fixed)
VI_{ij} represents the volume-interval interaction (fixed)
VS_{ik} represents the volume-shape interaction (fixed)
IS_{jk} represents the interval-shape interaction (fixed)
VIS_{ijk} represents the volume-interval-shape interaction (fixed)
ε_{ijkl} (l=1,5) represents the residual error for replicate I of the ijk factor combination.

Table 23.4 Late peaked triangle puff profile

Puff Volume (cm^3)	Puff Interval (sec)	Number of Puffs	Butt Length (mm)	Butt TPM (mg)	Butt Nicotine (mg)	Cambridge Filter TPM (mg)	Cambridge Filter Nicotine (mg)	Carbon Monoxide (mg)
23	19	20.4	27.8	22.6	0.91	27.7	2.07	30.3
23	33	15.0	28.2	22.5	0.82	22.5	1.79	29.7
23	58	10.2	28.0	16.5	0.57	14.3	1.25	21.8
23	102	6.4	27.3	9.0	0.34	8.0	0.77	8.4
35	19	17.4	28.0	28.2	1.04	40.8	2.96	45.7
35	33	13.4	27.8	26.0	0.87	34.0	2.49	45.1
35	58	9.0	27.7	19.0	0.66	22.5	2.02	28.2
35	102	6.0	28.0	9.6˙	0.33	11.7	0.99	18.3
52.5	19	15.8	28.8	31.4	1.06	58.1	3.03	64.4
52.5	33	12.6	28.4	26.1	0.97	48.3	2.67	49.6
52.5	58	8.8	28.2	20.7	0.79	33.0	2.23	44.5
52.5	102	5.8	27.2	15.5	0.52	20.8	1.58	23.7
78.8	19	14.0	28.5	27.7	0.96	70.9	3.46	51.9
78.8	33	11.2	27.8	29.6	0.93	52.6	3.00	42.6
78.8	58	7.6	29.0	26.8	0.72	36.8	2.06	39.0
78.8	102	5.4	27.7	13.3	0.39	25.2	1.48	31.0

It has been assumed that the residual error terms for replicates are random and have independent normal distributions with zero mean and variance σ^2.

The analysis of variance tables for the eight analyses indicate that each of the three factors, puff volume, puff shape and interval between puffs has a highly significant effect on each of the deliveries and delivery ratios. Volume and shape affect the filtration efficiency for nicotine and volume and interval affect the filtration efficiency for TPM.

The presence of highly significant interaction terms indicates that the effect of a factor on a response is not independent of the values of the other two factors.

The main effects are illustrated in Figures 23.1 to 23.8. The error bars represent the standard errors on the mean values, estimated using the residual error variance shown in the analysis of variance tables.

In each Figure the response is averaged over all levels of two of the factors and plotted against the third factor showing the main effect of each of the three factors on the deliveries, delivery ratios and filtration efficiencies studied.

An orthogonal polynomial breakdown was made for each response as a function of puff volume and as a function of puff interval. The percentage of the total sum

Table 23.5 Square puff profile

Puff Volume (cm^3)	Puff Interval (sec)	Number of puffs	Butt			Cambridge Filter		Carbon monoxide (mg)
			Length (mm)	TPM (mg)	Nicotine (mg)	TPM (mg)	Nicotine (mg)	
23	19	20.6	28.1	23.9	0.89	27.1	1.99	17.4
23	33	16.0	28.8	21.0	0.61	19.2	1.27	17.7
23	58	10.6	27.6	14.3	0.48	13.3	0.98	11.8
23	102	6.4	27.5	9.5	0.32	6.1	0.63	6.7
35	19	17.2	27.6	32.8	1.37	38.9	3.18	19.4
35	33	12.6	28.2	21.5	1.09	29.7	2.58	26.3
35	58	9.0	27.5	18.0	0.74	20.7	1.78	22.2
35	102	5.8	27.6	14.6	0.48	12.2	1.10	10.8
52.5	19	14.8	27.5	30.5	1.44	53.3	3.62	34.2
52.5	33	11.4	28.0	26.0	1.15	40.3	3.13	30.2
52.5	58	8.2	28.0	20.8	0.78	28.5	2.29	31.8
52.5	102	5.6	28.2	11.9	0.57	18.4	1.49	19.0
78.8	19	12.4	28.9	27.9	0.90	60.6	3.25	54.8
78.8	33	10.2	28.6	27.1	0.98	58.7	3.15	49.9
78.8	58	8.0	28.0	25.8	0.78	41.8	2.41	41.9
78.8	102	5.0	27.9	14.7	0.40	24.1	1.57	29.6

of squares of deviations about the mean response value for which the linear component of the polynomial breakdown accounts is shown on each of the appropriate graphs.

The effect of puff interval

It can be seen from the figures that, on average, each of the three deliveries reaches a maximum at one of the two intermediate intervals but for TPM the maximum is reached at a shorter interval than for carbon monoxide or TNA.

The delivery of carbon monoxide has been shown to increase as the interval between puffs increases up to a maximum interval of 1 minute and then to decrease again. It can also be seen that the TPM to nicotine ratio decreases systematically with increasing puff interval; 88% of the sum of squares being explained by the linear component of the orthogonal polynomial breakdown. The TPM to carbon monoxide ratio also shows a systematic decrease with increasing intervals between puffs whilst the carbon monoxide to nicotine ratio was fairly constant with increasing intervals between puffs.

MAIN EFFECTS FOR TPM

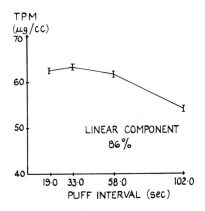

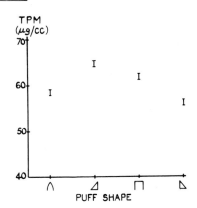

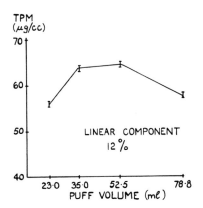

Fig. 23.1

It can be seen that the filtration efficiency of the filter to nicotine does not change with increasing intervals between puffs, whereas the filtration efficiency to TPM increases almost linearly with increasing intervals between puffs, 99% of the sum of squares being explained by the linear component. This effect may be due to the absorption of water by the cigarette filter during the interval between puffs.

The effect of puff volume
The figures indicate that increasing puff volume has a similar effect on deliveries as does increasing interval between puffs; that is the deliveries again rise to a maximum and then start to decrease.

Examination of the delivery ratios reveals some previously unreported effects. It can be seen that the TPM to nicotine and carbon monoxide to nicotine ratios increase with increasing puff volume while the TPM to carbon monoxide ratio is approximately constant.

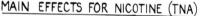

MAIN EFFECTS FOR NICOTINE (TNA)

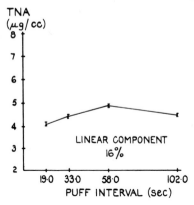

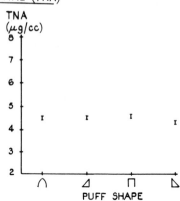

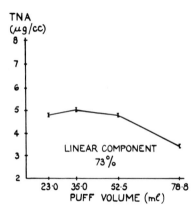

Fig. 23.2

For the TPM to nicotine ratio 96% of the sum of squares may be accounted for by the linear component of the orthogonal polynomial breakdown and for the carbon monoxide to nicotine ratio 99% is explained.

The filtration efficiencies for both nicotine and TPM decrease logarithmically with increasing puff volume, 99% of the sum of squares being accounted for by the log relationship. Since the puff duration was constant at 2 seconds, increasing puff volume is equivalent to increasing puff velocity and the inverse relationship between filtration efficiency and puff velocity previously reported (Overton, 1973) has been confirmed.

The effect of puff shape
The nicotine delivery is almost independent of puff shape at least when averaged over all levels of interval and volume. For TPM and carbon monoxide the deliveries are greatest from the late triangle shape and least for the early triangle

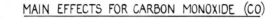

MAIN EFFECTS FOR CARBON MONOXIDE (CO)

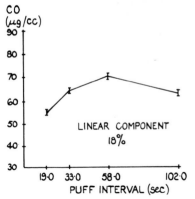

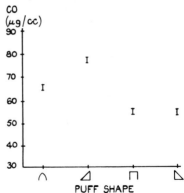

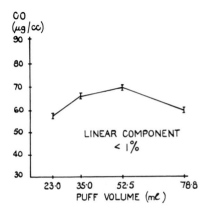

Fig. 23.3

shape puffs. This was also observed by Frisch and Spivey (1968) and Seehofer and Wennberg (1971) for TPM.

On average the bell or sine shaped puff gave higher carbon monoxide deliveries and lower TPM deliveries than the square shaped puff.

The filtration efficiency for TPM was not dependent on puff shape but for nicotine the filtration efficiency for the square puff was significantly higher than for the late peaked triangular puff. The early peaked triangle and bell shaped puffs were intermediate.

The interaction effects

In order to examine the two factor interactions for each response, the response values must be averaged over the third factor for each combination of levels of the factors in the interaction. The response is then plotted against each of the factors for all levels of the other factor. These plots are not shown, but it was clear that although the description of the main effects given above is also broadly

MAIN EFFECTS FOR TPM TO NICOTINE RATIO

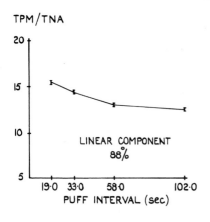

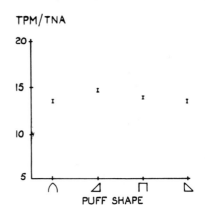

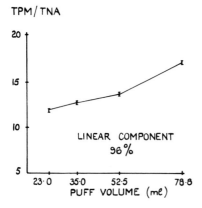

Fig. 23.4

correct for the interaction plots, there are small but significant differences in the shapes of the distributions.

Discussion

The analysis shows that the actual deliveries of smoke components and the ratios of the deliveries of smoke components are not primarily dependent on a single factor such as the volume of smoke drawn, the interval between puffs or the shape of the puffs. All three factors have their own influence on the deliveries and ratios of deliveries as well as having an interaction effect.

From a practical point of view this means that it is not possible to predict with accuracy the deliveries or ratios of the deliveries of a cigarette simply from a knowledge of the volume of smoke drawn by a human smoker and the deliveries when the cigarette was smoked under standard conditions (unless the

MAIN EFFECTS FOR CARBON MONOXIDE TO NICOTINE RATIO

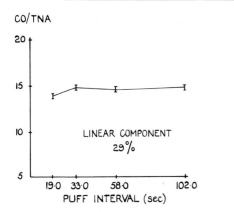

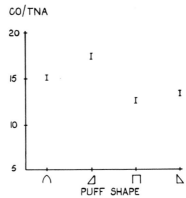

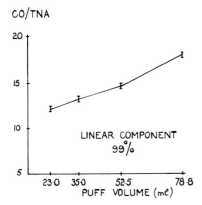

Fig. 23.5

smoker used exactly the same smoking pattern as a standard smoking machine).

We have observed that the volumes of smoke drawn from a cigarette by a human smoker tend to decrease as successive puffs are taken, and the intervals between puffs tend to increase. The puff shape tends to be characteristic for an individual but some subjects use a variety of puff shapes. Few subjects could be said to have an invariate puff profile. It is unlikely that the deliveries or ratios of the deliveries of a cigarette for a human smoker could be readily calculated mathematically even with a knowledge of the complete smoking pattern. The league table deliveries only apply to one arbitrary smoking pattern.

The most common way of estimating actual deliveries of nicotine and some particulate matter components for human smokers is to analyse the filter tips from their discarded butts. This method has the disadvantage of assuming a constant filtration efficiency based on standard machine smoking which may lead to systematic as well as random errors in delivery estimates. No estimate of carbon monoxide delivery may be obtained in this way.

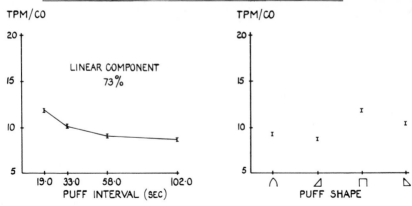

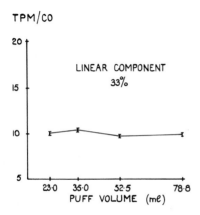

Fig. 23.6

The data presented in this report indicates the importance of exact duplication of the smoking patterns of human smokers when attempting to estimate deliveries obtained by human smokers.

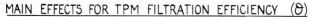

MAIN EFFECTS FOR TPM FILTRATION EFFICIENCY (θ)

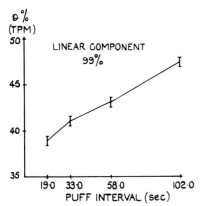

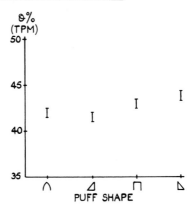

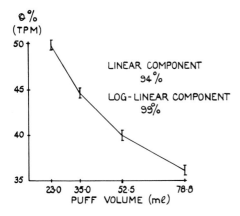

Fig. 23.7

Acknowledgement

The authors gratefully acknowledge the technical assistance of Mrs. U.C. Hopkins, Mr. M.J. Derrick and Mr. S. Basevi.

References

Creighton, D.E. & Lewis, P.H. (1978) The effect of different cigarettes on human smoking patterns. *This volume.*

Creighton, D.E., Noble, M.J. & Whewell, R.T. (1978) Instruments to measure, record and duplicate human smoking patterns. *This volume.*

Frisch, A.F. & Spivey, R. (1968) The effect of puff shape on smoke deliveries. *22nd Tobacco Chemists' Conference.* Richmond, V.A.

Overton, J.R. (1973) Filtration of cigarette smoke: Relative contributions of

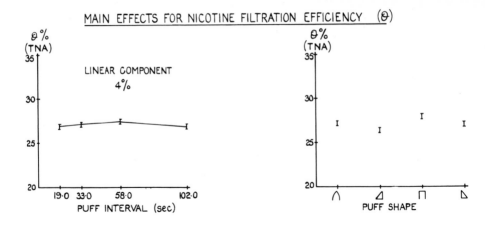

MAIN EFFECTS FOR NICOTINE FILTRATION EFFICIENCY   (θ)

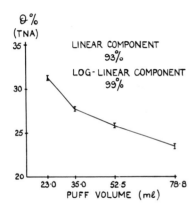

Fig. 23.8

inertial impaction, diffusional deposition and direct interception. *Beiträge zur Tabakforschung,* **7**, 117-120.

Seehofer, F. & Wennberg, D. (1971) Einfluss verschiedener zugvolumenprofile aug ausbeute und zusammensetzung des rauches beim maschinellen abrauchen von cigaretten. *Beiträge zur Tabakforschung,* **6**, 7-11.

24. Smoking behaviour and nicotine intake in smokers presented with a 'two-thirds' cigarette

HEATHER ASHTON, ROBERT STEPNEY AND J W THOMPSON

Introduction

The present study was designed to contribute to an understanding of the role of nicotine in smoking motivation. Various experimental approaches (outlined in Table 24.1) have been used in the investigation of this question, but none, so far, has produced unequivocal results. Animal studies using the rat (Clark, 1969) and the monkey (Deneau & Inoki, 1967; Jarvik, 1967) have shown that nicotine has some intrinsic reward value for these animals and the pattern of use of nicotine-containing substances, together with the effects of their withdrawal, suggest this is also the case for man.

Table 24.1 Experimental approaches used in the investigation of the role of nicotine in smoking motivation.

A. Animal studies:

    (i)   voluntary self-administration

    (ii)   use as reward

B. Man:

    (i)   patterns of tobacco use

    (ii)   withdrawal effects

    (iii)   self regulation of nicotine intake

            i.e. apparent adaptation of smoking behaviour with

            (a)   provision of nicotine from an alternative source - gum; intravenous injection.

            (b)   blocked nicotine effect.

            (c)   altered availability of nicotine from the cigarette - manipulation of nicotine content of tobacco, filter efficiency, cigarette length.

The main concern of human behavioural research into smoking, however, has been to demonstrate experimentally the self-regulation of nicotine intake, on the assumption that if smoking is primarily a form of nicotine self-administration, compensatory changes in behaviour will be produced by altering the availability of nicotine either from the cigarette or from alternative sources.

The reduction of the availability of nicotine from cigarettes by manipulating the nicotine content of the tobacco, or by increasing the extraction efficiency of the filter, has repeatedly been found to increase the rate of smoking (Ashton & Watson, 1970; Finnegan, Larson & Haag, 1945; Frith, 1971; Goldfarb, Jarvik & Glick, 1970; Kozlowski, Jarvik & Gritz, 1975; Russell et al, 1975; Turner, Sillett & Ball, 1974).

Pharmacologically blocking nicotine's central action has a similar effect (Stolerman et al, 1973).

The provision of nicotine in orally administered nicotine-containing chewing gum was shown by Russell et al (1976) to decrease the rate of smoking. This result has also been found by Lucchesi, Schuster & Emley (1967) following intravenous injection of nicotine although the most recent study to use this alternative source of nicotine (Kumar et al, 1977) has failed to find this effect.

Although the behavioural changes found to follow this experimental manipulation of nicotine availability demonstrate an often significant degree of regulation of nicotine intake, the changes are generally not large enough to prove convincingly that the self-administration of nicotine is the major factor in the maintenance of the smoking habit.

Altering the length of cigarette available to be smoked is a further experimental approach to the problem. The present study takes as its starting point work by Gritz, Baer-Weiss & Jarvik (1976) who showed that subjects smoking half-length cigarettes obtained proportionately more nicotine from the half cigarettes than from the whole ones. Nicotine intake was measured in terms of the amount of nicotine excreted in the urine, which is a rather indirect measure of intake and one subject to various uncontrolled variables such as urinary pH. No behavioural measures were used during this essentially non-laboratory investigation and the authors pointed out that measurement of such variables should play a part in any subsequent study.

In the present experiment subjects smoked two-thirds of their normal length of tobacco rod. The amount of nicotine drawn into the mouth was estimated on the basis of the analysis of residual nicotine in smoked filter tips, and the change in plasma nicotine levels before and after smoking provided direct measures of nicotine intake. Certain variables of smoking behaviour were also measured and these were related to any apparent self-regulation of nicotine intake.

The effects of smoking full and 'shortened' cigarettes on heart rate and fingertip temperature change and on subjective ratings of cigarette satisfaction were also compared.

Method

Subjects

The study involved 14 paid subjects (seven male and seven female) with ages ranging from 18-40 years, but concentrated in the 18-22 age group (mean age 22.9 years). All subjects had smoked 10-25 middle tar cigarettes per day for two or more years. All inhaled.

Throughout the experiment, subjects smoked their own regular brand of cigarettes. Subjects agreed to participate in an experiment 'investigating some of the physiological responses to smoking' and remained unaware that we were interested in their smoking behaviour and in the regulation of nicotine intake.

Procedure

Subjects were randomly assigned to two groups, differing in the order in which they experienced the experimental conditions. The detailed procedure for each group is set out in Table 24.2.

Table 24.2 Procedure

	Group I subjects n = 8	Group II subjects n = 6
Stage 1	Normal smoking	Smoke normal cigarettes over 24 hours and collect butts.
2	Smoke full cigarette over 24 hours and collect butts	Smoke two-third cigarettes over 24 hours and collect butts.
3	Smoke one full length cigarette in laboratory	Smoke one two-third cigarette in laboratory
4	Smoke two-third cigarettes over 24 hours and collect butts.	Smoke full cigarettes over 24 hours and collect butts
5	Smoke one two-third cigarette in laboratory	Smoke one full length cigarette in laboratory.

The experiment involved two conditions: *the full cigarette condition* in which subjects smoked cigarettes in their usual way, and *the two-thirds cigarette condition* in which subjects smoked only two-thirds of the length of tobacco rod normally consumed.

Each subject attended the laboratory on two successive days, at the same time of day. On each attendance subjects smoked either a full cigarette or a two-thirds cigarette. Subjects also smoked full and two-thirds cigarettes over 24 hour periods, during which they collected their cigarette butts in an air-tight tin.

Before two-thirds cigarettes were encountered by the subjects (and before they were mentioned) members of both groups had collected the butts from a 24 hour period of normal smoking. These butts, unrestricted as to length and number, were counted and the mean butt length calculated. The mean butt length, subtracted from the total length of the cigarette, indicated the length of tobacco rod normally consumed. Two-thirds of this length measured from the distal end of the cigarette then indicated the length of tobacco rod to be consumed in the 'shortened' cigarette condition (Fig. 24.1).   The point beyond which subjects were not to smoke was shown by a red line (dotted in Fig. 24.1) drawn on the cigarette. The two-thirds cigarettes were thus 'tailor-made' for individual subjects - who differed considerably in the length of tobacco rod normally consumed - to ensure a uniform degree of 'deprivation'.

To prevent subjects simply increasing the number of cigarettes smoked to compensate for their decreased size, subjects were issued with precisely the same number of two-thirds cigarettes as the full cigarettes they had smoked in the

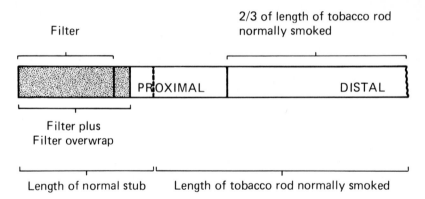

Fig. 24.1 The two-thirds cigarette.

previous 24 hours, and they were asked, and agreed, not to supplement their 'issue' of cigarettes from other sources.

The experimental procedure outlined in Table 24.2 allowed smokers of both groups 24 hours experience with the two-thirds cigarettes in which to adjust their smoking behaviour to the unusual length (if any adjustment was to be made) before the two-thirds cigarette was smoked in the laboratory. The time-table for Group II subjects also required a similar period for adjustment on their return to normal, full-length, cigarettes.

Measures

The butts collected by subjects from cigarettes smoked over the 24 hour periods were counted, their length measured, and their nicotine content assayed. Butts from laboratory-smoked cigarettes were also measured and assayed for nicotine. On each attendance subjects were asked to rate on a 100 mm bipolar scale the 'degree of enjoyment and satisfaction' they had experienced from the previous 24 hours' cigarettes, and the degree of enjoyment and satisfaction they had experienced from the laboratory-smoked cigarette.

Unknown to the subjects, the smoking of each laboratory cigarette was observed through a one-way screen and the duration of each puff and interpuff interval marked on an event recorder.

Heart rate and fingertip temperature were recorded during the smoking of each laboratory cigarette, and for five minutes pre and post smoking. The ECG was recorded from chest electrodes and fingertip temperature by a thermistor (linked to a digital thermometer) strapped to the second finger of the nondominant hand.

Blood samples (20 ml) were taken via an indwelling cannula one to two minutes pre-smoking and one to two minutes post-smoking on both laboratory attendances.

Plasma nicotine concentrations were measured by combined capillary column gas chromatography-mass spectrometry according to the method described by Dow and Hall (1977).

Results

Subjective ratings

When asked to rate the enjoyment and satisfaction they had been given by the full
and two-thirds cigarettes, the subjects produced no very clear picture of preference.
The majority of subjects found the full cigarettes more enjoyable and satisfying
both in the laboratory and over the full 24 hours' smoking, but no statistically
significant differences in the ratings were found.

Heart rate and fingertip temperature

Since both heart rate and fingertip temperature are very responsive to nicotine
intake, comparison of the effects of the full and two-thirds cigarettes on these
variables should provide information on the dose of nicotine taken by subjects
in the two experimental conditions.

Table 24.3 Heart rate and fingertip temperature change with full and two-thirds
cigarettes.

Heart rate increase:		beats/min.		%	
		full	2/3	full	2/3
$\bar{x}$		12.86	13.26	16.91	16.95
se		2.14	1.76	2.87	2.23
t		.3 ns		.03 ns	
Fingertip temperature decrease:		$^{\circ}C$		%	
		full	2/3	full	2/3
$\bar{x}$		1.18	.71	3.74	2.31
se		.33	.21	.99	.61
t		1.85 $p < .05$		1.77 $p < .05$	

n = 14

The heart rate figures shown in Table 24.3 are based on the difference between
the mean heart rate over five minutes immediately pre-smoking and the mean
heart rate during smoking.

The fingertip temperature figures are based on the difference between fingertip
temperature at the time the cigarette was lit and the time it was extinguished.

The increase in heart rate during smoking was almost exactly the same in the
full and the two-thirds cigarette condition, there being a very slight (non significant)
tendency for the heart rate increase to be greater (in both absolute and percentage
terms) in the two-thirds cigarette condition. This could be accounted for on the
basis of a faster *rate* of nicotine intake in the two-thirds cigarette condition, even
if the total dose of nicotine is lower.

Table 24.3 also shows the way smoking affected fingertip temperature. In both conditions temperature fell during smoking and here (in contrast to changes in heart rate), there is a significant difference ($p < .05$) between the full and two-thirds conditions, the greater effect being found in the full condition.

Smoking behaviour

From the smoking variables measured it was possible to calculate the mean puff duration and mean interpuff interval for the smoking of each laboratory cigarette.

Thirteen out of the 14 subjects responded to the two-thirds cigarettes either by increasing their puff duration or by lessening the interval between puffs, or by doing both. Since either method would serve to make possible a greater than usual rate of nicotine intake the most convenient way of expressing behavioural change is by combining them, considering the total time the subject spent puffing as a percentage of the total time the cigarette was lit.

Table 24.4 Smoking behaviour with full and two-thirds cigarettes.

	Mean puff duration (secs)		Mean interpuff interval (secs)		% puff time	
	full	2/3	full	2/3	full	2/3
$\bar{x}$	1.47	1.6	24.0	19.11	5.46	7.61
se						
t		1.5 ns		2.6 p$<$.05		3.4 p $<$.005

n = 14

The mean percent time spent puffing, for the group as a whole, increased from 5.46 in the full cigarette condition to 7.61 in the two-thirds cigarette condition - a difference significant at the .005 level and indicating the much more intensive smoking of the reduced-length cigarettes (Table 24.4).

There were, however, considerable individual differences in the extent of behavioural compensation. Figs. 24.2 (a) and (b) show puffing profiles plotted for the smoking of the full and two-thirds cigarettes by two subjects.

Fig. 24.2 (a) is the puffing profile for subject E.J., who shows a doubling in percent puff time, indicating a considerably more intense smoking of the two-thirds cigarette. This is reflected in the compressed pattern of the lower puffing profile.

Subject M.J., however, (Fig. 24.2 (b)) showed very little behavioural change. Both the mean puff duration and the mean interpuff interval are almost unaltered, and the pattern of the puffing profile shows no compression of puffs into the shorter period of time taken to smoke the two-thirds cigarette.

Nicotine intake: butt analysis

Since the amount of nicotine retained by the filter tip of a cigarette is proportional to the amount which passes through it, the amount of nicotine drawn into the mouth of the smoker can be estimated by measuring the nicotine left in the smoked filter tip. The filter efficiency of cigarettes differs according to brand and to take account of this the following formula is used:

$$NS = \frac{Nr\,(1 - TR)}{TR}$$

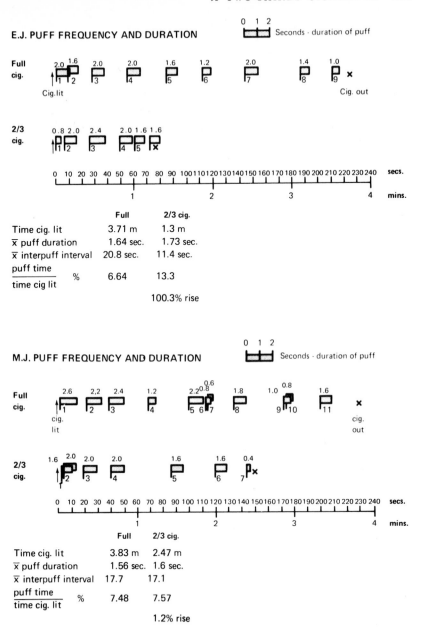

Fig. 24.2 (a) Puffing profile for subject E.J. showing marked behavioural adaptation. The duration of each puff is represented graphically by the length of the stippled rectangles and numerically by the values (in seconds) above each rectangle. The interpuff intervals are shown as the distance between the numbered vertical lines, measured along the bottom scale.

Fig. 24.2 (b) Puffing profile for subject M.J. showing little behavioural change.

where   TR = tip retention efficiency
          NS = nicotine presented to smoker
          Nr = nicotine retained in tip

Analysis of the nicotine retained in the filters of both laboratory-smoked cigarettes and the 24 hour cigarette samples was carried out at the B.A.T. Group Research and Development Centre, Southampton. On the basis of this information the estimates of nicotine presented to the smoker by the full and two-thirds cigarettes were as shown in the left hand columns of Table 24.5.

Table 24.5 Mean nicotine delivery from full and two-thirds cigarettes. Estimates of nicotine delivery are based on analysis of the nicotine retained in smoked filter tips (butt analysis). The expected deliveries are based on smoking machine data.

	Actual deliveries m/g/cig. $\pm$ s.e.		Two-thirds full %	Expected deliveries mg/cig. $\pm$ s.e.		Two-thirds full %
	full	2/3		full	2/3	
Laboratory smoked cigarette	$1.122\pm.07$ (1)	$0.811\pm.04$ (3)	72.3	$1.006\pm.07$	$0.665\pm.03$	66.1
Mean value for 24 hrs. cigarettes	$0.969\pm.05$ (2)	$0.732\pm.04$ (4)	75.5	$1.003\pm.05$	$0.666\pm.03$	66.4

(1)	vs (3)	6.78	<.001
(2)	vs (4)	16.82	<.001
(1)	vs (2)	3.71	<.005
(3)	vs (4)	2.12	<.05

Gritz *et al*(1976) found that when smoking the half cigarette nearer the filter, subjects were able to obtain a dose of nicotine not significantly different from that obtained when smoking full cigarettes. By contrast, in the present experiment, subjects obtained significantly less nicotine from the two-thirds cigarettes than from the full ones both in the laboratory and over 24 hours' smoking. Thus despite the behavioural changes observed the subjects' nicotine intake from the two-thirds cigarettes did not even approximate to that from the full cigarettes. Subjects obtained, on average, 75.5% of the full cigarette yield when smoking the two-thirds cigarettes over a 24 hour period, and 72.3% of the full cigarette yield when smoking them in the laboratory.

Figures presented by Gritz *et al* (1976) suggest that 61% of the nicotine-in-smoke delivered by a typical American cellulose acetate filter cigarette comes from the half of the cigarette nearer the filter tip (the 'proximal half') and only 39% from the 'distal half'. Although these figures are based on the standardised puff volume, duration, velocity and interpuff interval of a smoking machine, the smoker experiences a similar effect of rod filtration. The ability of Gritz' subjects to extract from the proximal half of a cigarette a dose of nicotine not significantly different from that obtained from the full cigarette, and their failure to do this when smoking the distal half, is evidence that this is in fact the case.

The filtration of smoke is exponentially related to the length of tobacco rod and the confounding influence of any rod filtration effects in the present experiment can be taken into account either by calculation or by direct measurement. Using a smoking machine it is possible to obtain a figure for the expected delivery of nicotine for any length of cigarette smoked. These expected deliveries, based on the actual length of tobacco rod smoked by individual subjects in each experimental condition are shown in the right hand columns of Table 24.5.

On the basis of the standardised behaviour of a smoking machine, we would expect subjects smoking two-thirds cigarettes to have obtained 66.1% of the full cigarette dose in the laboratory, and 66.4% of the full cigarette dose over the 24 hour period. The fact that these percentages are close to the 66.7% expected by simple comparison of lengths is coincidental and is due to subjects leaving slightly different butt lengths for the whole and two-thirds length cigarettes.

As stated earlier, subjects obtained 72.3% and 75.5% of the full cigarette dose - a slightly greater proportion than expected.

The same small but consistent self-regulation effect can also be seen when the actual delivery in each condition is expressed as a percentage of the expected delivery for that condition (Table 24.6).

Table 24.6 Nicotine delivery actually obtained in each condition as a percentage of the expected delivery. Figures are means based on the difference between actual and expected deliveries for each subject.

	full	%	2/3
Laboratory smoked cigarette	114.9		122.7
		t 1.3 p $<$.2	
Mean value for 24 hours' cigarettes	99.8		112.3
		t 5.49 p$<$.001	

(n = 14)

Over the 24 hour period subjects obtained 99.8% of the expected delivery of the full cigarettes but 112.3% of the expected delivery of the two-thirds cigarettes. The difference between these values is significant (p $<$.001), indicating that subjects obtained proportionately more of the available nicotine when smoking the reduced-length cigarettes.

In the laboratory, the difference between the full and two-thirds conditions is in the same direction, but does not achieve significance.

An interesting subsidiary point to emerge from the figures for actual and expected nicotine delivery concerns the difference between the laboratory and non-laboratory conditions. Subjects obtained significantly more nicotine from their laboratory cigarettes than they obtained, on average, from cigarettes smoked over 24 hour periods away from the laboratory. This difference appears with both full and two-thirds cigarettes (Table 24.5, (1) vs (2) and (3) vs (4)).

   This greater apparent nicotine dose in the laboratory presumably reflects the abnormality of that particular smoking environment and may relate either to the period of cigarette deprivation constituted by the pre-experiment procedure, or to the stressfulness involved in the taking of blood samples before and after smoking.

Nicotine intake: plasma nicotine levels

The most direct way of measuring the dose of nicotine obtained from a cigarette is by assaying blood nicotine levels before and after smoking. However, such a procedure is not without problems.

   Work in both animals and man indicates that nicotine is rapidly eliminated from the blood in the period immediately following administration. Timing of the post smoking blood sample is consequently of critical importance. Moreover, it is possible that the peak blood levels of nicotine are actually achieved by a smoker some time before the cigarette is extinguished, and that, if the distribution of puff frequency, inhalation depth, etc. during the period of smoking is not constant from cigarette to cigarette, the time of extinguishing of a cigarette may bear no constant relationship to the time blood nicotine levels actually peak.

   Until more information is available about these factors, interpretation of blood nicotine levels ought to be approached with caution. Nevertheless some pattern does seem to emerge from the present study when the blood nicotine levels of the six subjects for whom we have a complete set of data are considered (Table 24.7).

Table 24.7 Blood plasma nicotine levels pre- and post-smoking.

	Full cigarette			Two-thirds cigarette		
Subject	pre	post	difference	pre	post	difference
L.C.	16.6	35.3	18.7	18.7	22.1	3.4
F.H.	19.6	31.64	12.04	15.85	29.59	13.7
E.H.	19.05	33.32	14.27	25.28	20.49	-4.79
R.K.	12.5	19.2	6.7	9.3	29.9	20.6
T.D.	18.1	29.3	11.2	25.3	40.3	17.0
L.W.	11.6	15.5	3.9	19.3	17.3	-2.0
$\bar{x}$	16.24	27.38	11.14	18.62	26.61	7.99
se	1.39	3.31	2.16	2.32	3.42	4.31
t	(1)	(2)	(3)	(4)	(5)	(6)
n = 6				all figs. ng/ml		

				t	$\bar{p}$
(1)	vs	(2)	- 5.1565		< .0025
(4)	vs	(5)	- 1.8539		ns
(3)	vs	(6)	0.6091		ns
(1)	vs	(4)	- 1.1907		ns
(2)	vs	(5)	0.1738		ns

After smoking a full cigarette, subjects' mean blood nicotine levels are, as expected, significantly higher than pre-smoking ($p < .0025$). In the two-thirds cigarette condition, the pre-post smoking difference approaches but does not achieve significance.

The full and two-thirds cigarette conditions do not differ in the pre and post-smoking nicotine levels (1 vs 4, 2 vs 5) and in the pre and post-smoking rise in nicotine levels (3 vs 6).

The differences between pre and post-smoking levels should directly reflect the differences in the doses of nicotine obtained from smoking the full and two-thirds cigarettes. In the case of the full cigarettes the mean difference is 11.14 ng/ml; for the two-thirds cigarettes it is 7.99 ng/ml., or 71.7% of the former figure. This suggests, in agreement with the estimates of nicotine dose derived from the analysis of the filter tips, that subjects obtained from the two-thirds cigarettes slightly more than two-thirds of the full cigarette dose.

Correlation of behavioural change with apparent self-regulation of nicotine intake
It was expected that those subjects who had adapted their smoking behaviour most to the two-thirds cigarette would have approached nearest to the full cigarette nicotine yield. In fact, the relationship between behavioural change (measured by increase in percent time spent puffing) and apparent self-regulation of intake (i.e. the two-thirds cigarette yield as a percentage of the full cigarette yield) shows no correlation ($r = .07$).

The reason for the absence of an association between behavioural change and change in nicotine intake becomes clear when aspects of smoking behaviour are separately correlated with nicotine intake from the full and the two-thirds cigarettes. The picture is similar for both butt analysis-derived estimates of nicotine intake and those based on blood plasma levels (Table 24.8).

Table 24.8 Correlation of inferred nicotine dose and puffing variables.

Correlation of nicotine dose (estimated from filter tip analysis) with	Mean puff duration	Mean inter-puff interval	Percent time spent puffing
Full cigarette condition	$p < .05$ .5083	.0955 ns	$p < .025$ .5172
2/3 cigarette condition	.2213 ns	− .0372 ns	.0145 ns
n = 14			

Correlation of blood nicotine rise with	Mean puff duration	Mean inter-puff interval	Percent time spent puffing
Full cigarette condition n = 6	.5253 ns	− .0029 ns	.4191 ns
2/3 cigarette condition n = 7	− .0061 ns	− .5707 ns	.1963 ns

In the full cigarette condition there is a good correlation between nicotine intake and mean puff duration and the percent time spent puffing, i.e. those subjects who took longer puffs and who spent a greater percentage of time puffing obtained a greater nicotine delivery, as measured by butt analysis, and obtained a larger nicotine dose, as indicated by the rise in blood plasma nicotine concentrations. However, this entirely expected relationship does not hold when subjects smoked the two-thirds cigarettes. It is presumably because of the breakdown of the expected association between the puffing variables and nicotine intake in the two-thirds cigarette condition that there is no correlation between change in those variables and apparent regulation of intake. Presumably aspects of smoking behaviour other than those measured (such as puff volume and velocity and, especially, depth of inhalation) are playing a critical role in determining nicotine intake in this situation.

Effects of experience with the 'shortened' cigarette
The time-table for Group II subjects called for the collection of two samples of 24 hours' normal cigarette butts, one sample before, and one after, experience with the two-thirds cigarettes.

The samples collected after smoking the 'shortened' cigarettes had a significantly longer mean butt length than those smoked before indicating that subjects had been encouraged by experience with the two-thirds cigarettes to smoke less of the tobacco rod (Table 24.9).

Table 24.9 Effects of experience with the two-thirds cigarettes on return to normal smoking.

	mean butt length mm		mean nicotine yield mg	
	pre 2/3	post 2/3	pre 2/3	post 2/3
$\bar{x}$	6.22	8.03	1.043	.982
se	.976	1.298	.088	.117
t	2.77 p $<$.05		1.06 ns	

n = 6

However, the nicotine deliveries before and after experience with the two-thirds cigarettes were not significantly different suggesting that even though a slightly shorter length of tobacco rod had been consumed this had not been accompanied by a reduced demand for nicotine.

Discussion

The present study has succeeded in demonstrating a degree of self-regulation of intake by smokers when the availability of nicotine from a cigarette is experimentally manipulated.

However, in common with most other studies of the same phenomenon, the effect, although consistent, was relatively small, and whilst providing evidence that nicotine may be important in the maintenance of the smoking habit it certainly does not go far in demonstrating that dependence on nicotine is its prime motivation. Indeed, the thesis that cigarette smoking is used essentially as a peculiarly effective form of nicotine self-administration has been singularly difficult to prove experimentally.

Restricting the length of tobacco rod subjects are permitted to smoke is a complementary approach to that used in studies in which nicotine availability is reduced by increasing filter efficiency and cigarette ventilation. Such alterations affect the 'character' of a cigarette (taste, draw resistance etc.) in ways not affected by an alteration in effective cigarette length. Using 'shortened' cigarettes thus presents smokers, in effect, with less of his usual cigarette rather than with a completely new kind of cigarette.

Whilst avoiding some confounding variables (such as difference in taste and ease of draw), reducing cigarette length does not surmount all difficulties. In reducing the length of cigarettes we are reducing the availability of oral gratification, taste, tar, carbon monoxide and a host of other factors as well, and at the same time as, nicotine. Any behavioural change consequent on these experimental manipulations cannot therefore be unequivocally attributed to altered nicotine availability.

The difference between the way in which cigarettes are smoked in the laboratory and over a 24 hour period is worthy of further consideration. The comparisons we were able to draw were not ideal, being between single cigarettes smoked in the laboratory and *mean* values obtained from 15-20 cigarettes smoked over 24 hours. Nevertheless, the differences were striking and consistent. Research into the regulation of nicotine intake usually involves considering subjects' behaviour either wholly in the laboratory or wholly outside it. Where both environments are used, the variables measured in one are different from those measured in the other. The comparison of butt analysis estimates of nicotine dose from cigarettes smoked in the laboratory with those obtained from cigarettes smoked outside the laboratory is therefore of considerable interest. The finding of significant differences between the two suggests firstly that people smoke differently in different situations and, secondly, that findings in the laboratory (including those relating to self-regulation of nicotine intake) cannot necessarily be used to draw conclusions about smokers' behaviour in other situations. This must be especially so where the laboratory situation has involved interference in the subject's smoking behaviour itself - having the subject smoke through a special cigarette holder or exhale smoke into a collection apparatus, for example.

It is of course the smoker's behaviour in the non-laboratory context which is of primary concern, and, unfortunately, the most difficult to observe and measure. The use of butt analysis would seem to be a very valuable tool in this connection since for a subject to collect butts in a small tin is not a great inconvenience, and the method appears capable of providing a measure of nicotine intake which, when used with large enough subject samples, is sensitive to changing conditions. Butt analysis, of course, estimates the nicotine drawn into the smoker's mouth, and not the dose of nicotine actually obtained after inhalation and as such provides suggestive rather than conclusive evidence relating to nicotine dose.

The absence of a correlation between those aspects of smoking behaviour which were measured and nicotine intake in the two-thirds cigarette condition is also interesting. It suggests that other behavioural variables, which were not measured, played a crucial role. Most important amongst these were probably depth and duration of inhalation.

Those who cannot give up smoking have been advised, amongst other things, to decrease the length of tobacco rod smoked by leaving longer butts. This measure would be of no help if it led to proportionately more intensive smoking of the rest of the cigarette. Although subjects in this experiment smoked the reduced length cigarettes more intensively there was a substantial fall in nicotine intake. Since nicotine and tar are closely allied in the cigarette this would suggest their tar intake also fell and that moulding smoker's behaviour in the direction of leaving longer butts might be an effective way of progressively reducing the health risks of smoking.

Acknowledgements

The authors wish to acknowledge the invaluable assistance of Dr. J. Dow and Mr. E. Meredith for G.C.M.S. analysis of blood plasma nicotine levels and of Dr. R.E. Thornton (British American Tobacco) for arranging the assaying of butt nicotine levels and for calculating the expected deliveries of nicotine.

We also wish to thank Mrs. V. Wright for data processing and Mr. V.R. Marsh and Mr. A. Johnson for technical assistance.

The work reported here was supported by a generous grant from the Tobacco Research Council.

References

Ashton, H. & Watson, D.W. (1970) Puffing frequency and nicotine intake in cigarette smokers. *British Medical Journal, 3*, 679-681.

Clark, M.S.G. (1969) Self-administered nicotine solutions preferred to placebo by the rat. *British Journal of Pharmacology, 35*, 367 P.

Deneau, G.A. & Inoki, R. (1967) Nicotine self-administration in monkeys. *Annals of the New York Academy of Sciences, 142*, 277-279.

Dow, J. & Hall, K. (1977) Estimation of plasma nicotine by combined capillary column gas chromatography - mass spectrometry. *British Journal of Pharmacology, 61*, 159P.

Finnegan, J.K., Larson, P.S. & Haag, H.B. (1945) The role of nicotine in the cigarette habit. *Science, N.Y., 102*, 94-96.

Frith, C.D. (1971) The effect of varying the nicotine content of cigarettes on human smoking behaviour. *Psychopharmacologia, 19*, 188-192.

Goldfarb, T.L., Jarvik, M.E. & Glick, S.D. (1970) Cigarette nicotine content as a determinant of human smoking behaviour. *Psychopharmacologia, 17*, 89-93.

Gritz, E.R., Baer-Weiss, V. & Jarvik, M.E. (1976) Titration of nicotine intake with full-length and half-length cigarettes. *Clinical Pharmacology and Therapeutics, 20*, 553-556.

Jarvik, M.E. (1967) Tobacco smoking in monkeys. *Annals of the New York Academy of Sciences, 142*, 280-294.

Kozlowski, L.T., Jarvik, M.E. & Gritz, E.R. (1975) Nicotine regulation and cigarette smoking. *Clinical Pharmacology and Therapeutics, 17*, 93-97.

Kumar, R., Cooke, E.C., Lader, M.H. & Russell, M.A.H. (1977) Is nicotine important in tobacco smoking? *Clinical Pharmacology and Therapeutics, 21*, 520-529.

Lucchesi, B.R., Schuster, C.R. & Emley, G.S. (1967) The role of nicotine as a determinant of cigarette smoking frequency in man with observations of certain cardiovascular effects associated with the tobacco alkaloid. *Clinical Pharmacology and Therapeutics,* **8,** 789-796.

Russell, M.A.H., Wilson, C., Feyerabend, C. & Cole, P.V. (1976) Effects of nicotine chewing gum on smoking behaviour and as an aid to cigarette withdrawal. *British Medical Journal,* **2,** 391-393.

Russell, M.A.H., Wilson, C., Patel, U.A., Feyerabend, C. & Cole, P.V. (1975) Plasma nicotine levels after smoking cigarettes with high, medium and low nicotine yields. *British Medical Journal,* **2,** 414-416.

Stolerman, I.P., Goldfarb, T., Fink, R. & Jarvik, M.E. (1973) Influencing cigarette smoking with nicotine antagonists. *Psychopharmacologia,* **28,** 247-259.

Turner, J.A.McM., Sillett, R.W. & Ball, K.P. (1974) Some effects of changing to low-tar and low-nicotine cigarettes. *Lancet,* **2,** 737-739.

25. Smokers' response to dilution of smoke by ventilated cigarette holders

S R SUTTON, M A H RUSSELL, C FEYERABEND AND Y SALOOJEE

In April 1976 a new smoking withdrawal aid was introduced in the U.K. Known as MD4, it consists of four cigarette holders each with an air-hole which increases in diameter from the first to the fourth holder producing a progressive dilution of the cigarette smoke from about 20% on the first holder to about 80% on the fourth holder. The smoker is supposed to wean himself off cigarettes by using each holder in turn for two weeks.

The study reported here was designed to examine not the effectiveness of this device as a smoking withdrawal aid but the extent to which smokers who were *not* trying to stop smoking would compensate for the dilution of smoke which it produced. This paper is a preliminary report in which the main findings are presented briefly; a fuller report will be published elsewhere (Sutton *et al*, in press).

Method

The MD4 holders were supplied by Miles Laboratories Ltd., Stoke Poges, Slough. Only the first two holders from the set of four were used. On standard machine smoking of one brand of cigarette (regular sized filter tipped) Holder 1 has been found to reduce nicotine yield by 23% and carbon monoxide yield by 15%; reductions on Holder 2 were 58% for nicotine and 52% for carbon monoxide (Miles Laboratories, personal communication).

Eighteen cigarette smokers took part in the study. There were 16 women and two men aged 23 to 55 years around a mean of about 38 years. Their average cigarette consumption was about thirty cigarettes a day. They attended six times over a three-week period. On the first day all subjects smoked normally without using a holder. They then spent two days on one holder followed by two days on the other, with the order of holders balanced. They continued using their second holder for a further five days before switching again to their first holder for the following seven days. For the remaining five days they reverted to smoking without a holder. Subjects smoked their usual brand of cigarette and were instructed throughout to smoke as much or as little as they felt inclined.

All attendances were in the late afternoon or early evening and each subject was seen at the same time on all six occasions. The procedure on each attendance day was exactly the same. Subjects kept a record of the number of cigarettes they smoked up to the time of arrival. On arrival they were asked to smoke a cigarette and a venous blood sample was taken two minutes after the cigarette was completed. The blood samples were analysed for carboxyhaemoglobin (Russell, Cole and Brown, 1973) and for plasma nicotine (Feyerabend, Levitt and Russell, 1975).

Results

Cigarette consumption
The number of cigarettes smoked up to the time of arrival on each attendance day was remarkably constant, averaging about 16 cigarettes (see Table 25.1).

Plasma nicotine
The mean plasma nicotine levels under the various conditions are shown in Table 25.1 and in Figure 25.1. Table 25.2 gives the t values and significance levels of the main comparisons.

Table 25.1 Cigarette consumption, plasma nicotine, and COHb levels of 18 smokers when using MD4 holders and when smoking without a holder (Means $\pm$ SEM)

	No Holder (before)	Holder 1 2 days	Holder 1 7 days	Holder 2 2 days	Holder 2 7 days	No Holder (after)
Cigarette Consumption	15.8 (2.4)	14.7 (2.0)	14.7 (1.6)	15.8 (2.3)	13.7 (1.4)	16.3 (2.0)
Plasma nicotine (ng/ml)	29.0 (4.1)	22.0 (2.9)	24.1 (2.8)	16.9 (2.4)	16.3 (2.5)	25.9 (2.7)
COHb (%)	8.5 (0.5)	6.5 (0.4)	7.7 (0.4)	5.7 (0.4)	5.8 (0.4)	8.5 (0.5)

Cigarette consumption refers to the number of cigarettes smoked up to the time of attendance. The SEM's are in parenthesis. The "expected" levels (i.e. those predicted from the degree of smoke dilution assuming that there was no change in smoking pattern) on Holders 1 and 2 respectively were 21.3(2.3) and 11.4(1.3) for nicotine and 7.2(0.4) and 4.1(0.2) for COHb.

Table 25.2; t values and significance levels of the main comparisons. All tests were two-tailed with 17 df.

Comparison		Plasma Nicotine t	Plasma Nicotine p	COHb t	COHb p
No Holder vs. Holder	1-2 days	3.0	.01	4.7	.001
	-7 days	1.4	NS	2.3	.05
No Holder vs Holder	2-2 days	5.4	.001	7.1	.001
	-7 days	5.5	.001	8.1	.001
Holder 1 vs Holder	2-2 days	3.0	.01	2.2	.05
	-7 days	5.0	.001	4.8	.001
2 days vs 7 days -	Holder 1	1.0	NS	3.3	.005
-	Holder 2	0.4	NS	0.4	NS
Observed -	Holder 1 at 2 days	0.4	NS	1.8	NS
vs Expected -	Holder 1 at 7 days	1.4	NS	1.6	NS
-	Holder 2 at 2 days	3.2	.005	4.6	.001
-	Holder 2 at 7 days	2.8	.02	5.3	.001

The mean levels on the two days when subjects were smoking normally without a holder did not differ significantly, showing that the experience of being on the holders for two weeks or so had little or no effect on subsequent smoking. The average of the levels on the two 'No Holder' days was computed for each subject, and the mean of these was used as the basis for comparison with the levels obtained when using the holders.

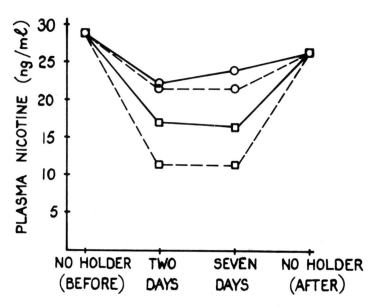

Fig. 25.1 Observed and expected changes in mean plasma nicotine levels.

On Holder 1 the reduction at two days was significant on a paired t-test ($p < .01$) but the reduction at seven days was not. Much greater reductions were obtained on the second holder; these were highly significant ($p < .001$) at both two days and at seven days. The changes in levels from two days to seven days were not signif- icant for either holder but the differences between Holders 1 and 2 were significant at both times ($p < .01$ and $p < .001$). Our subjects, then, failed to maintain their no-holder levels on Holder 2 and, initially, on Holder 1. After seven days on Holder 1, however, they obtained levels that approached their no-holder levels.

In order to see whether or not they compensated for the reduced smoke delivery it is necessary to compare the observed nicotine and COHb levels with the 'expected' levels predicted from the degree of smoke dilution. If a smoker responds to the dilution of smoke by smoking in exactly the same way as he does normally then one would expect his blood levels to fall roughly in proportion to the reduction in delivery from the cigarettes. So if a holder reduces nicotine delivery by 20% then the smoker's blood nicotine level would also be expected to fall by about 20%. If, however, he compensates for the reduction by modifying his smoking pattern so as to take in more smoke then his blood level should fall by less than 20%. In other words, if a subject's observed level is higher than his expected level this would indicate at least partial compensation. For each subject we calculated expected levels on the two holders and the means are shown in Figure 25.1.

On Holder 2 the observed levels were significantly greater than expected at two days and at seven days ($p < .005$, $p < .02$), indicating that partial compensation occurred on Holder 2: in fact, subjects obtained levels on Holder 2 that were about 60% of their no-holder levels instead of the expected 42%. By contrast, on Holder 1 the observed levels were not significantly greater than expected even after seven days, showing that they modified their smoking behaviour little if at all.

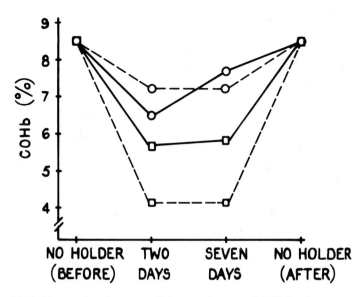

Fig. 25.2 Observed and expected changes in mean COHb levels.

Carboxyhaemoglobin

The mean COHb levels are shown in Table 25.1 and in Figure 25.2. COHb levels reflect the total amount of smoke inhaled over the day; they are less dependent than are the peak nicotine levels on when and how the last cigarette was smoked.

Expected COHb levels were calculated and compared with the observed levels. The results are basically the same as for nicotine, with one interesting exception: After two days on Holder 1 the observed level was actually *lower* than the expected level, though the comparison was significant only at $p < .1$. Our subjects, then, did modify their smoking on Holder 1 but they did so in the 'wrong' direction, that is, in the direction of taking in *less* smoke than they did normally. This effect was not apparent after seven days on Holder 1 nor was it apparent on Holder 2.

Compensators and Non-compensators

The data presented so far refer to mean levels. But there was marked individual variation, some subjects compensating fairly effectively, some compensating partially and some not compensating at all. On Holder 1 there were eight subjects who had observed levels that were higher than expected at both two days and seven days. All these eight subjects also had observed levels on Holder 2 that were higher than expected at two days and at seven days. In other words, we were able to identify eight subjects who seemed to compensate consistently throughout the study. We compared these eight subjects with the remaining ten who did not consistently compensate on the two holders but we found no differences between these two groups with regard to their normal smoking plasma nicotine and COHb levels, their cigarette consumption and the nicotine yields of their cigarettes.

Discussion

On Holder 2, then, subjects compensated partially, managing to obtain levels that were about 60% of their no-holder levels instead of the expected 42%. They did not achieve this compensation by smoking more cigarettes, so they must have somehow increased the amount of smoke inhaled from each cigarette. Compensation was not complete. In order to achieve this on Holder 2 they would have had to have more than doubled the amount of smoke they inhaled. This would have been difficult without greatly increasing the number of cigarettes smoked.

The picture is less clear in the case of Holder 1. After two days on Holder 1 there was no compensatory increase in the amount of smoke inhaled: observed levels were virtually identical to the expected levels for nicotine, and in the case of COHb the levels were actually lower than expected. Although the levels were higher at seven days they were still not significantly different from expected. However, even with this very minimal compensation they still managed to obtain levels that approached their no-holder levels - at least after seven days. This was possible because of the small reduction in smoke yield produced by Holder 1.

The COHb results indicate a tendency for subjects to reduce rather than increase their smoke intake at two days on Holder 1. What factor or factors were producing this inhibitory effect we do not know, but it was not apparent after seven days on Holder 1 or on Holder 2 where it was possibly 'swamped' by the greater need for nicotine. Interestingly, the effect was not mediated by a reduction in cigarette consumption; subjects must have reduced their smoke intake in other more subtle ways.

There was a wide degree of individual variation in compensation. However, we could find no differences between compensators and non-compensators with regard to their usual cigarette consumption and their normal smoking plasma nicotine and COHb levels. This is rather surprising to those who believe nicotine to have an important role in smoking since those with higher no-holder levels would potentially suffer the largest absolute drop in blood levels when on the holders and might therefore have been expected to be more likely to compensate, or to try to compensate, than those with lower no-holder levels.

In conclusion, our subjects were clearly compensating on Holder 2. But we cannot conclude from this study that they were compensating for the reduction in nicotine delivery rather than some other factor. After all, the holders affected taste, tar yield, the feel of the smoke in the mouth and so on, and subjects may have been compensating for the change in these other factors rather than the change in nicotine delivery.

Acknowledgement

We would like to thank Miles Laboratories Ltd., for their advice and for supplying the cigarette holders for the study.

References

Feyerabend, C., Levitt, T. & Russell, M.A.H. (1975) A rapid gas-liquid chromatographic estimation of nicotine in biological fluids. *Journal of Pharmacy and Pharmacology,* **27**, 434-436.

Russell, M.A.H., Cole, P.V. & Brown, E. (1973) Absorption by non-smokers of carbon monoxide from room-air polluted by tobacco smoke. *Lancet,* **1**, 576-579.

Sutton, S.R., Feyerabend, C., Cole., P.V. & Russell, M.A.H. Adjustment of smokers to dilution of tobacco smoke by ventilated cigarette holders. *Clinical Pharmacology and Therapeutics,* in press.

26. Addiction Research Unit[*] nicotine titration studies

M A H RUSSELL, S R SUTTON, C FEYERABEND AND P V COLE

Introduction

It is widely believed that a change to low-tar and low-nicotine cigarettes will reduce the health hazards of cigarette smoking. It is not known, however, to what extent the benefits of such a change are offset by a tendency for smokers to compensate for the reduction in tar and nicotine yields by smoking more cigarettes or increasing inhalation. At present the evidence is conflicting (Russell, 1976a). Short-term studies have shown that some smokers appear to modify their smoking pattern to maintain a constant intake of nicotine and/or tar (Ashton & Watson, 1970; Cherry & Forbes, 1972; Frith, 1971; Russell, Wilson et al, 1973; Russell, Wilson et al, 1975; Schachter, 1977; Turner, Sillett & Ball, 1974), but the only long-term study suggested that some smokers would adapt without compensation to a reduction in nicotine yield from 1.4 to 1.0 mg (Friedman & Fletcher, 1976).

At the Addiction Research Unit of the Institute of Psychiatry we have done four nicotine titration studies. The first, a study of smokers' response to changing to high and low nicotine cigarettes, has been published elsewhere as has the second which is a study of smokers' response to nicotine chewing-gum. Our third study, the response of smokers to dilution of smoke by ventilated cigarette holders, though not yet analysed completely, has been presented as a preliminary report at this conference. The fourth of our nicotine titration studies, the response of smokers to shortened cigarettes, will be presented here, also in a preliminary and incomplete form. Indeed, a fifth study done in collaboration with Dr. R. Kumar and Dr. M. Lader, which Dr. Kumar has presented to this conference (Kumar et al, 1978) was intended to examine nicotine titration among other things. Unfortunately, at the pilot stage, we found that blood sampling interfered excessively with the psychophysiological and puffing measures so that blood nicotine and COHb measures were sacrificed.

Compensatory increase in inhalation

Before going on to outline the findings of our nicotine titration studies mention should be made of the relationship of inhalation increase to compensation. The nature of this relationship is important and seems to have been overlooked. Since nicotine intake from cigarette smoking depends almost entirely on inhalation the only way the smoker can titrate nicotine intake is by regulating inhalation. Thus, when he is trying to compensate for a dilution of smoke, whether he does this by increasing the number of cigarettes smoked, or the amount of smoke inhaled

---

[*] Addiction Research, Unit, Institute of Psychiatry, The Mandsley Hospital, London. S.E.5.

from each cigarette, or the rate of smoking the cigarette, or a combination of all three, compensation for smoke dilution depends ultimately on increasing the overall amount of diluted smoke inhaled over a given period of time. Furthermore, it requires proportionally more of the diluted smoke to make up for a given loss of "stronger", less dilute smoke. For example, if the mainstream smoke is diluted to half its strength, to maintain intake it is necessary to inhale twice as much. In other words, a 50% dilution requires a 100% increase in inhalation. The form of this reciprocal relationship is demonstrated in Figure 26.1.

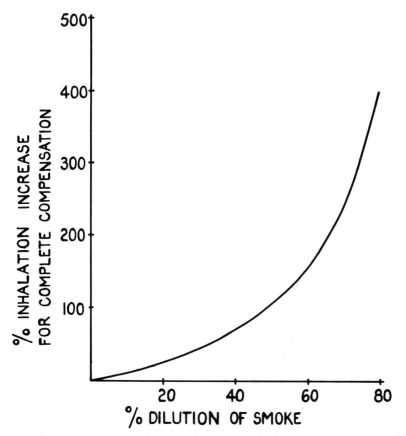

Fig. 26.1 Percentage increase in inhalation necessary for complete compensation. The relationship is expressed by the formula $Y = \frac{X}{100-X} \cdot 100$ where Y is the % increase in inhalation necessary to compensate for a given % dilution (X) of mainstream smoke. This produces a hyperbolic curve from which it can be seen how a smoker must increase inhalation in geometric fashion to compensate for progressive dilution of mainstream smoke (from Sutton et al, (1978a).

The relationship shown in Figure 26.1 may partly explain why so many smokers have switched so easily from smoking untipped cigarettes with nicotine yields above 2 mg to filter-tipped cigarettes with nicotine yields around 1.2 mg., but find it far more difficult or even impossible to gain satisfaction from cigarettes with nicotine yields below about 0.8 mg. The situation is illustrated in Table 26.1 using the hypothetical starting point of a 2 mg nicotine cigarette. Clearly a point must be reached where it is impossible to obtain a higher total puff volume from a cigarette however intensively it is smoked.

Table 26.1 Inhalation increase necessary to compensate for progressive reduction in nicotine yields of cigarettes from an arbitrary starting point of 2.0 mg per cigarette. The arbitrary volume of 350 ml is the amount which would be obtained from ten standard 35 ml machine-smoked puffs. The estimates are derived from the formula in Figure 26.1.

Nicotine yield of cigarette (mg)	Dilution of nicotine (%)	Inhalation increase for complete compensation (%)	Volume of mainstream smoke it would be necessary to inhale for complete compensation (ml)
2.0	--	--	350
1.2	40	66.7	583
1.0	50	100	700
0.8	60	150	875
0.5	75	300	1400

Adjustment of smokers to cigarettes with lower tar and nicotine yields depends, therefore, on a complex interaction of many factors. These include (i) Initial nicotine intake which may be very much more or far less than the standard yield of the cigarette smoked. (ii) 'Maximum nicotine yield' as opposed to 'Standard nicotine yield' of the lower nicotine cigarettes. (iii) The extent to which nicotine yields are reduced by deposition on the filter vs ventilation. (iv) Degree of tolerance to a reduced nicotine intake. (v) The extent to which the smoker seeks a given nicotine effect from a single cigarette as opposed to the maintenance of a certain 'trough' plasma nicotine level (see below). The latter, but not the former, can be maintained equally well by increasing the number of cigarettes smoked. (vi) Numerous other factors such as pleasure from the flavour, tolerance to irritancy, draw resistance and the discomfort of large increases in puff volume etc.

Nicotine Titration Study I: Response of smokers to changing to high and low nicotine cigarettes.

The results of this study are shown in Table 26.2. The subjects were studied before and after a five-hour period spent smoking under natural conditions at work. We went to their place of work to collect the blood samples. It will be seen that there was a 38% decrease in consumption on switching from the usual to the high-nicotine brand ($p < .01$). The 17% increase in the number of low-nicotine cigarettes smoked was not statistically significant. Average plasma nicotine levels were similar after smoking medium and high-nicotine cigarettes, but on the low-nicotine cigarettes the levels were substantially reduced (p .001). Unfortunately the yield of the low-nicotine brand was too extreme to test the titration hypothesis. To have obtained the same level on these cigarettes would have been impossible. Furthermore, they were aversive in having an excessively high draw resistance. The study should be repeated using low-nicotine cigarettes with a yield around 0.5 to 0.8 mg.

Table 26.2 Relation of nicotine yield to cigarette consumption and carbon monoxide and nicotine intake (means of ten subjects—

Brand of Cigarette	Mean nicotine yield (mg)	Mean carbon monoxide yield (mg)	Mean number smoked in 5 hr test period	Weight smoked in 5 hr test period (gm)	Mean COHb change in 5 hr test period (%)	Plasma nicotine after 5 hr test period (ng/ml)
Usual	1.34	17.2	10.7	6.0	+1.79	30.1
Low nicotine	0.14	5.0	12.5	6.5	−0.34	8.5
High nicotine	3.2	16.7	6.7	4.2	−1.04	29.2

Abstracted from Russell, Wilson et al (1973, 1975). The mean CO yields are derived from Russell, Cole et al (1975). The order of taking the high and low nicotine cigarettes was balanced within the group. The data for the usual brand are the means of two 5-hr test periods. COHb (%) is a unit of measure not a percent change.

Nicotine Titration Study II: Smokers' response to nicotine chewing-gum

A chewing-gum containing nicotine has been developed which is buffered at an alkaline pH to enable buccal absorption of nicotine (Ferno, Lichtneckert & Lundgren, 1973). The fact that nicotine absorption from this gum is satisfactory (Russell, Cole et al, 1975 (Russell et al, 1977) provided an opportunity to test the nicotine-titration hypothesis. This study has been reported more fully elsewhere (Russell, Wilson et al, 1976).

Table 26.3 Effect of nicotine chewing-gum on plasma nicotine levels during *ad libitum* smoking (means of 41 subjects).

	No gum	Placebo gum	Nicotine gum
Cigarettes per day	33.3	23.0	20.9
COHb %	8.5	7.2	6.3
Plasma nicotine ng/ml	30.1	24.7	27.4

Note: One piece of gum containing 2 mg nicotine was chewed hourly for 30 min to a total of ten pieces per day. The specific effect of nicotine (as opposed to the effect of placebo gum) accounted for 17% of the reduction in daily cigarette consumption $(23.0 - 20.9) \div (33.3 - 20.9) \times 100 = 17$. By similar calculation it accounted for 41% of the reduction in COHb and hence degree of inhalation. Abstracted from Russell, Wilson et al, (1976).

A group of 43 smokers were instructed to take the nicotine chewing-gum and to continue smoking as much or as little as they felt inclined. Despite an extra 20 mg nicotine from the gum, the nicotine intake from smoking was diminished just sufficiently to ensure a constant plasma level; the average plasma nicotine peak just after a cigarette was 27.4 ng/ml when the subjects were taking the gum and smoking *ad libitum*, compared to 30.1 ng/ml when smoking normally without the gum (Table 26.3). The difference is not statistically significant and this supports the view that it is nicotine rather than tar intake which is being titrated. On the other hand, when taking placebo gum and smoking *ad libitum*, the average plasma nicotine peak just after a cigarette was a little lower (24.7 ng/ml, p<0.05) suggesting that nicotine intake was not maintained completely constant possibly due to time-out from smoking during the chewing. This does not support the nicotine-titration hypothesis. These findings suggest that the self-regulation of nicotine intake downwards to avoid excessively high levels may be more sensitive and complete than compensation upwards to avoid unduly low levels.

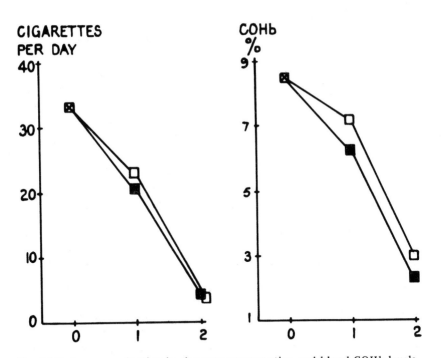

Fig. 26.2 Average reduction in cigarette consumption and blood COHb levels. The effect of nicotine in the gum, though significant, is small compared with the overall reduction in smoking achieved by other factors.
0 = Initial levels before taking gum; 1 = Taking gum but smoking as inclined; 2 = Taking gum and trying to stop smoking. ⊠ No gum; □ Placebo gum; ■ 2 mg Nicotine gum. The difference in consumption for Nicotine and Placebo gums on **condition** 1 is significant, p<.05; the COHb differences on conditions 1 and 2 are significant p<.01 and <.02 respectively.

Another finding of this study was the marked reduction of *ad libitum* smoking on both placebo and nicotine gum (Table 26.3, Figure 26.2). The specific effect of the nicotine was significant (p .05 for cigarette consumption, p .01 for COHb differences) but it was small; probably because the nicotine content of the gum was only 2 mg per piece, whereas a stronger 4 mg gum is necessary to produce plasma nicotine levels comparable to smoking (Russell *et al,* 1976; Russell *et al,* 1977). Nevertheless, the significant inhibitory effect is supportive evidence that nicotine is a determinant of smoking. The fact that nicotine accounted for only 17% of the reduction in cigarette consumption but 41% of the reduction of COHb in the *ad libitum* smoking condition indicates that the smokers were titrating their nicotine intake by reducing inhalation as well as the number of cigarettes smoked.

Nicotine Titration Study IV*: Smokers' adjustment to shortened cigarettes

This study was designed to see whether smokers would compensate for the reductions in smoke yields produced by shortening their usual brand of cigarette to 75% and 50% of the smokable length. The first shortened cigarette study was that reported by Goldfarb and Jarvik (1972). In their study, 18 subjects spent a week smoking cigarettes that had been cut to half the original length and another week smoking only the distal half of each cigarette which had a red line drawn around the half-way mark. Although the average number of these half-cigarettes smoked per day by the group as a whole was not significantly higher than on the control weeks with whole cigarettes, 12 of the subjects did increase the number of lined cigarettes smoked by an average of five per day and the number of cut cigarettes by an average of seven per day, suggesting that these 12 subjects were trying to compensate. It is probable that further compensation was also achieved by deeper inhalation, as is suggested in a subsequent study by Jarvik's group (Gritz, Baer-Weiss & Jarvik, 1976).

Another 'shortened' cigarette study has been reported by Ashton, Stepney and Thompson (this volume) and elsewhere (Stepney & Thompson, 1977). Their 14 subjects were studied after part of one day of smoking cigarettes which they were instructed not to smoke beyond a line at 'two-thirds of the tobacco rod normally consumed'. The proportion of the time spent puffing the lined cigarettes was increased by 39% compared to full cigarettes (7.61% vs 5.46% respectively of the time taken to smoke the cigarette, p .005). Butt nicotine levels after smoking the two-thirds cigarettes varied between 66% and 95% of the full cigarette levels, and plasma nicotine levels averaged 71.7% of the full cigarette levels. There was no significant reduction in subjective ratings of enjoyment/satisfaction, though the decrease in fingertip temperature during smoking was significantly reduced.

In our study, 14 subjects attended on three occasions over one week - on the Monday, Wednesday and Friday. At each attendance subjects had been smoking either full, three-quarters or half length cigarettes balanced in a 3 x 3 latin square design. All attendances were in the afternoon and each subject attended at approximately the same time on all three days. The shortened cigarettes were provided by the British American Tobacco Co. Ltd., and consisted of the subjects' usual brand which were shortened by cutting them to half or three-quarters of the length of the tobacco rods. They were then re-packed in the original packs.

---

*Nicotine Titration Study III: 'Smokers' response to dilution of smoke by ventilated cigarette holders' is presented as a preliminary report (Sutton *et al*, this volume).

The number of cigarettes smoked was carefully recorded on a card. Cigarette butts were collected, the lengths were measured and they were analysed for nicotine content in the laboratories of B.A.T.   At each attendance, subjects were asked to smoke a cigarette. The pulse rate was measured with a finger pulsemeter and the puff rate and number of puffs were counted. Venous blood samples were then taken approximately two minutes after finishing the cigarette and analysed for COHb (Russell, Cole & Brown, 1973) and plasma nicotine (Feyerabend, Levitt & Russell, 1975).   Subjective ratings of mood and of satisfaction derived from the cigarettes were also obtained.

The preliminary results are shown in Table 26.4   For various reasons tar and nicotine deliveries are not reduced in exact proportion to the degree of shortening of the tobacco rods. Our estimates of the reduction in nicotine deliveries, shown in the table as 'estimated' nicotine deliveries, were based on the machine-smoked deliveries of the shortened cigarettes smoked in 35 ml, 2 sec puffs at a rate of one per min to the individual butt lengths of the subjects when smoking their usual full length cigarettes (rather than to the standard butt length).   On this basis shortening the cigarettes reduced the nicotine yields by an average of 23.1% and 38.0% for the three-quarters and half length cigarettes respectively. We have not yet assessed the reductions in CO yields of the shortened cigarettes.

Table 26.4 Changes in smoking behaviour in response to shortened cigarettes expressed as the means with the % change from full length cigarettes shown in parenthesis.

	Full length	¾ length (%)	½ length (%)
Consumption (No. cigs)	13.6	14.8 (+8.8%)	17.6 (+29.4%)
Puffs per min	1.8	2.1 (+17.0%)	2.5 (+39.0%)
Butt length (mm)	27.8	26.4 (−5.0%)	23.5 (−15.5%)
Nicotine delivery (mg/cig)			
'Estimated'	1.08	0.83 (−23.1%)	0.67 (−38.0%)
'Observed'	1.25	0.99 (−20.8%)	0.80 (−36.0%)
Total mouth level intake			
of nicotine (mg)	17.0	14.7 (−13.5%)	14.1 (−17.1%)
Plasma nicotine (ng/ml)	35.8	28.3 (−20.9%)	17.6 (−50.8%)
COHb (%)	7.7	6.4 (−16.9%)	5.2 (−32.5%)
Satisfaction rating	3.5	3.1 (−11.4%)	2.0 (−42.9%)

Note: 'Estimated' nicotine deliveries per cigarette are based on the machine-smoked deliveries of the subjects' usual brands (full length and shortened) smoked in 35 ml, 2 sec puffs, at a rate one per min, to the individual butt lengths of the subjects when smoking their usual full length cigarettes (rather than to the standard butt length). 'Observed' nicotine deliveries were calculated from the butt nicotine content. Total mouth level intake of nicotine is the product of the delivery per cigarette and the number of cigarettes smoked.   The data for this preliminary presentation refer only to those nine subjects who smoked standard or king size filter-tipped cigarettes and for whom complete data were available.

The main preliminary findings of this study are as follows:

(i)   There was a systematic and highly significant increase in the number of cigarettes smoked as the cigarettes were shortened. This is contrary to the overall findings and conclusions of the Goldfarb and Jarvik study (1972). It also differs from the MD4 Study (Sutton *et al*, this volume) which showed no change in cigarette consumption in response to smoke dilution.

(ii)   There was a systematic and highly significant increase in the rate of puffing at the shorter cigarettes which were also smoked to a shorter butt. This is in keeping with Stepney and Thompson's (1977) finding of 39% more puffing time on two-thirds length cigarettes. However, these changes did not appreciably increase the nicotine deliveries, and the percentage reduction in 'observed' nicotine deliveries due to the shortening were similar to those 'estimated' with a smoking machine.

(iii)   It is worth noting in passing that the subjects abstracted more nicotine from their usual full-length brand when smoking normally than occurred with standardised machine-smoking to the same butt length (1.25 vs 1.08 mg).

(iv)   There is evidence of compensation in the total mouth level intake of nicotine in that the percentage reductions due to shortening are substantially less than the estimated reductions in deliveries of the shortened cigarettes. This compensation was due to the increase in the number of cigarettes smoked. Although the subjects attempted to compensate by increasing puff rate, this did not seem to increase the delivery per cigarette.

(v)   Despite the compensatory increase in total mouth level intake of nicotine, there is no evidence whatsoever of compensation in the plasma nicotine levels. The 21% reduction on three-quarter cigarettes is similar to the 23% estimated reduction in nicotine deliveries (based on reduction in smoking-machine yields). On the half length cigarettes the 51% reduction in plasma nicotine is considerably more than 38% reduction in 'estimated' nicotine deliveries of the half cigarettes. This suggests some factor with an inhibitory **effect** on inhalation – possibly related to the higher temperature of the smoke from the very short half length cigarettes. Despite the increase in consumption, peak plasma nicotine levels on the shortened cigarettes were not higher than might be expected from the estimated reductions in nicotine yields. This is because peak levels are related more to the intake from the preceding cigarette rather than the number of cigarettes smoked that day. The plasma nicotine data agree with the Stepney and Thompson study (1977). which showed a 28% reduction on 2/3 length cigarettes, but disagree with the study of Gritz *et al* (1976) whose subjects excreted proportionately more nicotine in their urine when smoking half length cigarettes than on full length cigarettes.

(vi)   Though the CO yields of the shortened cigarettes have not yet been estimated, the fact that COHb levels were substantially reduced despite the increase in cigarette consumption is in keeping with the plasma nicotine data and confirms the lack of compensatory increase in inhalation.

(vii)   Satisfaction and enjoyment derived from the shortened cigarettes was systematically and significantly reduced, possibly due to the failure to maintain smoke intake other than at mouth level.

Finally, it should be emphasised that the MD4 study (Sutton *et al*, this volume) was concerned with the response of smokers to a *dilution* of mainstream smoke.

M*

The situation with shortened cigarettes is very different. It involves, not a dilution of smoke, but a *reduction in volume* of the smoke available from each cigarette. With smoke dilution in the MD4 study there was no change in cigarette consumption but there was a significant compensatory increase in inhalation. In contrast, with shortened cigarettes there was an increase in consumption but not inhalation. To use an alcohol analogy, the double scotch drinker whose drink is diluted with water can get just as inebriated by drinking a larger volume of the diluted scotch. But if the amount of scotch is halved by giving him singles, the only way for him to maintain his alcohol intake is to take more drinks. This is in part how the smokers have responded to MD4 and shortened cigarettes.

Concluding remarks

How important is nicotine?
The picture is still far from clear and many questions remain unanswered. Our purpose at this conference has been to present the findings of those of our studies that are relevant to this question and we have not attempted an overall review. Such reviews have been published by one of us elsewhere (Russell, 1976a, 1978) but these are now clearly outdated by some of the new data presented at this conference. A brief summary of the evidence and its limitations would seem to be as follows:

1. There is circumstantial historical evidence that nicotine is an important factor in tobacco smoking. Throughout history people have used tobacco only in ways that enable nicotine to exert a pharmacologic effect and smoking has never been practised as a habit in the absence of a pharmacologically active alkaloid.

2. Numerous short-term studies have shown that many smokers modify their smoking patterns in response to changes in the tar and nicotine yields of their cigarettes, with self-regulation downwards to avoid excessive intake appearing to be more sensitive and complete than compensation upwards to avoid a reduced intake of nicotine and/or tar or vapour phase constituents (Ashton & Watson, 1970; Cherry & Forbes, 1972; Finnegan, Larson & Haag, 1945; Frith, 1971; Russell Wilson *et al*, 1973; Russell, Wilson *et al*, 1975; Schachter, 1977; Turner *et al*, 1974).   There is a remarkable lack of adequate long-term studies (Friedman & Fletcher, 1976).

3. Evidence that this modification of smoking pattern is mediated by a need to titrate the intake of nicotine rather than some other factor is slender and conflicting. There is no adequate report of the response of smokers to cigarettes in which the yields of nicotine and other components are independently varied (Goldfarb *et al*, 1976). The importance of nicotine is suggested by (i) A single, uncontrolled almost anecdotal report of the capacity of nicotine injections to relieve the craving of cigarette withdrawal and to induce dependence (Johnston, 1942). (ii) A single study showing changes in puffing and cigarette consumption when the central effects of nicotine are blocked by mecamylamine (Stolerman *et al*, 1973). (iii) Evidence that smokers regulate their cigarette consumption systematically in response to manipulation of their urinary nicotine excretion (Schachter, Kozlowski & Silverstein, 1977). (iv) Some evidence that inhalation and the number of cigarettes smoked are reduced when nicotine is administered via chewing-gum, but some countering of this evidence by lack of positive correlation between the plasma

nicotine levels it produces and its ability to relieve the subjective sense of missing cigarettes (Kozlowski *et al*, 1975; Russell *et al*, 1977; Russell, Wilson *et al*, 1976). (v) Suggestive statistical differentiation of self-reported reasons for smoking into pharmacological vs non-pharmacological motives (Russell *et al*, 1974). (vi) One study showing a reduction of cigarette smoking during slow intravenous infusion of nicotine (Lucchesi, Schuster & Emley, 1967) but another study showed no effect on puffing behaviour during and just after intravenous bolus injections of nicotine (Kumar *et al*, 1977).

   4. On balance, the evidence suggests that nicotine is an important factor. The questions which arise are how important it is, to what proportion of smokers, and to what type of smoker. Such questions are not merely academic but have crucial implications for the design of safer cigarettes. For if nicotine is the primary factor the present worldwide campaign for low tar, low nicotine cigarettes is misguided; to expect people who appear unable to stop smoking to smoke cigarettes with virtually no nicotine is illogical. A more logical approach would be to develop a cigarette low in tar and carbon monoxide, but with a medium or even high, rather than low, nicotine yield (Russell, 1976b). Functional autonomy and secondary reinforcement by stimuli such as taste and smell compete with the response to nicotine to reduce its influence in short-term studies. The lack of animal studies of nicotine self-injection to determine its potency as a primary reinforcer is lamentable.

'Peak-seekers' and 'Trough-maintainers'

If people do smoke for nicotine, we are still nowhere near the stage of knowing to what extent they smoke for some positive effects of the plasma nicotine peaks or to avoid whatever the pharmacological effects may be of falling below a certain plasma nicotine trough. Nevertheless, it would seem from preliminary pharmacokinetic findings (Russell & Feyerabend, 1978) that for those smokers who smoke less than one cigarette per hour and are inhalers the predominant plasma profile is one of repeated high nicotine peaks, whereas the accumulation of nicotine in the body would suggest that those who smoke at least one cigarette every thirty minutes would tend to show peaks which are smaller relative to the absolute level. They might, therefore, be more likely to be motivated by the need for 'trough maintenance'. Very tentatively we would suggest that trough maintenance is the main motive for the addicted heavy smoker while optimal peak effects are more important to indulgent smokers who smoke less heavily.

   There is no way that Schachter's (Schachter *et al*,1977) urinary pH manipulations would have altered the plasma nicotine peaks obtained by his subjects after each cigarette. But the alterations in redistribution and excretion rate could have affected the trough levels. Indeed, we have shown that urinary pH manipulations do affect trough levels of plasma nicotine (Feyerabend & Russell, 1978). The fact that Schachter's findings were so strikingly positive is, we suggest, because his subjects were heavy addicted smokers, i.e. 'trough-maintainers'. We would predict that his findings would have been negative in less heavy, indulgent smokers, i.e. 'peak-seekers'. Furthermore, we would suggest that 'peak-seekers' would titrate nicotine intake by modifying the way they smoke each cigarette but would be less likely to alter the number of cigarettes smoked. 'Trough-maintainers,' on the other hand, probably use both mechanisms. Differences of this kind may account for some of the discrepancies between the results of different nicotine titration studies.

In conclusion, it seems that at least 50% of smokers modify their smoking patterns to regulate their nicotine intake. At present, there is no indication whether 'trough maintainers' are more likely than 'peak-seekers' to be the more avid 'self-titrators'.

Acknowledgements

We thank Jean Crutch for secretarial help, our colleagues Colin Taylor, Martin Raw and J. Richard Eiser for helpful advice and comments, British-American Tobacco Company for supplying cigarettes and the analysis of butts for the shortened cigarette study, and the Medical Research Council and Department of Health and Social Security for financial support.

References

Ashton, H., Stepney, R. & Thompson, J.W.(1978) Smoking behaviour and nicotine intake in smokers presented with a "two-thirds" cigarette. *This volume.*

Ashton, H. & Watson, D.W. (1970) Puffing frequency and nicotine intake in cigarette smokers. *British Medical Journal, 3,* 679-681.

Cherry, W.H. & Forbes, W.F. (1972) Canadian studies aimed towards a less harmful cigarette. *Journal of the National Cancer Institute, 48,* 1765-1773.

Ferno, O., Lichtneckert, S.J.A. & Lundgren, C.E.G. (1973) A substitute for tobacco smoking. *Psychopharmacologia, 31,* 201-204.

Feyerabend, C., Levitt, T. & Russell, M.A.H. (1975) A rapid gas-liquid chromatographic estimation of nicotine in biological fluids. *Journal of Pharmacy and Pharmacology, 27,* 434-436.

Feyerabend, C. & Russell, M.A.H. (1978) Effect of urinary pH and nicotine excretion rate on plasma nicotine during cigarette smoking and chewing nicotine gum. *British Journal of Clinical Pharmacology, 5,* 293-297.

Finnegan, J.K., Larson, P.S. & Haag, H.B. (1945) The role of nicotine in the cigarette habit. *Science, 102,* 94-96.

Friedman, S. & Fletcher, C.M. (1976) Changes in smoking habits and cough in men smoking cigarettes with 30% NSM tobacco substitute. *British Medical Journal, 1,* 1427-1430.

Frith, C.D. (1971) The effect of varying nicotine content of cigarette on human smoking behaviour. *Psychopharmacologia, 19,* 188-192

Goldfarb, T.L., Gritz, E.R., Jarvik, M.E. & Stolerman, I.P. (1976) Reactions to cigarettes as a function of nicotine and tar. *Clinical Pharmacology and Therapeutics, 19,* 767-772.

Goldfarb, T.L. & Jarvik, M.E. (1972) Accommodation to restricted tobacco smoke intake in cigarette smokers. *International Journal of the Addictions, 7,* 559-565.

Gritz, E.R., Baer-Weiss, V. & Jarvik, M.E. (1976) Titration of nicotine intake with full-length and half-length cigarettes. *Clinical Pharmacology and Therapeutics, 20,* 552-556.

Johnston, L.M. (1942) Tobacco smoking and nicotine. *Lancet,* **2,** 742.

Kozlowski, L.T., Jarvik, M.E. & Gritz, E.R. (1975) Nicotine regulation and cigarette smoking. *Clinical Pharmacology and Therapeutics,* **17,** 93-97.

Kumar, R., Cooke, E.C., Lader, M.H., Russell, M.A.H. (1977) Is nicotine important in tobacco smoking? *Clinical Pharmacology and Therapeutics,* **21,** 520-529.

Kumar, R., Cooke, E.C., Lader, M.H. & Russell, M.A.H. (1978) Is tobacco-smoking a form of nicotine dependence? *This volume.*

Lucchesi, B.R., Schuster, C.R. & Emley, G.S. (1967) The role of nicotine as a determinant of cigarette smoking frequency in man with observations of certain cardiovascular effects associated with the tobacco alkaloid. *Clinical Pharmacology and Therapeutics,* **8,** 789-796.

Russell, M.A.H. (1976a) Tobacco Smoking and Nicotine Dependence. In *Research Advances in Alcohol and Drug Problems.* Volume III, ed. Gibbins, R.J. *et al,* pp. 1-47. New York: Wiley and Sons.

Russell, M.A.H. (1976b) Low-tar medium-nicotine cigarettes: A new approach to safer smoking. *British Medical Journal,* **1,** 1430-1433.

Russell, M.A.H. (1978) Self-regulation of nicotine intake by smokers. In *Behavioural Effects of Nicotine.* ed. Battig. K., pp 108-122. Basel: S. Karger.

Russell, M.A.H., Cole, P.V. & Brown, E. (1973) Absorption by non-smokers of carbon monoxide from room-air polluted by tobacco smoke. *Lancet,* **1,** 576-579.

Russell, M.A.H., Cole, P.V., Idle, M.S. & Adams, L. (1975) Carbon monoxide yields of cigarettes and their relation to nicotine yield and type of filter. *British Medical Journal,* **3,** 71-73.

Russell, M.A.H., Feyerabend, C. (1978) Cigarette smoking: A dependence on high-nicotine boli. *Drug Metabolism Reviews.* **8,** 29-57.

Russell, M.A.H., Feyerabend, C. & Cole, P.V. (1976) Plasma nicotine levels after cigarette smoking and chewing nicotine gum. *British Medical Journal,* **1,** 1043-1046.

Russell, M.A.H., Peto, J. & Patel, U.A. (1974) The classification of smoking by factorial structure of motives. *Journal of the Royal Statistical Society, A.* **137,** 313-333.

Russell, M.A.H., Sutton, S.R., Feyerabend, C., Cole, P.V. & Saloojee, Y. (1977) Nicotine chewing gum as a substitute for smoking. *British Medical Journal,* **1,** 1060-1063.

Russell, M.A.H., Wilson, C., Feyerabend, C. & Cole, P.V. (1976) Effect of nicotine chewing-gum on smoking behaviour and as an aid to cigarette withdrawal. *British Medical Journal,* **2,** 391-393.

Russell, M.A.H., Wilson, C., Patel, U.A., Cole, P.V. & Feyerabend, C. (1973) Comparison of the effect on tobacco consumption and carbon monoxide absorption of changing to high and low nicotine cigarettes. *British Medical Journal,* **4,** 512-516.

Russell, M.A.H., Wilson, C., Patel, U.A., Cole, P.V. & Feyerabend, C. (1975) Plasma nicotine levels after smoking cigarettes with high, medium and low nicotine yields. *British Medical Journal,* **2,** 414-416.

Schachter, S. (1977) Nicotine regulation in heavy and light smokers, *Journal of Experimental Psychology: General,* **106,** 5-12.

Schachter, S., Kozlowski, L.T. & Silverstein, B. (1977) Effects of urinary pH on cigarette smoking. *Journal of Experimental Psychology: General,* **106,** 13-·19.

Stepney, R. & Thompson, J.W. (1977) Behavioural regulation of nicotine intake in cigarette smokers presented with a 'shortened' cigarette. *British Journal of Clinical Pharmacology,* **4,** 653P.

Stolerman, I.P., Goldfarb, T.L., Fink, R. & Jarvik, M.E. (1973) Influencing cigarette smoking with nicotine antagonists. *Psychopharmacologia,* **28,** 247-259.

Sutton, S.R. Feyerabend, C., Cole, P.V. & Russell, M.A.H. (1978a) Adjustment of smokers to dilution of tobacco smoke by ventilated cigarette holders. Clinical Pharmacology and Therapeutics, In press.

Sutton, S.R., Russell, M.A.H., Feyerabend, C. & Saloojee, Y. (1978b) Smokers' response to dilution of smoke by ventilated cigarette holders. *This volume.*

Turner J.A.McM., Sillett, R.W. & Ball, K.P. (1974) Some effects of changing to low-tar and low-nicotine cigarettes. *Lancet,* **2,** 737-739.

27. The influence of cigarette smoke yields on smoking habits

P I ADAMS

Introduction

It is a matter of great interest to any product manufacturer to know how his product is consumed. In the case of a tobacco manufacturer it is relatively easy to conduct market research surveys to discover who smokes cigarettes - how many, which brand and on what occasion. It is less easy to obtain data on subjective opinions about cigarettes - their quality, flavour, and the satisfaction given. It is very difficult indeed to investigate how a cigarette is actually smoked.

Each person has a variety of ways in which he can smoke his cigarette differently from someone else. The method of drawing smoke from a cigarette in terms of the flow rate/time profile of the puff may differ. The puff volumes and spacing of the puffs during the life of the cigarette may differ. These factors have been shown to affect the smoke yield from the cigarette. Given the smoke drawn from the cigarette there are two further ways in which the smokers can alter their dose - by losing some smoke before the act of inhaling and changes in the act of inhalation itself.

In theory all these factors are susceptible to measurement but in practice efforts to do so sometimes intrude unacceptably into the normal smoking behaviour.

Experimental methods

We have for many years been using a method for recording the smoking habits of our panels (Adams, 1972, 1976). It is somewhat similar to that described in the paper by Creighton, Noble and Whewell (1978). There are disadvantages to the procedure which we mention:- intrusion into the habit by the use of a cigarette holder and the tubes necessary to make flow measurement; increased resistance to puffing presented by the measuring orifice. As tests of the validity of our experiments, we have compared recordings of smokings made by different methods. We have filmed smokers and subsequently analysed the film frame by frame to obtain puffing data (Adams, 1972). We have also unobtrusively observed panel members smoking in situations other than in our lounge - laboratory. A pressure sensitive transmitter of the type originally described by Mackay and Jacobson (1957), has been used to avoid the physical linkage between the cigarette holder and the transducers. Comparisons of the data have shown a satisfactory agreement between the different methods of measurement.

In addition there are effects due to the test surroundings. We have made efforts to provide a relaxed atmosphere; the lounges have carpets, easy chairs, pictures, magazines are available and the tests are administered by pleasant people. Conditions for different panels are as similar as we can make them.

Tests must also be made when the recording apparatus is available rather than when a smoker wishes to smoke. Any effect this may have has not been revealed by experiments in which the time since last smoking and the number of cigarettes smoked before the test have been considered as experimental variables. In addition, we have invited smokers to come and be measured when they felt they would like to smoke. We have not been able to show any significant differences associated with this procedure.

Our methods stop short of measurement of any smoke lost before inhalation and of measurement of inhalation itself. Puff volumes are therefore only deliveries from the end of the cigarette and not necessarily volumes which are inhaled by the smoker.

Findings: Experiments 1 and 2

We have conducted three major experiments in our attempts to determine whether changes in cigarette smoke yield (measured by standard analytical methods) influence personal smoking habits. In 1970, smokers at Research Department of Imperial Tobacco at Bristol tested three types of filter cigarette. These were the cigarettes being used by Dr. C.M. Fletcher at Hammersmith Hospital in his studies supported by the Tobacco Research Council. The PM (wnf) (particulate matter, water and nicotine free) yields were 17 to 23 mg and the nicotine levels were 1.6 to 1.7 mg. The nicotine level is high and the differences between the yields of the cigarette small by 1977 standards. One cigarette type had a carbon filter and therefore about 50% reduction in vapour phase delivery. The smokers took significantly larger puffs from the vapour phase reduced cigarettes and therefore showed some change in habit despite otherwise fairly similar particulate matter and nicotine levels. If a compensation mechanism exists, this experiment suggests that the sensory factor in the control of smoking includes detection of the vapour phase. Other factors must include particulate matter and nicotine yields and, perhaps, the overall draw resistance of the cigarette.

The second experiment in 1972/3 (Adams, 1976) was designed to include these factors, to measure subjective opinions and to show whether the results from the panel at our Research Department represented smoking by the general public. We studied the results from three panels at non-tobacco subsidiaries of Imperial Tobacco Group (Sutton-in-Ashfield, Manchester and Bristol). We concluded that when nicotine and PM (wnf) are reduced simultaneously the smokers took an increased volume of smoke. For a low yielding ventilated cigarette in which yield reduction was about 40%, the amount of compensation by puffing was 10% and the possible increase in cigarette usage was a further 5%. The smokers responded to higher pressure drop cigarettes by lowering their puffing flow rate so as to lower the perceived draw resistance. The data on cigarette usage was unsatisfactory. The weekly consumptions of the free issues of cigarettes was 20 to 25% higher than the panels stated before the experiment began. The data failed to confirm significantly, the known result that males smoke more than females. In all this work, we took steps not to tell the smokers when their supplies of cigarettes were changed. Comments received showed that some changes were detected, others were not and some were thought to have been detected when no changes were made.

Experiment 3

Our third experiment attempted to answer three questions:

1. Do smokers increase their consumption when changing from a middle to a low tar brand?
2. Does it matter whether they are informed about the change or not?
3. Are the changes in puffing habits seen previously reproducible?

Experimental Design

Two panels each of 32 smokers at different locations in Bristol took part in a ten week smoking test beginning in March 1977. One panel was composed of Research Department personnel and the other from Imperial Tobacco Limited Head Office personnel. The panels were chosen from volunteers to give a balance between male and female, high and low consumption smokers.

Each panel was divided into three groups:

A) Ten smokers who changed from a middle tar to a low tar brand and were told about the change.

B) Ten smokers who changed from a middle tar to a low tar brand and were not told about the change.

C) Twelve smokers who acted as a control panel.

  C(i) Eight smoked the middle tar brand throughout.

  C(ii) Four smoked the low tar brand throughout.

Where possible they were also balanced across groups to allow for differences in age and normal cigarette brand. Of all these variables, cigarette consumption was treated as most important. In addition, the panellists were selected so that as far as possible those in groups A, B and C (i) were middle tar regular length filter cigarette smokers and those in group C (ii) were low tar filter smokers.

The plan of the smoking changes is shown in Table 27.1.

Table 27.1 Calendar of smoking changes

Week	1	2	3	4	5	6	7	8	9	10	11
Panel Group											
A	--	OB	M	M	M	M	M	L	L	L	L
B	OB	M	M	M	M	M	L	L	L	L	—
C(i)	OB	M	M	M	M	M	M	M	M	M	M
C(ii)	OB	L	L	L	L	L	L	L	L	L	L

Note: OB - Own Brand; M - Middle Tar; L - Low Tar

Cigarettes

The regular size (70mm long, 24.5mm circumference) tipped cigarettes manufactured by ITL, were supplied in white 20's packs stamped with the Government Health warning. Cigarettes for Group A were labelled 'Middle Tar' or 'Low Tar'; for Groups B and C they were coded with the panellist's personal number and the test week.

The analytical data for the test cigarettes is given in Table 27.2.

Table 27.2 Analytical data

	Middle tar	Low tar
TPM	25	12
Nicotine	1.4	0.8
Water	5.2	1.4
PM (wnf)	18	9.3
Number of puffs	8.4	9.0
Filter retention % (for nicotine)	48	62
Pressure Drop mmH$_2$O	105	105

(TPM, Nicotine, Water, PM (wnf) in mg)

Conduct of the experiment

Smokers were asked to visit the smoking lounges to smoke their cigarettes on two occasions in each week. During the first test the smokers filled in a questionnaire about their cigarettes and during the second they were normally reading magazines or newspapers. Measurements of puff volumes, durations and the intervals between puffs were made on each occasion.

Cigarette butts were collected after each test so that butt length could be measured and the amount of nicotine retained in the filter tip estimated.

The first two test weeks formed a running-in period to acclimatise the smokers to the test procedure. Test weeks began and cigarettes were issued to panel members on Wednesdays. This enabled us to make one test on each smoker during the calander week of issue and a second test after the weekend. When smokers came to collect their weekly issue they were asked to return any remaining cigarettes of the previous week's supply. They were also asked how many cigarettes they had given away or received during the previous week so that their weekly consumption could be calculated.

Smokers who complained that cigarettes were too strong were given exchange packets of the same type. Smokers who complained that cigarettes were too mild were reminded that they could smoke as many cigarettes as they liked. In this experiment we again decided to make a free gift of as many cigarettes as were required by the members of the panels. Control groups C (i) and C (ii) were used in an attempt to measure the effect due to the free gift when it was not confounded with a change of type of cigarette.

Subjective and objective variables

The following objective variables were measured:
Weekly Cigarette Consumption.
Number of Puffs taken.
Total puff volume per cigarette: ml (Total Volume).
Sum of the puff durations per cigarettes: s (Total Duration).
Duration of the test smoking: s (Total Time Alight).

Butt Length: mm.

Nicotine retained in filter: mg.

The questionnaire measured subjective opinions about Strength, Smoothness, Hotness, Amount of Flavour, Flavour, Satisfaction and Quality. It also offered space for recording unspecified comments about the cigarettes.

Results of the statistical analyses

The data were examined by an analysis of variance for groups A and B separately and then jointly in the two panels, having shown that any differences were statistically non-significant. Data from Groups C (i) and C (ii) were considered separately.

The data for each individual week were treated as a replicate after checking for absence of systematic effects.

Objective variables

Knowledge about the type change. The analysis first showed that any changes in the smoking habit which can be associated with being told about the change from one type of cigarette to the other were statistically non-significant. The data for groups A and B have not subsequently been considered separately.

Puffing variables. The analysis shows that cigarette type had a significant effect (at the 0.01 level or higher) on all the variables named above except Total Time Alight. The mean values for all the results combined are given below (Table 27.3) and show clearly what happened.

Table 27.3 Puffing data

Variable	Period	1 Middle Tar	2 Low Tar
Total Volume (ml)		364 (8)*	469 (8)
Total Duration (s)		17.0 (0.4)	22.6 (0.4)
Total Time Alight (s)		390 (4)	387 (4)
Number of Puffs		11.1 (0.2)	12.0 (0.2)
Filter Nicotine (mg)		1.5 (0.03)	1.9 (0.03).

*Standard errors given in ( ).

The panels responded to the change from middle tar to low tar by increasing the volume of smoke taken from the cigarette. This has been done by taking more puffs of longer duration at slightly higher puff frequency (total time alight is unchanged) keeping the average puff flow rates similar.

There is other significant evidence (Table 27.4) of the effects due to the panel and to a panel/cigarette interaction.

Butt length. The data show that smokers at ITL Head Office (HO) left a longer butt length than those at Research Department (RD). The reason for this is not known but it might be associated with greater familiarity and longer use of the apparatus by

Table 27.4 Butt length and cigarette consumption.

Variable	Period Cigarette Panel	Research Dept. 1 M	L	2 M	L	ITL Head Office 1 M	L	2 M	L	Standard Error
Butt	Main (A&B)	4.8			5.4	8.5			6.5	(0.2)
Length										
(mm)	Control C (i)	5.0		5.4		9.2		8.4		(0.5)
	Control C (ii)		6.3		6.8		6.3		6.8	
Cigarette	Main (A&B)	206			237	162			168	(4)
Consump-										
tion (per	Control C (i)	200		206		197		197		(High
week)	Control C (ii)		193		206		136		133	23-61)

Note: 1. Butt length is measured from the forward edge of the cork joining paper.

2. Standard errors on control consumptions are high because of the small size of the panel. Actual values depend on the actual period studied between the limits quoted.

the panel at RD.   The fact that HO smokers leave a shorter butt length with low tar cigarettes might be expected from the possible methods of compensation. This is the first clear evidence of this effect but it is made less clear by the opposite response of the RD panel.

Cigarette consumption. Table 27.4 shows several interesting facts:
(i)   The Research Department consumptions were the greater.
(ii)   The control groups smoked consistently.
(iii)   Consumption did not increase due to the change to low tar at HO but it did at RD.

Table 27.5 repeats the data from Table 27.4 and adds the consumption as stated before the experiment.

Table 27.5 Stated versus actual consumption (cigarettes/week)

	RD Stated in advance Period	Actual 1	2	HO Stated in advance Period	Actual 1	2
Main (A&B) 148		206	237	143	162	168
Control C(i) 162		200	206	179	197	197
Control C(ii) 144		193	206	103	136	133

There are very considerable difficulties in obtaining a true picture of cigarette consumption. In a survey it is usually found that an unexplained difference of about 5% exists between the integrated stated consumption of a representative population of smokers and the number of cigarettes known to have been sold. Sales are greater.

Table 27.5 shows that the HO panel results were not much in excess of the 5%. RD on the other hand showed a greater discrepancy. The overall level is inflated by some of the panel members who took vastly more cigarettes than they previously stated.

It is possible that the members of the panel did not know how many cigarettes they smoked before the experiment began. It is possible that they do not want to know and this may be because of personal psychological barriers regarding money spent or the number of packets consumed.   There is also the problem in asking for daily or weekly consumptions with regard to the errors involved in scaling from the former to the latter. Some of the panel normally smoke King Size cigarettes at weekends, replacing these with smaller regular size cigarettes could contribute to the observed increase in consumption.

In an experiment in which panels of people are asked to smoke brands different from their normal choice, it is difficult to decide whether they should be given cigarettes or pay for them. We have chosen the gift because this provides some incentive to the smokers to smoke only test cigarettes during the course of the experiment. Table 27.5 shows that the HO panel, which was least familiar with the experimenters and their apparatus, was more inhibited in its demands for cigarettes. We think that this inhibition is akin to that which might operate in the market place because of a reluctance to buy additional cigarettes.

Cigarette Yields   The filter nicotine values in Table 27.3 need some qualification and interpretation. We can calculate the smoke nicotine delivery from these data and the efficiency of the filters on the cigarettes. We assume that efficiency is the same for human and machine smoking.

The efficiency of filtration of particulate matter is also assumed to be the same as that for nicotine. This is known not to be quite true but it is a reasonable assumption for the average results from a large panel (Creighton and Lewis, 1978a, b).   These are assumptions which can only be tested by the use of a puff duplicating machine, (Creighton *et al*, 1978), i.e. a machine which smokes a cigarette with the same sequence and shapes of puff as a human smoker.

Our data suggest that the flow rates during puffs for our panels are higher than those in the standard analytical regime. These could lead to reductions in filter efficiency and consequent increases in smoke yield to the human smokers of up to 5% for these types of cigarettes. We have made no allowance for this possible error in the dose calculations below.

The dose of PM (wnf) for a particular panel is therefore calculated by use of the expression

$$\text{Dose} = \frac{\text{analytical PM(wnf)}}{\text{analytical nicotine}} \times \text{cigarette consumption} \times \text{panel smoke nicotine}$$

Further, as an upper limit, we assume that all smoke passing the filter enters the human smoker and is totally retained. Table 27.6 shows these data.

Table 27.6 Smoke doses

	Middle Tar	Low Tar
Cigarette consumption		
Head Office	162	168
Research Department	206	237
Smoke nicotine (mg)		
Analysis	1.4	0.8
Head Office	1.6	1.1
Research Department	1.8	1.3
PM (wnf) (mg)		
Analysis	18.2	9.3
Dose nicotine (mg/week)		
Head Office	257	188
Research Department	360	298
Dose PM (wnf) (mg/week)		
Head Office	3328	2090
Research Department	4658	3318

Clearly the smoker's dose of nicotine and PM (wnf) are much reduced when smoking low tar cigarettes. Note that the reduced dose at RD is equal to the normal dose at HO.

Even more interestingly is the result that the nicotine available to the smoker is proportionately more from the low tar than from the middle tar cigarette. In his smoking he does not therefore find quite the reduction in nicotine yield that the standard analytical values would suggest.

Subjective variables The questionnaire on which the smokers recorded their opinions about the subjective qualities of the cigarettes is reproduced in the Appendix. Their answers were measured by the use of the arbitrary scales shown on the questionnaire. These scales were not known to the smokers when they were answering the questions.

Mean values are given in Table 27.7.

We found that the effect of cigarettes was highly significant. With respect to the middle tar cigarette, the low tar cigarette was: slightly too mild, slightly too smooth, slightly too hot, fairly satisfying, and had less than usual amount of flavour.

The opinion of the control groups was reassuringly consistent throughout the experiment.

Table 27.7n Subjective data

Period			1		2
Variable	Panel				
			Cigarette type		Cigarette type
	A & B	M	3.7(0.1)	L	4.9(0.1)
Strength or	C (i)	M	3.9	M	4.0
mildness	C (ii)	L	3.9	L	3.8
	A & B	M	4.4(0.1)	L	3.6(0.1)
Smoothness	C (i)	M	4.6	M	4.4
/harshness	C (ii)	L	4.2	L	4.3
	A & B	M	3.7(0.1)	L	4.4(0.1
Hotness	C (i)	M	3.5	M	3.7
	C (ii)	L	3.9	L	3.9
	A & B	M	3.1(0.1)	L	2.7(0.1)
Amount of	C (i)	M	3.2	M	3.1
flavour	C (ii)	L	3.1	L	3.2
	A & B	M	3.0(0.1)	L	3.1(0.1)
Flavour	C (i)	M	3.2	M	3.1
	C (ii)	L	2.7	L	2.7
Satisfaction	A & B	M	3.5(0.1)	L	4.1(0.1)
from one	C (i)	M	3.7	M	3.6
cigarette	C (ii)	L	3.2	L	3.3
	A & B	M	3.2(0.1)	L	3.0(0.1)
Overall	C (i)	M	3.3	M	3.4
quality	C (ii)	L	3.3	L	3.4
Comparison	A & B	M	3.6(0.1)	L	3.6(0.1)
with usual	C (i)	M	3.6	M	3.5
cigarette	C (ii)	M	3.2	M	3.2
Comparison	A & B	M	3.0(0.1)	L	3.1(0.1)
with previous	C (i)	M	2.9	M	2.9
supply	C (ii)	L	3.0	L	2.9

( ) least significant difference

Comments by the panel.   These were recorded week by week and were also received in a meeting of the HO panel at the end of the experiment. The recorded comments reveal preconceived ideas about the changes or lack of them. They add little to the results from the questionnaire.

The panellists showed great interest to know what types of cigarettes they had been smoking and revealed that there had been very little association between the groups A and B. Most smokers said that they had noticed the change and that it had caused them to smoke more cigarettes. Two people who held this view most strongly were surprised to find that in fact, after one week of slightly increased consumption, they had actually returned almost exactly to their previous level. For this panel at least any subjective association between low tar cigarettes and increased consumption is not supported by the evidence.

Acknowledgement

The author is grateful to many colleagues in Imperial Tobacco Limited for their help in the conduct of the experiment, the analysis of the data, and the preparation of this paper.

Appendix

We would like to have your opinions of the latest supply of cigarettes.

Below are a number of statements about different aspects of the cigarettes. Please tick, under each heading, one of the statements which best describes your opinion about that aspect of the cigarettes.

1. THE STRENGTH OR MILDNESS

Much too strong for me	.... 1.
Too strong for me	.... 2.
Slightly on the strong side for me	.... 3.
Just right for me	.... 4.
Slightly on the mild side for me	.... 5.
Too mild for me	.... 6.
Much too mild for me	.... 7.

2. THE SMOOTHNESS OR HARSHNESS

Much too smooth for me	.... 1.
Too smooth for me	.... 2.
Slightly too smooth for me	.... 3.
Just right for me	.... 4.
Slightly too harsh for me	.... 5.
Too harsh for me	.... 6.
Much too harsh for me	.... 7.

3. THE HOTNESS

Much too hot for me	.... 1.
Too hot for me	.... 2.
Slightly on the hot side for me	.... 3.
Just right for me	.... 4.

Slightly on the cool side for me   .... 5.
Too cool for me   .... 6.
Much too cool for me   .... 7.

4. THE AMOUNT OF FLAVOUR

No flavour at all   .... 1.
A flavour I hardly noticed   .... 2.
About the usual amount of flavour .... 3.
Quite a noticeable amount of flavour .... 4.
A very noticeable amount of flavour............ 5.

5. THE FLAVOUR

Absolutely right for me   .... 1.
Would suit me quite well   .... 2.
It seemed reasonable enough   .... 3.
Not very suitable for me   .... 4.
Not what I would choose   .... 5.

6. THE SATISFACTION FROM ONE CIGARETTE

Extremely satisfying   .... 1.
Very satisfying   .... 2.
Sufficiently satisfying   .... 3.
Fairly satisfying   .... 4.
Only slightly satisfying   .... 5.
Not satisfying at all   .... 6.

7. THE OVERALL QUALITY

A very poor cigarette   .... 1.
A poor cigarette   .... 2.
A fair cigarette   .... 3.
A good cigarette   .... 4.
A very good cigarette   .... 5.

8. How do these cigarettes compare, overall, with your usual cigarette?

Much better   .... 1.
A little better   .... 2.
About the same   .... 3.
Not quite as good   .... 4.
Not nearly as good   .... 5.

9. Generally, how do these cigarettes compare with your previous supply?

Much better   .... 1.
A little better   .... 2.
About the same   .... 3.
Not quite as good   .... 4.
Not nearly as good   .... 5.

10. Finally, are there any other comments you would like to make about these cigarettes?

The numbers by each possible answer are arbitary values for analysis and are not shown on the copies given to the panellists.

References

Adams, P.I. (1972) Cigar smoking: measurement of the human smoking regime and its relationship to smoking machines. In *CORESTA Information Bulletin,* CORESTA/TCRC Joint Conference, Williamsburg, Virginia, **No. 1972 Special.**

Adams, P.I. (1976) Changes in personal smoking habits brought about by changes in cigarette smoke yield. *Proceedings of the Sixth International Tobacco Scientific Congress,* Tokyo, 102-108.

Creighton, D.E. & Lewis, P.H. (1978a) The effect of different cigarettes on human smoking patterns. *This volume.*

Creighton, D.E. & Lewis, P.H. (1978b) The effect of smoking pattern on smoke deliveries. *This volume.*

Creighton, D.E., Noble, M.J. & Whewell, R.T. (1978) Instruments to measure, record and duplicate human smoking patterns. *This volume.*

Mackay, R.S. & Jacobson, B. (1957) Endoradiosonde, *Nature,* **179,** 1239-1240.

28. Analysis of smoking pattern including intake of carbon monoxide and influences of changes in cigarette design

R GUILLERM AND E RADZISZEWSKI

A comparative analysis of the respiratory effects of substituting a low-irritant cigarette for the usual one in eighty heavy smokers over a five-week period seemed to show that changing the type of cigarette induced changes in smoking pattern (Guillerm *et al,* 1974). We had then come to the conclusion that referring only to the chemical composition of tobacco or smoke might lead us to make significant errors as regards the estimation of the biological effects of a cigarette. We have therefore developed an original method that enables the smoking pattern and its possible changes as a function of the type of cigarette smoked to be analysed with precision (Guillerm and Radziszewski, 1975). This paper deals with the results obtained by using this method and substituting a mild cigarette for the usual one over a period of one week.

Materials and methods

It may be recalled that our technique published in 1975 combines three techniques of investigation as follows: the measurement of puff parameters, the analysis of the smoker's ventilatory behaviour and the measurement of carbon monoxide intake. Two methods are involved in *the analysis of puff parameters,* a method using a flowmeter and a method using a pyrometer.

In the *flowmeter method* a miniature flowmeter is used (dead space : 2.5ml) which is made of two plastic parts enclosing a small disc of wire-gauze screen with fine mesh (0.063 mm). The flowmeter we used in a preliminary experiment was a cigarette-holder but it was found that the use of such a flowmeter induced changes in the smoking pattern (Guillerm and Radziszewski, 1975). In our latest study the flowmeter is incorporated into the cigarette (Fig. 28.1). The results obtained during our experiments have shown that this flowmeter does not disturb the smoker very much (low resistance : $\Delta p = 0.12$mm of water/ml/sec).

Figure 28.2 shows the whole system used during our measurements. The flow is measured by means of an Elema-Schonander differential pressure gauge (EMT 32) connected to the flowmeter through a small diameter tube made of flexible poly-vinyl; the flowmeter reading is linear over the range of flows usually observed for a smoker. The puff flow and puff volume (electronic flow integration) as well as the puff duration and puff frequency are recorded continuously during smoking by means of an ink-jet polygraph.

The *pyrometer technique,* which produces no constraints whatever on the subject, makes it possible to make a remote measurement (from three metres approximately)

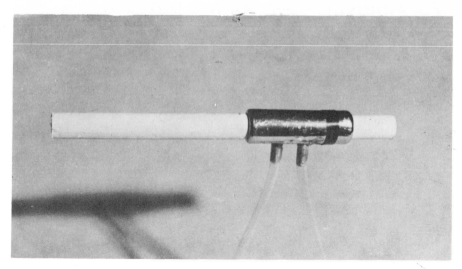

Fig. 28.1 View of the miniature flowmeter used to measure puff parameters.

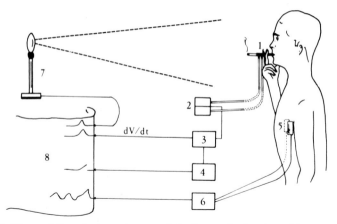

Fig. 28.2 View of the whole system used during analysis of smoking patterns.
1. Flowmeter
2. Differential pressure gauge
3. Galvanometer
4. Integrator
5. Pneumographic electrodes
6. Impedance pneumograph
7. Pyrometer
8. Polygraph

of the instantaneous temperature of the cigarette burning cone. By means of a special infra-red pyrometer the puff frequency and the number of puffs are determined. By comparing these results with those obtained with the flowmeter we could make sure that our experimental system did not induce any significant change in the smoking pattern.

The *smoker's ventilatory behaviour* is analysed by impedance pneumography. Two electrodes are placed in the upper mid-axillary position. Recording the changes in thoracic impedance due to ventilatory movements makes it possible, after calibration, to know the variations of tidal volume and respiratory frequency. The ventilation is thus recorded continuously enabling the determination of the location of the puffs in the ventilatory cycle to measure the duration of smoke-holding in the mouth before the next inspiration and to estimate the volume of smoke dilution in the smoker's lungs. The puff and ventilation parameters are recorded on magentic tape so that they can be computer-processed subsequently (HP2100).

Carbon monoxide intake is measured by determining the smoker's COHb level before and after smoking one cigarette, using a method that does not require the taking of blood samples (Guillerm *et al*, 1959). It is a pure-oxygen rebreathing technique; when blood and alveolar air are in equilibrium (which takes about six minutes) partial pressures of CO and oxygen are measured and the COHb level is determined. It should be stressed that such measurements are quite as accurate (accuracy of COHb $\pm$ 0.1%, on an average) and reproducible as direct measurements with blood sampling.

Finally, we used *liquid chromatography* to measure the quantity of urinary nicotine excreted by four subjects in the time interval between the measurements (8 a.m. to 4 p.m.).

The above techniques were used during a comparative analysis of the behaviour of eight smokers voluntarily changing from the usual cigarette (U.C.) to a less irritant cigarette (E.C.) over a seven-day period. The characteristics and composition of these two types of cigarette are listed in Table 28.1. These cigarettes have nearly similar nicotine contents, however the E.C. is provided with an active charcoal filter which decreases its irritating power; in fact, the ciliostatic activity of the E.C. is about one third of that of the U.C.

Table 28.1 Details of the two brands of cigarette smoked in the experiment

	Usual Cigarette (UC)	Experimental Cigarette (EC) ventilated charcoal filter
NICOTINE (mg)	1.66	1.31
pH	7.30	7.45
TAR (mg)	30.9	15.9
CO (ml)	15	14
ACROLEIN (μg)	102	27
PHENOLS (μg)	110	58

The experimental schedule included two investigations: the first one at 8 a.m. in subjects deprived of cigarettes, and the second one in the afternoon at about 4 p.m.   In the time interval between the investigations the subjects were allowed to smoke an unrestricted number of cigarettes of the type prescribed by the experimental schedule and the number of cigarettes smoked was carefully noted.

Each investigation included two cases: one measurement with the flowmeter and one without the flowmeter (pyrometer) with a time interval of about thirty minutes between them. Such measurements were balanced so as to avoid the influence of the measurement sequences. In both cases the COHb level was measured first, then the smoker entered the examination room in order to smoke. The subjects were allowed to smoke the U.C. up to a mark placed at 23 mm from the proximal pa (standard butt length) and the E.C. up to 29 mm (including the filter). The COHb level was measured again precisely five minutes after smoking.

In order to prevent the smoker from being disturbed by factors other than those to be measured the environmental conditions were controlled (background music, subjects sitting beyond the visual field of the experimenter). The sequence of smoking (U.C./E.C.) as well as the sequence of measurements (with restraint/ without restraint) were matched for each subject.

Results

An example of a record obtained during smoking is shown in Figure 28.3. The complete analysis of the diagram takes into account the following parameters: flow, volume and duration of each puff, number of puffs, interval between puffs, tidal volume between puffs, tidal volume immediately following the puffs and represent- ing the volume of smoke dilution and location of the puff in the ventilatory cycle. The results obtained are then analysed statistically using Student's t test applied to paired values.

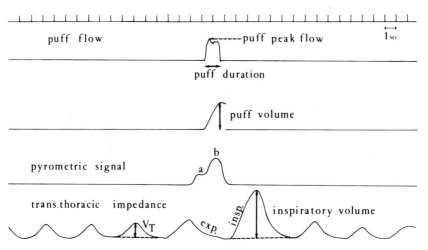

Fig. 28.3 A sample recording of smoking act parameters.

Smoking pattern with the usual cigarette (U.C.)
The values of the various puff parameters are given in Table 28.2 together with the CO intake.

Table 28.2 Puff parameters & CO intake values during smoking usual cigarette.

Parameters	Mean (8 subjects)	Limit of variation
Puff volume	38.5 ml	15 - 80 ml
Puff peak flow	35 ml/sec	15 - 50 ml/sec
Puff duration	1.85 sec	0.8 - 2.9 sec
Time between puffs	40.7 sec	23 - 115 sec
Number of puffs	12	5 - 16
CO intake (first cigarette of the morning)	1.22%	0.3 - 2.21%
CO intake at 4.00 p.m.	0.61%	0 - 1.56%

As can be seen from the last column, inter-individual variations are very significant. It was found, on the other hand, that intra-individual variations are very small. Only the mean values (middle column) will be taken into consideration and compared with those obtained with the experimental cigarette (E.C.) It is to be noted that the carbon monoxide intake significantly decreases during the day; in fact the increase in COHb level measured after smoking one cigarette is 1.22% on average at 8 a.m. in a subject deprived of cigarettes and only 0.6% in the afternoon after smoking under the same experimental conditions. On the other hand, all other smoking pattern parameters measured (puff parameters, ventilation) do not vary very much between the morning and the afternoon. Such findings will be analysed in detail and discussed.

As far as the *location of the puff in the ventilatory cycle* is concerned we found that all subjects located 80% of their puffs during an expiratory pause. The corresponding expiratory cycle is twice as long as the expiration during cycles between puffs. The inspiration volume that follows a puff (therefore representing, as a rule, the volume of air which dilutes the smoke inhaled), as twice as large on average as the inspiration during normal cycles.   It should be stressed here that we have always observed the same profiles during other experiments with other subjects. In Figure 28.4 the ventilatory profile has been schematised at the time of the puff taking into account the mean values obtained in the eight subjects.

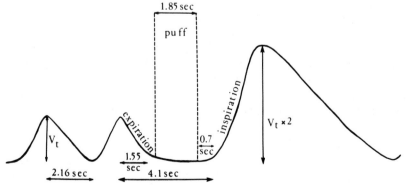

Fig. 28.4 Puff position on the ventilatory cycle during usual cigarette smoking (mean values in eight subjects).

The time interval between the end of the puff and the beginning of the inhalation is shown in Figure 28.4; it is equal to 0.7 s on average.

All these values are only indicative because of the small number of subjects and of the wide inter-individual variations. However, an experiment now in progress with a greater number of subjects will make it possible to generalise our results.

As already mentioned above, it is of interest to note that intra-individual variations are small for all parameters measured. As a matter of fact, each subject has his own distinctive way of smoking with the result that the experimenters can identify the subjects by their smoking behaviour records in the same way that fingerprints are used. Figure 28.5 shows an example of a record obtained in three different subjects. It is obvious that for each subject the puff profile and the corresponding ventilatory profile can be superimposed, but that each subject differs from the others by one or the other of the above mentioned parameters.

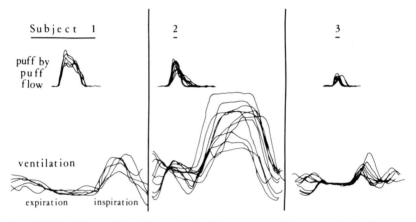

Fig. 28.5 Puff by puff profiles and simultaneous ventilatory cycles in three subjects during usual cigarette smoking.

Effects of substituting the E.C. for the U.C.
The mean values obtained with the U.C. and E.C. at 8 a.m. and 4 p.m. are given in Figure 28.6. Changing from the U.C. to the E.C. results in significant changes in some parameters of the smoking pattern. Thus, with the E.C. the puff peak flow falls by 31% (p =.001), the number of puffs is increased by two puffs (p =.001) the puff duration is 27% longer (p =.001) and, last of all, the total smoking duration increases from 390 sec. to 455 sec. (p =.01). The variations of the other parameters are more discrete and without any statistical significance. This is the case for the puff volume (34.8 ml with the E.C.; 38.5 ml with the U.C.), the total volume of smoke inhaled (485 ml with the E.C.; 452 ml with the U.C.), the puff frequency and the inspiratory volume following the puff (918 ml with both types of cigarettes). It may be noted that the values obtained for all parameters with E.C. and U.C. differ significantly from the CORESTA standards.

The mean values for the COHb level are given in Figure 28.7. In the morning the CO intake after smoking one cigarette is significantly greater with the E.C. (ΔCOHb = 1.36%) than with the U.C. (ΔCOHb = 1.09%) (p. = .05). On the other hand, in the

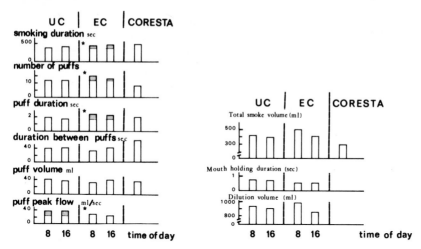

Fig. 28.6 Puff parameter values during smoking usual (U.C.) or experimental (E.C.) cigarette (mean of eight subjects) (*statistically significant).

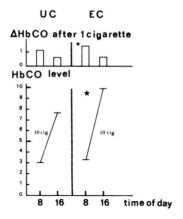

Fig. 28.7 Mean COHb intake/cigarette (upper part of the figure) and COHb level while smoking U.C. or E.C. at 8.00 a.m. and 4.00 p.m. (*statistically significant).

evening the CO intake is identical with both types of cigarette ($\Delta COHb = 0.6\%$) but appreciably lower than in the morning. The COHb level at the end of the day is significantly higher with the E.C. (9.9% on an average) than with the U.C. (7.7%) (p = .001); it should be noted here that cigarette consumption remains absolutely unchanged (ten cigarettes between 8 a.m. and 4 p.m.).

Discussion

The method and experimental schedule we used have provided qualitative and quantitative information about the smoker's behaviour during the day as a function of the type of cigarette smoked.

It is clear that each subject has his own way of smoking which is mainly charac-

N

acterised by the puff location in the ventilatory cycle, but also by the puff volume, the puff duration and puff frequency as well as by the ventilatory profile at the time of the puff.

The important decrease in carbon monoxide intake observed between the morning and the evening measurements after the smoking of one cigarette is not associated with any significant change in the puff or ventilation parameters. The assumption that such a decrease might be due to a change in the CO alveolo-arterial gradient has been confirmed by our laboratory experiments. In fact, in subjects deprived of cigarettes whose COHb levels were raised to 6% within a few minutes by means of a rebreathing technique, we observed a decrease in CO intake during the smoking of a cigarette similar to our experimental cigarette (Figure 28.8). This result also shows that the alveolar CO concentration during smoking should be low (a few hundred ppm compared with more than 4% in the smoke) since CO intake is influenced by relatively low venous COHb levels.

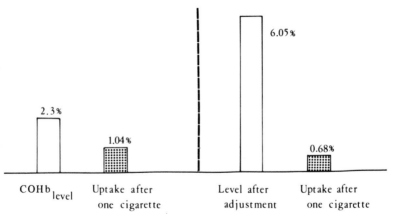

Fig. 28.8 Relationships between COHb level and CO intake (mean of 12 values)

Consequently, the coefficient of smoke inhalation (that is the ratio between the observed CO intake and the CO volume indicated by the smoking machine) will have to be determined in the morning. The differences between subjects and between cigarette types may indeed be reduced and not very discriminative in the evening.

It is interesting to calculate and compare the inhalation coefficient for different cigarettes. In our experiment with the U.C. the average increase of 1.22% in COHb level corresponds to a CO intake of about 12 ml in a subject with an average weight of 70 kg. The CO volume given by the smoking machine with this same type of cigarette is 15 ml. This means that all the CO would be retained if the subject smoked in accordance with the CORESTA standards. This cannot be possible and may be explained by the fact that our subjects do not smoke in accordance with the standards. This result was not a great surprise to us since other authors, such as Keith (1962) in particular, have observed with different means of investigation that the smoking pattern parameters are appreciably different from those generally accepted for smoking machines.

We will now discuss the changes in smoking pattern parameters when substituting the low-irritant cigarette for the usual cigarette. Certainly the most important finding is the 26% increase in CO intake observed in the morning with the E.C. together with the significant increase in COHb level in the afternoon (in comparison with the results obtained with the U.C.). This is not easily explained. In fact the CO values indicated by the smoking machine are similar for both types of cigarette (refer to Table 28.1). On the other hand, there is no correlation between the COHb level and the main parameters of the smoking pattern. However, Figure 28.9 shows that the CO intake is correlated with the total volume of smoke inhaled (puff volume x number of puffs). In such a case the total volume of smoke inhaled, which is 20% greater on average with the E.C., may account to a large extent for the increase in COHb level.

Finally, the multiple-factor analysis of the smoking behaviour does provide interesting qualitative and quantitative information but the essential data is the carbon monoxide intake which gives the best indication of the quantity of smoke actually inhaled.

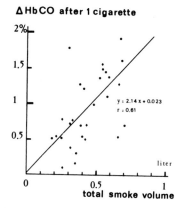

Fig. 28.9 Relationship between COHb uptake after smoking one cigarette and total smoke volume inhaled.

We will now examine the factor (or factors) that contributes to changes in the increase in carbon monoxide intake observed with the E.C.

Russell (1976) considers that smokers generally alter their smoking behaviour so as to regulate the nicotine intake. In our experiment the nicotine contents of the U.C. and the E.C. are almost identical (1.66 mg and 1.33 mg) and one may think that this factor has no significant effects particularly since the cigarette consumption per day does not vary. On the other hand, the urinary excretion of nicotine measured for each subject under identical pH conditions is greater with the E.C.

In our opinion the main contributing factor is the decrease in tar content, and, above all, in the irritating power of the two smoke phases. This finding is regrettable because investigations by Guillerm et al, (1974) have shown that the smoking of a cigarette having a low irritating power results in a spectacular regression or disappearance of any signs of bronchial intolerance from both the clinical and functional points of view.

Conclusions

Our results show that the subjects increase their inhalation coefficients and thereby their COHb levels when smoking a low-irritant cigarette. It may be concluded that knowing the chemical composition of the smoke given by the smoking machine is not enough and that it is essential to know the two principal parameters (CO intake and total smoke volume inhaled) of the smoker's behaviour towards any new cigarette. The information thus obtained is necessary in order to make use of the results of the chemical analysis of the smoke.

Acknowledgements

We thank J. Moreni for her technical help. This study was carried out in collaboration with SEITA.

References

Guillerm, R., Badré, R., Dupoux, J., Porsin, M. & Colin, B. (1959) Sur une méthode d'évaluation de l'oxycarbonémie à partir des concentrations d'oxyde de carbone mesurées dans l'air alvéolaire. *Revue de Médecine Navale,* **14**, 237-259.

Guillerm, R., Masurel, G., Broussolle, B., Hyacinthe, R., Simon, A. & Hée, J. (1974) Effets cliniques et fonctionnels respiratoires de la substitution d'une cigarette peu irritante à la cigarette habituelle dans un groupe de grands fumeurs. *Les Bronche* **24**, 209-231.

Guillerm, R. & Radziszewski, E. (1975) Une nouvelle méthode d'analyse de l'acte du fumeur. *Annales du tabac,* **1**, 101-110. Paris: SEITA.

Keith, C.H. (1962) Laboratory measurements of the smoking characteristics of human beings. (Abstract) *16th Tobacco Chemists' Research Conference,* Richmond, 14-15.

Russell, M.A.H. (1976) Low-tar medium-nicotine cigarettes: a new approach to safer smoking. *British Medical Journal,* **1**, 1430-1433.

29. Metabolic aspects of smoking behaviour

HELMUT SCHIEVELBEIN, GUNTER HEINEMANN, KARIN LOSCHENKOHL,
CHRISTIAN TROLL AND JOACHIM SCHLEGEL

Introduction

McDonough *et al* (1965) reported elevated haematocrit values in cigarette smokers in contrast to non smokers but did not observe any connection with the amount of cigarettes smoked. Other authors (Andrus *et al*, 1968; Sagone *et al*, 1973) were able to confirm this finding. Okuno, moreover observed that smokers had a higher erythrocyte count, higher haemoglobin content, an elevated erythrocyte volume (MCV = mean cell volume) and an increased mean haemoglobin concentration (MCHC = mean cell haemoglobin content) than non-smokers. Enhancement of the leucocyte count in smokers was reported by Okuno (1973), Fisch and Freedman (1975) and Corre, Lellouch and Schwartz (1971). Okuno compared smokers with a consumption of less than one pack of cigarettes per day with those who smoked more than one and a half packs and found that smokers who were in the higher consumption group showed a rise in white blood cell count of about 18% (Okuno, 1973).

The investigations mentioned above were performed with respect to haematological differences between smokers and non smokers with the exception of Okuno's (1973) finding with regard to the white cell count in medium and heavier smokers. Apart from this no results are known with regard to metabolic differences between smokers of different brands of cigarettes. We decided therefore, to evaluate, whether there are differences of metabolic systems in humans by smoking cigarettes with different concentrations of smoke components. We were partly encouraged by the work of Sagone who found that smokers have a lower level of ATP in the serum than non smokers.

In a preliminary investigation we therefore tested the concentration of some enzymes and metabolites of different organ systems in smokers of cigarettes with low and high total particular matter (TPM) and nicotine content in the smoke. These investigations showed that acute differences are only to be expected in the metabolism of the red blood cells and we decided to measure indicative parameters in the two experiments described in this paper. The parameters measured are registered in Table 29.1.

Materials and methods

Subjects

Smokers were healthy medical students who underwent a physical and laboratory examination before and at the end of the experiments. The control group of non-

371

Table 29.1 Parameters measured with abbreviations used in the text.

1.	Red Blood Count	RBC
2.	Mean Cell Volume	MCV
3.	Haemoglobin	Hb
4.	Mean Cell Haemoglobin	MCH
5.	Mean Cell Haemoglobin Content	MCHC
6.	Haematocrit	HC
7.	White Blood Count	WBC
8.	Glucose-6-Phosphate Dehydrogenase in Erythrocytes	G-6-PDH
9.	Adenosinetriphosphate in Erythrocytes	ATP
10.	2,3-Diphosphoglycerate	2,3-DPG
11.	Nicotine*	N
12.	Cotinine*	C
13.	Carboxyhaemoglobin*	COHb

* only in the second experiment

smokers in the second experiment underwent the same procedure. Further experimental conditions can be seen from Table 29.2 and Table 29.3.   All volunteers had to deliver a record of the amount of cigarettes smoked and the smoking pattern during the day; furthermore they were requested to collect the butts. At the change from one brand to another a so called 'profile smoking' was performed to evaluate the smoking behaviour with respect to number of puffs, length of puffs and intensity of drawing (for details see Schulz and Seehofer, 1978). All cigarettes were brands on the German market. To estimate the intake of smoke components, the excretion of nicotine and cotinine in the urine was measured in the second experiment.

Table 29.2 Experimental conditions (first experiment) 14 days smoking of the usual brand, length of subsequent smoking periods 14 days.

Subjects	Cigarettes		
		TPM, dry (mg)	N (mg)
15 male	A:	12	0.5
15 female	B:	19	1.2
	C:	9	0.4
	D:	12	0.6

Abbreviations in the tables:

TPM	=	Total Particular Matter
N	=	Nicotine
S	=	statistically significant
NS	=	not statistically significant
m	=	male
f	=	female

Table 29.3 Experimental conditions (second experiment) 14 days smoking of the usual brand, length of subsequent smoking periods 14 days.

Subjects	Cigarettes	
	TPM, dry (mg)	N (mg)
15 smokers, m.	E*: 15	0.8
15 smokers, f.	F: 14	0.7
5 non-smokers, m.	B: 19	1.2
5 non-smokers, f.	C: 9	0.4

*usual brand, weighted mean.

Haematological and biochemical methods
The estimation of haemotological parameters was performed with the 'Coulter Counter, Model S' (Coulter Inc., Krefeld). The concentration of ATP was estimated after Gruber, Möllering and Bergmeyer (1970), of 2,3-DPG after Ericson and de Verchier (1972) and Michal (1974), the estimation of the activity of G-6-PDH after Löhr and Waller (1970). The estimation of COHb was performed with the 'Co-Oximeter' (Instrumentation Boskamp) using the three wavelength method (Malenfant et al, 1968). Determination of nicotine and cotinine was performed in principle after Beckett and Triggs (1966) with modifications.

Statistical method
All parameters measured in our experiments showed normal distribution and inasmuch as each subject smoked each sort of cigarette we felt justified to compare the mean values with the Student's t test for statistical analysis. All significance values in the Tables are at the 95 per cent level.

Results

In Table 29.4 the number of cigarettes smoked per day in the first experiment is recorded. Very probably there are no significant differences between the number of cigarettes consumed.

Table 29.4 Number of cigarettes smoked per day (first experiment)

Brand	Subjects n	TPM, dry (mg)	N (mg)	Number $\bar{x}$
Usual brand	30	15*	0.8*	20
A	30	12	0.5	22
B	30	19	1.2	20
C	30	9	0.4	24
D	30	12	0.6	23

* mean

Haematological parameters in the first experiment and the second experiment were in the normal range and did not differ significantly between the different brands; neither were any trends in these parameters observed.

Metabolic values at the end of each smoking period of the first experiment are shown in Table 29.5. Table 29.6 contains the statistically significant differences and the trends, even if they are not statistically significant.

To confirm these findings we repeated the experiment with certain variations. The experimental conditions have already been described in Table 29.3.

Table 29.5 Values at the end of each smoking period (first experiment)

Parameter	A TPM: 12 N: 0.5	B TPM: 19 N: 1.2	C TPM: 9 N: 0.4	D TPM: 12 N: 0.6
G-6-PDH m U/10^{10} erythrocytes	1179 ± 169	1211 ± 259	673 ± 143	700 ± 172
2,3-DPG mmol/1 erythrocytes	4.07 ± 0.64	4.35 ± 0.68	3.74 ± 0.59	4.12 ± 0.68
ATP μmol/1 blood	495 ± 89	410 ± 91	460 ± 89	442 ± 71

Table 29.6 Presentation of significant values and trends of Table 29.5

Parameter	A TPM 12 N 0.5	→ B → 19 → 1.2	C 9 0.4	D 12 0.6
G-6-PDH	$p < 0.30$ ↑	NS	$p < 0.0005$ ↓ S	$p < 0.30$ ↑ NS
2,3-DPG	$p < 0.10$ ↑	NS	$p < 0.0005$ ↓ S	$p < 0.01$ ↑ S
ATP	$p < 0.005$ ↓	S	$p < 0.05$ ↑ S	$p > 0.25$ ↓ NS

The number of cigarettes smoked daily in the second experiment are shown in Table 29.7. There is no significant difference in cigarette consumption. The metabolic values obtained in this experiment can be seen from Table 29.8. There are some significant differences between the different brands, but no clear cut pattern of change could be observed. It seems striking that almost all values of the smokers are higher than those of the non-smokers.

Table 29.9 shows the values at the end of each smoking period, male smokers versus female smokers. There are also some statistical differences, but again no clear cut pattern can be seen.

Table 29.7 Number of cigarettes smoked per day (second experiment)

brand	number**	TPM, dry mg	N mg
E*:	20.4	15*	0.8*
F:	23.1	14	0.7
B:	21.6	19	1.2
C:	22.3	9	0.4

*   usual brand, weighted mean
**   number of cigarettes per day.

Table 29.8 Values at the end of each smoking period. Smokers versus non smokers. Upper line in each compartment: smokers, lower line in each compartment: non smokers (second experiment)

Parameter	E TPM: 15 N: 0.8		F TPM: 14 N: 0.7		B TPM: 19 N: 1.2		C TPM: 9 N: 0.4	
G-6-PDH mU/10^{10} erythrocytes	719 ± 195 700 ± 114	NS	$1433*\pm425$ 816 ± 262	S	$895*\pm302$ 692 ± 115	S	$1211*\pm171$ 1401 ± 290	S
2,3-DPG mmol/l erythrocytes	4.16 ± 0.70 3.32 ± 0.40	S	4.29 ± 0.53 3.87 ± 0.49	S	4.14 ± 0.73 3.94 ± 0.42	NS	4.24 ± 0.68 3.69 ± 0.34	S
ATP mol/l blood	617 ± 60 541 ± 55	S	$580*\pm86$ 568 ± 95	NS	$728*\pm47$ 776 ± 84	NS	696 ± 63 692 ± 83	NS
COHb %	4.2 ± 1.47 –		$5.26*\pm1.49$ 3.72 ± 0.64	S	4.47 ± 1.73 2.73 ± 0.52	S	$5.56*\pm2.11$ 2.52 ± 0.56	S

*Statistically significant to the previous smoking period.

Table 29.9 Values at the end of each smoking period. Male smokers versus female smokers. Upper line in each compartment: male smokers; lower line in each compartment: female smokers (second experiment)

Parameter	E TPM: 15 N: 0.8		F TPM: 14 N: 0.7		B TPM: 19 N: 1.2		C TPM: 9 N: 0.4	
G-6-PDH mU/10^{10} erythrocytes	799 ± 182 639 ± 179	S	1267 ± 468 1575 ± 335	S	824 ± 281 956 ± 316	NS	1261 ± 179 1173 ± 172	NS
2,3-DPG mmol/l erythrocytes	4.5 ± 0.62 3.79 ± 0.56	S	4.7 ± 0.33 3.90 ± 0.36	S	4.67 ± 0.66 3.72 ± 0.56	S	4.53 ± 0.46 3.69 ± 0.31	S
ATP μmol/l blood	623 ± 57 612 ± 64	NS	562 ± 96 597 ± 74	NS	747 ± 105 711 ± 56	NS	692 ± 59 700 ± 68	NS
COHb%	4.56 ± 1.20 3.93 ± 1.63	NS	5.35 ± 1.01 21 ± 1.76	NS	4.55 ± 1.71 3.95 ± 0.88	NS	6.64 ± 2.05 4.55 ± 1.68	S

In tables 29.10, 29.11 and 29.12 the excretion of nicotine and cotinine in the urine of the subjects is shown.   As can be seen from Table 29.10 there are only a few significant differences in the results obtained in the second experiment, but there is a striking difference between male and female smokers with the exception of brand F (Table 29.11). Female smokers excrete far less nicotine and cotinine than male smokers.

Table 29.10 Nicotine and cotinine excretion in the urine of male and female smokers. Each brand tested against the following brand.

Substances μmol/24 h		E	F	B	C
Nicotine	m	11.582	12.309 NS	14.454 NS	11.514 NS
Cotinine		9.057	7.162 NS	8.887 NS	5.607 S
Nicotine	f	5.486	8.642 NS	7.162 NS	5.819 NS
Cotinine		5.243	7.298 NS	4.455 S	3.479 NS
Nicotine	m + f	8.432	10.411 NS	10.818 NS	8.568 NS
Cotinine		7.082	7.235	6.486	4.557 S

Table 29.11 Nicotine and cotinine excretion in male and female smokers at the end of each smoking period. Male versus female smokers.

Substances μmol/24 h	E	F	B	C
Nicotine				
m	11.582	12.309	14.454	11.514
f	5.486 S	8.642 NS	7.162 S	5.819 S
Cotinine				
m	9.057	7.162	8.887	5.607
f	5.243 S	7.298 NS	4.455 S	3.479 S

Table 29.12 Nicotine + cotinine excretion in the urine of male and female smokers each brand tested against the following brand.

Substances μmol/24 hr		E	F	B	C
Nicotine + Cotinine	m	10.270	9.632 NS	11.783 NS	8.441 NS
Nicotine + Cotinine	f	5.363	6.925 NS	5.770 NS	4.052 NS
Nicotine + Cotinine	m + f	6.737	7.633 NS	7.489 NS	5.645 NS

This difference can also be observed by calculating the excretion of nicotine and cotinine together (Table 29.12).   There again is no change between the different brands, but the difference between male and female smokers becomes again evident.

From Table 29.13 can be seen that the number of cigarettes smoked was equal in male and female smokers. The volume of urine collected in 24 hr was the same for male and female smokers.

Table 29.13 Number of cigarettes smoked during the different smoking periods. Male versus female smokers.

Cigarettes	E TPM: 15 N: 0.8	F TPM: 14 N: 0.7	B TPM: 19 N: 1.2	C TPM: 9 N: 0.4
m	309.0 ± 107.6	330.1 ± 112.3	323.2 ± 86.8	348.8 ± 97.9
	NS	NS	NS	NS
F	284.1 ± 71.4	319.1 ± 105.1	300.9 ± 84.2	299.9 ± 116.5

Discussion

It seems possible to demonstrate an acute influence of cigarette smoke on erythrocyte metabolism, as shown in the first experiment. No data are available for intake of cigarette smoke components by the volunteers. But indirectly, it can be concluded from the KIPA-Analysis (see Schulz and Seehofer, 1978, Table 20.9 - nicotine intake in test smokers, 1976) that the intake of smoke was different for the different brands.

The results of the second experiment favour this conclusion. There was less variation in the intake of smoke components than in the first experiment (see Schulz and Seehofer, 1978, Table 20.9 - nicotine intake in test smokers, 1977). Furthermore the excretion of nicotine and cotinine did not differ significantly during the experiment (Tables 29.9 and 29.10), so the intake of nicotine could not have been very different. Also, the COHb content in the blood of the smokers did not differ significantly.

Most striking is the difference of nicotine and cotinine excretion of male and female smokers (Tables 29.11 and 29.12) (with the exception of the results for cigarette F).   The female smokers excreted much less of the alkaloid and its main metabolite than the male smokers. As all smokers, males and females smoked nearly the same amount of cigarettes per period (Table 29.13), differences in smoking behaviour between men and women must be the cause of this difference. Probable sex differences in the metabolic pathway of nicotine have to be considered too.

Glucose-6-phosphate dehydrogenase is the key enzyme in the oxidative pathway of red blood cell metabolism. The metabolite 2,3-diglycerophosphate occurs solely in erythrocytes during the glycolytic breakdown of glucose. This latter compound facilitates the release of oxygen from the red blood cells to the tissues according to the following formula:

$$HbO_2 + 2,3\text{-}DPG \rightleftharpoons Hb - 2,3\text{-}DPG + O_2$$

The unexpected result that the concentrations of most of the compounds measured are higher in smokers than in non smokers may be explained by compensation for the elevated level of COHb in smokers.

The same explanation may hold true for the elevated level of ATP in smokers (in contrast to non smokers), but such elevated levels of ATP are in contrast to the findings of Sagone *et al*, (1973).

Further experiments will show whether these findings can be confirmed. In this paper we described an attempt to link smoking behaviour with metabolic processes in humans and therefore the results should be regarded as such.

References

Andrus, L.H., Miller, D.C., Stallones, R.A., Ehrlich, S.P. & Jones, J.P. (1968) Epidemiological study of coronary disease risk factors. 1. Study design and characteristics of individual study subjects. *American Journal of Epidemiology*, 87, 73-86.

Beckett, A.H. & Triggs, E.J. (1966) Determination of nicotine and its metabolite, cotinine, in urine by gas chromatography. *Nature, London*, 211, 1415-1417.

Corre, F., Lellouch, J. & Schwartz, D. (1971) Smoking and leucocyte-counts. Results of an epidemiological survey. *Lancet*, 2, 632-634.

Ericson, S. & de Verdier, C.H. (1972) A modified method for the determination of 2,3-diphosphoglycerate in erythrocytes. *The Scandinavian Journal of Clinical and Laboratory Investigation*, 29, 85-90.

Fisch, I.R. & Freedman, S.H. (1975) Smoking, oral contraceptives, and obesity. Effects on white blood cell count. *Journal of American Medical Association*, 234, 500-506.

Gruber, W., Möllering, H. & Bergmeyer, H.U. (1970) Analytische differenzierung von purin - und pyrimidin-nucleotiden. Bestimmung von ADP, ATP sowie summe GTP + ITP in biologischem material. In *Methoden der Enzymatischen Analyse* Vol. II. ed. Bergmeyer, H.U., pp. 2011-2019. Verlag Chemie.

Löhr, G.W. & Waller, H.D. (1970) Glucose-6-phosphat-dehydrogenase. In *Methoden der Enzymatischen Analyse*, Vol. I ed. Bergmeyer, H.U., pp. 599-606. Verlag Chemie.

McDonough, R., Hames, C.G., Garrison, G.E., Stulb, S.C., Lichtman, M.A. & Hefelfinger, D.C. (1965) The relationship of haematocrit to cardiovascular states of health in the negro and white population of Evans County, Georgia. *Journal of Chronic Diseases*, 18, 243-257.

Malenfant, A.L. *et al.*, (1968) Spectrophotometric determination of haemoglobin concentration and per cent oxyhaemoglobin and carboxyhaemoglobin saturation. *20th National Meeting of American Association of Clinical Chemists*. Washington, D.C., Aug. 19.

Michal, G. (1974) D-Glycerat-2,3-diphosphat. In *Methoden der Enzymatischen Analyse*, 3rd edn. ed. Bergmeyer, H.U., pp. 1478-1483. Verlag Chemie.

Okuno, T. (1973) Smoking and blood changes. *Journal of American Medical*

Association, **225**, 1387-1388.
Sagone, A.L. Jr., Lawrence, T. & Balcerzak, S.P. (1973) Effect of smoking on tissue oxygen supply. *Blood,* **41**, 845-852.

30. Ranking cigarette brands on smoke deliveries

S J GREEN

In 1952 tests of selected filter tipped brands were introduced by the American Medical Association. In 1957 'Readers' Digest' in the U.S.A. began publishing listings of brands showing the deliveries of 'tar' and nicotine. By 1977 some ten countries had introduced such brand rankings, although there were many variations in the procedures for measuring deliveries. There were and still are, for example, variations in the conditions under which cigarettes are smoked, the smoking machine used, the method of smoke collection and the analytical procedures followed. Most brand tables list the deliveries of tar and nicotine, although figures for additional compounds in smoke have been issued in certain countries.

In some respects it is unfortunate that cigarettes have been tested for so long by simulated smoking. There is no prima facie reason why such a method should be chosen. It might easily have developed differently. Cigarettes might have been crushed and the tobacco pyrolysed under some standard conditions. Several attempts were made to develop such techniques because the use of simulated human smoking entailed, for research work, the great burden of producing cigarettes. Because of the need to select such cigarettes to some constant properties (such as moisture content) they must be produced in considerable numbers. It would have been of great help in research if a standard laboratory technique could have been widely adopted which could be used on small samples of tobacco and paper without the need to go through to cigarettes. But apart from this it is doubly unfortunate that machine smoking under fairly arbitrary conditions, probably different from those of any known human smoker, should be so often and so wrongly regarded as equivalent to human smoking.

Presumably the main objective in publishing the ranking of cigarette brands, as shown in Table 30.1, is to encourage smokers to choose their cigarettes using better information. There is some evidence (Hammond *et al*, 1976; Dean *et al*, 1977; Bross and Gibson, 1968; Wynder, Mabuchi and Beattie, 1970) which some interpret to show that the incidence of diseases associated with smoking should be reduced when cigarettes with lower deliveries of some components are smoked. If this is correct it may be argued, therefore, that it is reasonable to encourage smokers to reduce the general level of tar available for inhalation. If the information in ranking tables helps smokers so to choose it may be considered that, as far as simple tables (such as the D.H.S.S. list in Table 30.1) are concerned, there is some degree of validity.

Table 30.1 U.K. DHSS Table: September, 1977

LOW TAR

Tar yield mg/cig		Nicotine yield mg/cig
-4	Embassy Ultra Mild	0.3
-4	Player's Mild de Luxe	0.3
-4	Silk Cut Extra Mild	0.3
6	Piccadilly Mild	0.4
7	Peter Stuyvesant Extra Mild King Size	0.6
8	Player's Special Mild	0.7
8	Silk Cut	0.8
8	Silk Cut International	0.8
8	Silk Cut King Size	0.8
8	Silk Cut No. 3	0.7
8	Silk Cut No. 5	0.7
9	Player's No.6 Extra Mild	0.7
9	Rothmans Ransom	0.7
9	Silk Cut No. 1	0.8

LOW–MIDDLE TAR

Tar yield mg/cig		Nicotine yield mg/cig
11	Consulate Menthol	0.7
11	Consulate No. 2	0.7
11	Embassy Extra Mild	0.9
11	Embassy Extra Mild King Size	0.9
12	Belair Menthol Kings	0.8
12	Black Cat Filter	0.8
12	Black Cat No. 9	0.7
12	Embassy Extra Mild No. 5	1.0
12	Everest Menthol	0.8
12	Piccadilly No. 7	0.7
12	St. Moritz	0.9
13	Gauloises Caporal Filter	0.7
13	Gauloises Disque Bleu	0.7
13	Gitanes Caporal Filter	0.9
13	Kent	1.0
13	Player's No. 10 Extra Mild	0.9
14	Benson and Hedges Sovereign Mild	1.3
14	Guards Select	0.8
14	Peter Stuyvesant King Size	1.3
14	Philip Morris International	1.2
15	Cadets	1.0

15	Cambridge	0.9
15	Camel Filter Tip	1.0
15	Kensitas Club Mild	1.2
15	Kensitas Corsair Mild	1.3
15	Lark Filter Tip	1.3
15	Marlboro	1.2
15	Three Castles Filter	1.2
16	Benson & Hedges Special Vending Size	1.3
16	Dunhill King Size	1.2
16	Embassy Envoy	1.2
16	Guards	1.1
16	John Player Carlton King Size	1.5
16	John Player Carlton Long Size	1.4
16	John Player Carlton Premium	1.3
16	Kensitas Mild	1.2
16	Peter Stuyvesant Long Size	1.1

MIDDLE TAR

\

Tar yield mg/cig		Nicotine yield mg/cig
17	Benson & Hedges Gold Bond	1.2
17	Embassy Regal	1.3
17	L & M Box Filter Tip	1.4
17	Piccadilly No. 3	1.0
17	Rothmans International	1.3
17	Slim Kings	1.2
17	Winston	1.3
18	Benson & Hedges Sovereign	1.3
18	Embassy American King Size	1.4
18	Embassy Filter	1.4
18	John Player King Size	1.4
18	John Player Special	1.4
18	Kensitas Club	1.2
18	Kensitas Corsair	1.3

18	Kensitas 2	1.3
18	Nelson	1.3
18	Park Drive Tipped	1.3
18	Piccadilly Filter de Luxe	1.1
18	Player's No. 6 King Size	1.4
18	Sobranie Virginia Int.	1.4
18	Weights Filter	1.3
19	Bachelor	1.4
19	Benson & Hedges King Size	1.4
19	Du Maurier	1.3
19	Dunhill Int.	1.4
19	Embassy American Regular	1.4
19	Embassy Gold	1.3
19	Embassy Kings	1.4
19	Kensitas King Size	1.4
19	Kensitas Plain (P)	1.5
19	Kensitas Tipped	1.3
19	Piccadilly King Size	1.3
19	Players No. 6 Filter	1.3
19	Players No. 10	1.3
19	Senior Service Tipped	1.4
19	Silva Thins	1.5
19	Sterling	1.3
20	Embassy Plain (P)	1.2
20	Gallahers De Luxe Mild (P)	1.6
20	Lambert & Butler Int. Size	1.7
20	More	1.6
20	More Menthol	1.6
20	Players Filter Virginia	1.4
20	Players Gold Leaf	1.5
20	Players Mild Navy Cut (P)	1.8
20	Rothmans King Size	1.4
20	Woodbine Filter	1.5
21	Pall Mall Filter	2.3
21	Players No. 6 Plain (P)	1.6
21	Solent	1.3

MIDDLE–HIGH TAR

Tar yield mg/cig		Nicotine yield mg/cig
23	Craven 'A' Cork Tipped (P)	1.3

23	Gauloises Caporal Plain (P)	1.3
23	Gitanes Caporal Plain (P)	1.5
23	Piccadilly No. 1 (P) 1.4	1.4
23	Richmond Filter	1.9
24	Lucky Strike Filter	2.4
24	Park Drive Plain (P)	1.9
24	Richmond Plain (P)	1.8
24	Weights Plain (P)	1.7
24	Woodbine Plain (P)	2.0
25	Lucky Strike Plain (P)	1.6
25	Senior Service Plain (P)	1.9
27	Capstan Medium (P)	2.0
27	Gold Flake (P)	2.2
27	Players Medium Navy Cut (P)	2.0

HIGH–TAR

Tar yield mg/cig		Nicotine yield mg/cig
31	Churchmans No. 1 (P)	2.3
31	Gallaher De Luxe Medium	2.5
32	Players No. 3 (P)	2.3
34	Pall Mall King Size	3.3
35	Capstan Full Strength	3.6

(P) indicates plain cigarettes

However, epidemiology, by its nature, can tell us nothing about individuals; it is concerned only with populations. And people do not smoke cigarettes like machines; they do not necessarily smoke successive cigarettes of the same brand in the same way and it is unlikely that different brands are smoked in the same way. Work in B.A.T. laboratories (Creighton and Lewis, 1978) shows this. The summary in Table 30.2 indicates that individual smokers take in very different amounts of tar from those indicated by machine smoking. We are also aware that the way in which individuals smoke can change the smoke chemistry of the same brand one from another. Nevertheless if an individual smoker retained exactly the same smoking behaviour he would receive less tar from a low tar cigarette than from a cigarette in, say, the middle tar range. Also, it is true that a smoker would find it difficult to get as much tar from low tar cigarettes as from those in the highest categories unless he increased the number of cigarettes he smoked. Certainly if he modified his smoking behaviour only slightly by moving from one brand to another, the finer differences in the D.H.S.S. Table would become meaningless or even misleading. For example, consider a smoker of a *Low-Middle tar* cigarette with a tar yield of 11 mg and nicotine of 0.9 mg. If this smoker changed to a *Low tar* cigarette with 9 mg tar and 0.7 mg. nicotine and increased his puff volume to receive the same nicotine he would be smoking a cigarette yielding nearer 12 mg tar. Throughout the Table it can be shown that any 'fine tuning' is readily defeated by quite realistic but small changes in smoking behaviour. A change by only one puff would readily reverse the positions of adjacent cigarettes and for those at the top and bottom of bands would shift cigarettes into different bands.

Table 30.2 Variations in human smoking behaviour

Cigarette Category (Machine Smoking) (U.K. D.H.S.S. Categories)	Range of Deliveries (Human Smoking)
	1 2 3 4 5
1. Low Tar	⊢X———
2. Low to Middle Tar	⊢———X———————————⊣
3. Middle Tar	⊢——— X———————⊣
4. Middle to High Tar	⊢———————X———⊣
5. High Tar	⊢—————————X—⊣

A change of one puff coupled with a ten per cent increase in puff volume could transpose the position between the middle of the *Low-Middle* band and the *Middle tar* band.

Furthermore, in addition to variations in the way in which cigarettes are smoked, we can infer that there are also differences in the way in which smoke from different cigarettes is inhaled. Guillerm and his colleagues at Toulon (Guillerm *et al*, 1974) compared the way in which a panel of smokers smoked two cigarettes, 'Gallia' and 'Gauloises'. The results are shown in Table 30.3 and suggest, if carboxyhaemoglobin measurements are related to depth of inhalation, that the smoke from the lower delivery cigarette ('Gallia') was inhaled differently from that from 'Gauloises'.

P*

Table 30.3 Carbon monoxide versus carboxyhaemoglobin (Guillerm, 1974)

	Machine Smoking Delivery of Carbon Monoxide (mg/Cig)	Human Smoking (% Carboxyhaemo- globin)	Daily Consumption (Cigs/Day)
Gallia	11.4	7.4	34
Gauloises	17.2	5.8	32

It is also well known that alkaline mainstream smoke is more difficult to inhale than acidic smoke and a continuous spectrum of smoking products in this respect could be produced from among known brands around the world.

Theoretically brand tables might be developed for a whole variety of known compounds in smoke. Brand ranking tables with measurements such as carbon monoxide or nitrogen oxides have already appeared. For these compounds the relationship with any particular disease is obscure and it is possible, and in some cases proven, that the effects of individual smoke compounds can be modified by synergistic or antagonistic effects of other compounds present in smoke.

If smokers adjust their smoking behaviour on the basis of a response to tar or nicotine the deliveries of compounds such as carbon monoxide, as measured by smoking machine, have even less relevance for individual smokers than do the corresponding figures for tar and nicotine.

Guillerm *et al* (1974) have shown that the retention of carbon monoxide by smokers is not determined solely by the carbon monoxide delivery of the cigarette. Somewhat similar findings have been reported by Wald, Idle and Smith (1977). Carboxyhaemoglobin levels in smokers who smoke unventilated filter cigarettes were on average, higher than in smokers of plain cigarettes, as expected on the basis of machine smoking. However, the mean carboxyhaemoglobin level in subjects who smoked ventilated cigarettes was 7% higher than in those who smoked plain cigarettes, although the ventilated filter cigarettes had deliveries 21% lower than the plain cigarettes when smoked by machine. Results for cigarettes containing added nicotine (Dunn and Freiesleben, 1978) also indicate that the intake of carbon monoxide is not simply related to machine smoked measurements of the delivery of carbon monoxide.

If smokers adjust their smoking behaviour on the basis of nicotine intake, there is the implication, as expressed by Russell (1976), and shown in Table 30.4, that the preferred index would be the ratio of nicotine to tar or the ratio of nicotine to carbon monoxide or maybe both. A 'merit index' which in some way added tar, nicotine and carbon monoxide together would, of course, be wholly misleading. Yet this is precisely what some have tried to do. The so-called Herzfeld index attempts to add together total particulate matter, nicotine, carbon monoxide and nitrogen oxides using inconsistent units!

The assumptions implied in putting forward such an index are quite unacceptable. There are assumptions about relating the toxicity of simple compounds such as nitrogen oxides, nicotine and carbon monoxide with such very complex mixtures as in tar. There are assumptions that various diseases are related simply to specific

Table 30.4 U.K. DHSS Table: June 1975 (modified to show tar:nicotine ratio)

Nicotine and tar yield of cigarettes available in Britain in 1975

Nicotine yield (mg/ cigarette)	Brand	Filter(F) or plain(P)	Tar yield (mg/ cigarette)	Tar: nicotine ratio
	Very low nicotine			
0.06	Embassy Ultra Mild	F	1.25	20.83‡
0.08	Players Mild De Luxe	F	1.37	17.13
0.18	Silk Cut Extra Mild	F	2.27	12.61*
0.49	Piccadilly Mild	F	7.52	15.35
	Low nicotine			
0.65	Players No. 6 Extra Mild	F	8.74	13.45
0.67	Players Special Mild	F	8.98	13.40
0.67	Silk Cut No. 3	F	8.29	12.37
0.68	Silk Cut	F	7.98	11.74*
0.68	Silk Cut No. 1	F	8.69	12.78
0.75	Piccadilly No. 7	F	13.19	17.59‡
0.75	Silk Cut King Size	F	8.67	11.56
0.76	Pall Mall Long Size	F	10.48	13.79
0.80	Belair Menthol Kings	F	12.67	15.84
0.80	Consulate Menthol	F	12.60	15.75
0.80	Embassy Extra Mild King Size	F	11.16	13.95
0.82	Rothmans Ransom	F	9.58	11.68*
0.86	Gauloise Disque Bleu	F	15.31	17.80‡
0.87	Embassy Extra Mild	F	11.77	13.53
0.87	Everest Menthol	F	13.41	15.41
0.88	Gauloises Caporal Filter	F	15.23	17.31±
0.92	St. Moritz	F	11.92	12.96
0.94	Kensitas Mild	F	13.69	14.56
0.94	Kent	F	14.91	15.86
	Medium nicotine			
1.01	Cambridge	F	16.74	16.57‡
1.03	Guards King Size	F	15.94	15.48
1.04	Gitanes Caporal Filter	F	15.74	15.13
1.06	Camel Filter Tip	F	16.86	15.91
1.06	Piccadilly Filter de Luxe	F	16.86	15.91
1.09	Crown Filter	F	18.16	16.66‡
1.11	Three Castles Filter	F	15.19	13.68
1.14	St. Michel Filter	F	21.51	18.87‡
1.16	Benson & Hedges Gold Bond	F	17.17	14.80
1.17	Cadets	F	17.89	15.29
1.17	Guards	F	17.25	14.74
1.19	Embassy Gold	F	17.74	14.91
1.19	Marlboro	F	15.89	13.35

Table 30.4 contd.

1.20	Benson & Hedges Sovereign	F	17.62	14.68
1.20	Embassy Regal	F	17.19	14.33
1.21	Embassy Plain	P	19.96	16.50‡
1.21	Kent de Luxe Length	F	17.92	14.81
1.22	Peter Stuyvesant King Size	F	15.24	12.49†
1.22	Slim Kings	F	17.99	14.75
1.22	Sobranie Virginia International	F	16.55	13.57
1.25	Woodbine Filter	F	18.13	14.50
1.26	John Player Carlton Premium	F	15.47	12.28†
1.26	Kensitas Club	F	18.81	14.93
1.26	Players No. 6 Classic	F	18.26	14.49
1.27	Nelson	F	18.47	14.54
1.28	Kensitas King Size	F	17.33	13.54
1.29	Cameron	F	19.13	14.83
1.29	Peter Stuyvesant Luxury Length	F	16.64	12.90
1.30	Dunhill King Size	F	18.27	14.05
1.31	Dunhill International	F	18.33	13.99
1.31	Embassy Filter	F	19.08	14.56
1.31	Kensitas Corsair	F	19.02	14.52
1.31	Players No. 6 Filter	F	19.58	14.95
1.32	Kensitas Tipped	F	18.97	14.37
1.32	Park Drive Tipped	F	18.09	13.70
1.32	Players No. 6 Kings	F	19.65	14.89
1.33	John Player Special	F	19.31	14.52
1.33	Louis Rothmans Select	F	16.80	12.63†
1.33	Senior Service Tipped	F	19.22	14.45
1.33	Solent	F	21.54	16.20‡
1.34	Benson & Hedges King Size	F	19.26	14.37
1.36	Embassy Kings	F	19.07	14.02
1.36	Gauloises Caporal Plain	P	23.90	17.57‡
1.36	Sterling	F	19.29	14.18
1.37	Players No. 10	F	19.75	14.42
1.38	John Player Carlton Long Size	F	15.59	11.30✱
1.39	Du Maurier	F	19.49	14.02
1.39	Players Gold Leaf	F	19.99	14.38
1.39	Rothmans Int.	F	17.26	12.42†
1.42	Bachelor	F	21.40	15.07
1.42	John Player Kings	F	20.58	14.49
1.42	Piccadilly King Size	F	20.25	14.26
1.43	Craven A Cork Tipped	P	23.23	16.24‡
1.44	John Player Carlton King Size	F	15.28	10.61✱
1.44	Lark Filter Tip	F	18.34	12.74†
1.48	Chesterfield Filter Tip	F	18.83	12.72†
1.48	Gitanes Caporal Plain	P	23.07	15.59
1.48	Players Gold Leaf King Size	F	20.17	13.63

Table 30.5 contd.

1.48	Rothmans King Size	F	21.08	14.24
1.49	Piccadilly No. 1	P	23.61	15.85
	High nicotine			
1.50	Weights Filter	F	19.03	12.69
1.51	Players Filter Virginia	F	21.85	14.47
1.52	L & M Box Filter Tip	F	18.85	12.40
1.55	Players Perfectos	F	21.55	13.90
1.58	Silva Thins	F	20.39	12.91
1.61	Richmond Plain	P	22.66	14.07
1.63	Lambert & Butler International Size	F	19.60	12.02
1.63	Players Mild Navy Cut	P	20.40	12.52
1.67	Players No. 6 Plain	P	24.41	14.62
1.68	Weights Plain	P	24.54	14.61
1.71	Kensitas Plain	P	22.79	13.33
1.73	Gallahers De Luxe Mild	P	23.70	13.70
1.80	Richmond Filter	F	24.58	13.66
1.83	Woodbine Plain	P	24.18	13.21
1.86	Senior Service Plain	P	26.08	14.02
1.87	Players Medium Navy Cut	P	26.16	13.99
1.89	Capstan Medium	P	26.84	14.20
1.95	Park Drive Plain	P	24.82	12.73
	Very high nicotine			
2.09	Gold Flake	P	27.12	12.98
2.11	Churchmans No. 1	P	31.67	15.01
2.16	Pall Mall Filter	F	20.66	9.56 †
2.18	Players No. 3	P	32.02	14.69
2.30	Gallahers De Luxe Medium	P	30.10	13.09
2.40	Lucky Filters	F	23.33	9.72 †
2.56	Lucky Strike Plain	P	29.92	11.69
3.18	Pall Mall King Size	P	34.53	10.86
3.38	Capstan Full Strength	P	33.97	10.02

The brands are grouped according to nicotine yield. Smokers should try to switch
to a low or very low nicotine brand and select the brand in that nicotine yield group
that has the lowest tar:nicotine. The least harmful and most harmful brands
in each group are marked as follows:
*Recommended brands.   †Less harmful brands.   ‡Most harmful brands

compounds and complex components, that these do not interact, that they are
linearly dose related, and that there are no thresholds. Further, it is assumed that
various diseases may be ranked against each other: in what way (social cost,
economic cost or loss of expectation of life) is not said. It is difficult to believe
that such indices can be seriously proposed. There is, of course, no scientific
basis whatever. They could readily be created to position any selected products
in any rank order. Yet amazingly a similar approach was published in Belgium
which did not include mainstream oxides of nitrogen but threw in sidestream carbon

monoxide - presumably for luck!

It is concluded that while simple brand ranking tables do give information which may be useful to some smokers and by and large may assist a drift towards lower tar cigarettes in general, nevertheless they may mislead individual smokers. In particular small differences in simple tables are meaningless and suggestions that single indices covering several factors have any scientific foundation at present must be totally rejected.

References

Bross, I.D.J. & Gibson, R. (1968) Risks of lung cancer in smokers who switch to filter cigarettes. *American Journal of Public Health,* 58, 1396-1403

Creighton, D.E. & Lewis, P.H. (1978) The effect of different cigarettes on human smoking patterns. *This volume.*

Dean, G., Lee, P.N., Todd, G.F. & Wicken, A.J. (1977) *Report on a Second Retrospective Mortality Study in North-East England. Part 1.* Factors related to mortality from lung cancer, bronchitis, heart disease and stroke in Cleveland County, with particular emphasis on the relative risks associated with smoking filter and plain cigarettes. Tobacco Research Council, Research Paper 14, Part 1. London: Tobacco Research Council.

Dunn, P.J. & Freiesleben, E.R. (1978) The effects of nicotine enhanced cigarettes on human smoking parameters and alveolar CO levels. *This volume.*

Guillerm, R., Masurel, G., Broussolle, B., Hyacinthe, R., Simon, A. and Hée, J. (1974) Effets cliniques et functionnels respiratoires de la substitution d'une cigarette peu irritante à la cigarette habituelle dans un groupe de grands fumeurs. *Les Bronches,* 24, 209-231.

Hammond, C.E., Garfinkel, L., Seidman, H. & Lew, E. (1976) Some recent findings concerning cigarette smoking. Presented at a meeting on "The Origins of Human Cancer" at Cold Springs Harbor Laboratory on September 14, 1976.

Russell, M.A.H. (1976) Low-tar medium-nicotine cigarettes: a new approach to safer smoking. *British Medical Journal,* 1, 1430-1433.

Wald, N., Idle, M. & Smith, P.G. (1977) Carboxyhaemoglobin levels in smokers of filter and plain cigarettes. *Lancet,* 1, 110.112.

Wynder, E.L., Mabuchi, K. & Beattie, E.J. (1970) The epidemiology of lung cancer. Recent trends. *Journal of the American Medical Association,* 213, 2221-2228.

31. Conference overview

M E JARVIK

There were thirty papers at this International Smoking Behaviour Conference dealing with determinants of smoking, effects of smoking on various types of behaviour, and upon related physiological functions. Particular attention was paid to nicotine and carbon monoxide because they are the components of smoke most likely to produce behavioural effects. Broadly speaking, this conference was concerned with three questions about smoking: why do people start, why do they continue, and why do they stop?

The initial talk by Professor Mills dealt with coping mechanisms in the brain. Although this material was not directly related to smoking it is clear that smoking is used by subjects as a means of coping with stress. The important point brought up by Professor Mills was that drugs are used by individuals to modulate the arousal level, and individuals 'adjust their nicotine intake according to the mental demands being made upon them'. A number of other papers in this symposium stress this very important hypothesis, namely that smokers may adjust their nicotine intake to achieve an optimally desired level of arousal, either stimulant or depressant.

In the papers by Cherry and Kiernan and by Warburton, we learned how extraversion and neuroticism are related to the tendency to smoke, and also to performance during vigilance tasks.

The study by Cherry and Kiernan was based upon a large sample of 2700 subjects. They found that the neurotic extroverts smoke more than other groups. The groups that were able to give up smoking most easily were the stable extroverts.

Warburton (Reading University) carried this personality scheme even further. His work is an attempt to factor out an important source of variance in vigilance performance, namely personality. Apparently, the reason why extroverts smoke more than introverts is that they have a lower cortical arousal level and desire the extra stimulation provided by the drug. It would be interesting to see in longitudinal studies of hyperactive children whether they smoked more or used more stimulant drugs in adulthood than a comparable group of normal individuals.

Warburton found that subjects seek an optimal dose of nicotine to adjust their level of arousal to the point where they can function best, and this is determined by their personality, the degree of extroversion, introversion and neuroticism that they bring to the situation.

Warburton speculates that anxiolytic drugs like the benzodiazepines act by decreasing the release of acetylcholine and 5-hydroxytryptamine and by causing a relative increase in the activity of catecholamines in the brain. Fuxe et al(1977) found that catecholamine levels in the brain were diminished by nicotine, but concluded that the effect was probably indirect and mediated by cholinergic neurones. The exact balance of steroids, neurotransmitters, and other substances responsible for or associated with anxiety and its relief is still not known, but the speculations of Warburton that such a balance does exist are very important for research on the reinforcing effects of drugs such as nicotine.

If extroversion and neuroticism are related to smoking as they appear to be, it would be interesting to know whether they are causally related or whether they are related through a third variable, perhaps genetically determined. Data from adoption studies in Denmark might help us if subjects could be induced to take the appropriately translated personality tests. Warburton's investigations showed that buccal tablets provided an interesting method of administering nicotine in a relatively painless manner to smokers and non-smokers and equally acceptable to both. The efficiency of absorption by this method should be measured utilising blood and urine determinations.

Dr. Izard expressed many nascent thoughts about tobacco in an inimitable Gallic manner. His speculations about motivation for smoking were quite interesting and certainly important enough to follow up with controlled studies. There is no question that the beneficial effects of smoking have not received the attention that the harmful effects have. Some of the other participants in the symposium support his suggestion that smoking can help to relive the effects of psychological stress, and can reduce aggressiveness and irritability. Campaigns aimed at eliminating smoking may have the effect of 'throwing out the baby with the bath water'. It would be preferable to improve the beneficial effects of smoking while diminishing possible harmful effects.

Ashton and her colleagues discussed the importance of dose-response curves in accounting for the stimulating and relaxing effects of nicotine. They used the contingent negative variation (CNV) as a sensitive and objective indicator of stimulant and depressant drug action. The contingent negative variation was first described by Walter et al (1964) as an event related to slow direct current potential recorded between the vertex and the mastoid or earlobe. Since it occurs during the time between a warning signal and a 'go' signal, it is generally considered an expectancy wave. Previous work from the Newcastle University Laboratories demonstrated that central depressant drugs decrease this potential, while central stimulants increase it.

Smoking produced significant changes in the CNV in 22 subjects, but the direction varied. Further study showed that the direction of change was consistent and could be accounted for by extroversion/introversion as measured by the Eysenck Personality Inventory. Extroverted subjects extracted a smaller amount of nicotine from their cigarettes and showed a mean increase in CNV, while introverted subjects took a larger dose and showed a mean decrease.

Cigarette smoking and intravenous nicotine injections produced similar effects in the same subjects. Intravenous nicotine caused dose-related biphasic effects, stimulating or increasing the CNV at low doses and depressing or decreasing it at high doses. It was proposed that smokers can adjust their level of arousal by regulating their nicotine intake. This study would seem to resolve the old paradox that smoking sometimes relaxes and sometimes stimulates the smoker.

Two other groups utilised the CNV in their work. Binnie and Comer also showed that smoking caused the CNV to increase in some subjects and to decrease in others, and it tended to reduce eye movement. They speculated that the reduction in eye movement might increase attention in some subjects. It would be important to repeat this study, in view of the results of Ashton *et al*, and see whether there might be a biphasic dose-response curve for these variables. Comer and Creighton found that subjects smoked with increased intensity during an experiment to record the CNV when compared with smoking in a relaxed laboratory condition.

Studies from the Oxford University Laboratory of Mangan showed little effect of self-regulation with three brands, but the range of nicotine was small (0.9, 1.3 and 1.7 mg per cigarette). Furthermore, number of cigarettes smoked may not be the only crucial variable since puffing parameters could play a role. There were some paradoxical findings which would have to be replicated in other laboratories to determine if they were generalisable. Habituation to the Archimedes' spiral after-effect was diminished by smoking, whereas habituation to a tone was facilitated by smoking. There was a decrease in spontaneous fluctuation caused by smoking. Performance in a vigilance task was improved by smoking, particularly by a diminution in false positive responses. Smoking caused slower learning, but better remembering in a verbal learning task, and when interference was increased, smokers remembered better. These results are similar to those of Andersson (1975). Smoking appeared to prevent the impairing effect of noise upon reaction time.

Knott presented some very interesting and important evidence that a true abstinence syndrome may be detected in smokers deprived of cigarettes. He found that the dominant alpha frequency of the resting EEG differed in non-smokers and deprived smokers. Non-deprived smokers showed dominant alpha frequencies similar to those of non-smokers, but the frequencies of the deprived smoker were slower. His analysis of phasic, stimulus-induced, average cortical evoked response activity showed that deprived smokers had shorter latencies and larger amplitudes than both non-smokers and non-deprived smokers. He proposed a 'filter model' similar in some respects to that of Nelsen, Pelley and Goldstein (1975) in which nicotine is hypothesised to diminish the disruptive effects of distracting stimuli on the reticular system via the hippocampus. This may explain why smokers so commonly explain that they work better when they are smoking, and, indeed, often cannot work when they are not smoking.

Wesnes, also from the Reading University Laboratory, presented additional evidence that nicotine tablets had similar effects to cigarette smoking upon the visual vigilance performance of smokers in both auditory and visual tasks. In more demanding perceptual tasks, nicotine tablets were also capable of increasing efficiency. In a visual vigilance task, smokers did much better than non-smokers, indicating that smoking had a facilitating effect in this task. Deprived smokers did a little worse than non-smokers, indicating a very slight abstinence effect. In auditory vigilance, nicotine in the cigarette prevented the decrement which occurred with non-nicotine cigarettes. Nicotine tablets reduced the Stroop interference effect and smokers did better on a number monitoring task when smoking high nicotine cigarettes. In a vigilance clock task, herbal cigarettes impaired performance as compared with regular cigarettes. All of these studies provide additional evidence that smoking may have a truly beneficial effect upon psychological performance.

Myrsten and Andersson summarised work which was done in the laboratory of Professor Marianne Frankenhaeuser. They found that cigarette deprivation in smokers prolonged reaction time performance. Smoking not only produces an inverted U relationship with arousal and behavioural efficiency, but has different effects upon different kinds of cognitive tasks. Thus, in the same subjects, smoking impaired performance on a complex task and improved performance in a simple task. The results of the effects of smoking upon memory were rather complex. Cigarette induced arousal impaired learning, but improved later recall.

Another line of research from this laboratory dealt with alcohol-tobacco inter-actions which proved to be complex. The impairing effects of alcohol upon reaction time and arithmetic were counteracted with cigarettes. There appeared to be a sobering effect of smoking, which again may account for some of the results obtained by Griffiths, Bigelow and Liebson (1976). Acute abstinence from cigarette smoking produced surprisingly few objective effects, but there were subjective effects, and these were greater when deprivation was carried out in the customary habitat of subjects than in a new locale.

A number of papers dealt with the possible effects of carbon monoxide upon performance. Guillerm and his colleagues utilised an actual automobile driving task in which subjects drove an experimental automobile in a circular course for five hours. Driving precision, visual reaction time, heart rate, and EEG were all measured. None of these variables were affected when levels of 7% and 11% carbon monoxide were maintained for the five hour period. It seems unlikely that carbon monoxide in cigarette smoke is responsible for the acute behavioural effects of smoking.

Nevertheless, carbon monoxide is an important physiologically active compound found in cigarette smoke. Professor Cumming and his colleagues examined the manner in which this gas is absorbed in the conducting airways of the human lung. Carboxyhaemoglobin is a useful measure in inhalation of cigarette smoke since negligible amounts of carbon monoxide are absorbed across mucosal surfaces. Dunn showed that alveolar resting levels of carbon monoxide may also be used as an indicator of depth of inhalation. When smokers were switched to cigarettes of 30% reduced draw resistance, there was a decrease in alveolar levels of carbon monoxide. There was no adjustment in number of cigarettes smoked, butt length or puff number. Therefore smokers regulated their nicotine intake by decreasing the depth of inhalation.

Rawbone and associates measured various smoking parameters, including cigarette characteristics, smoking habits, puff parameters, nicotine deliveries and extractions, filtration characteristics, respiratory variables and carbon monoxide, both in expired air and blood. They derived a smoke exposure index from the volume and time periods of inhalations and concluded that there was a significant correlation between this measure and smoke absorbed as measured by increments in alveolar carbon monoxide levels. Smoke absorbed, however, was not related to smoke presented as measured by butt nicotine analysis. It thus appears that smokers can engage in compensatory behaviour by rather subtle changes in their methods of inhalation. It would appear that more research with refined technology will be necessary to clarify these relationships in different types of smokers.

Green made the point that the way humans smoke cigarettes is quite different from the way machines, which have been designed for standardisation, do so. The machine does not compensate for any change in taste, harshness, or nicotine content, whereas humans probably do. It is very likely that alkaline mainstream smoke from a cigarette such as a Gauloise is not inhaled as readily as the acid mainstream smoke from a Camel. A machine, of course, pays no attention to the pH. Green has pointed out the difficulties in deriving a 'merit index' which in some way added tar, nicotine and carbon monoxide together, or other substances. The way in which individual smokers inhale or the puffing patterns can distort the ranking of cigarettes obtained by machines; thus, a great deal more research would have to do done and certain agreement reached about conventions to be adopted before decisions concerning the relative merit of cigarettes can be made.

Professor Schievelbein and colleagues considered the metabolic aspects of smoking. These are a result of chronic smoking, which has long term effects on many physiological variables including red blood count, mean cell volume, mean cell haemoglobin content, haematocrit, glucose 6-phosphate dehydrogenase content of the red blood cells, and adenosine triphosphate in red blood cells. They also examined the white blood count, nicotine, cotinine and carboxyhaemoglobin levels in the blood. Subjects smoked four kinds of cigarettes: (a) moderate tar, high nicotine; (b) high tar, moderate nicotine; (c) moderately low tar, low nicotine and (d) moderate tar, low nicotine. Cigarettes (a) and (b) were very similar in content, while (c) was the lowest in tar and nicotine, and (b) was highest in tar and nicotine. Subjects were 15 male and 15 female students who were smokers. Five male and five female non-smokers were used as controls. There appeared to be little change in the number of cigarettes smoked per day regardless of the tar and nicotine content. However, the range of tar and nicotine was small, and this restricts our conclusions. There is the suggestion, at least, that the lowest tar and nicotine subjects smoked slightly more. Similarly, the haematological parameters were not changed by changing the brands. Again, it may be that the range of tar and nicotine was not great enough nor the cigarettes smoked for long enough time to produce a difference. The most striking finding is the fact that female smokers excrete far less nicotine and cotinine than male smokers. It is possible that since the vital capacity of females is markedly lower than that for males, that there is less absorption by females of nicotine. Other possibilities are in sex-related metabolic processes. The differences between smokers and non-smokers must be explained by the chronic effects of smoking which preceded this experiment.

Schultz and Seehofer presented their studies dealing with analysis of cigarette butts. Butt analysis is a convenient method for estimating the amount of smoke taken by the smoker. However, the authors admit the puffing parameters and draw pressure and duration can influence the amount of residue which remains in the butt. It is interesting that butt lengths seem to correlate with economic conditions. Not surprisingly, people smoke cigarettes down to shorter butt lengths in times of recession, whereas in times of prosperity the opposite appears to be true. Observed smoking parameters showed some interesting differences. Women had shorter puff durations and men tended to shorten puff durations with increasing age. These parameters again may be related to differences in vital capacity between these groups.

The total puff duration, which was puff duration multiplied by puff number, tended to remain constant. Puff durations were longer with the cigarettes manufactured from air-cured tobaccos, and this may be due to a difference in irritation. Under conditions of stress, both puff duration and puff interval were shortened. This could imply that less nicotine was taken in during such situations, quite contrary to expectations.

These investigators measured puff flows and, by integration calculated the volume. Most smokers are said to reduce their puff volume after the first three or four of the ten to 19 puffs they take per cigarette. This may account for a fair amount of the variance. It would be useful to have measures of variability and of significance. Puff duplicators will be necessary to check this pattern of puffing. The percentage variation and nicotine retained in the butts of cigarettes smoked by different individuals was fairly high, ranging around 25% (a standard deviation might be a little more informative). In any case, the variation in nicotine content of the different brands tested ranged from a high of 1.09 mg to a low of 0.61 mg. This range was probably too small to produce significant differences in smoking behaviour. Furthermore, the different brands varied not only in nicotine but in flavouring agents, tar, and in types of filter. The question of whether compensatory smoking behaviour would occur when switching to a low nicotine product was brought up. In Table 20.9, it can be seen that there was some attempt at compensation, and the authors feel that this was accomplished primarily by increasing or decreasing the puff volume. There is a suggestion that heavy, normal and light smokers may react differently to changes in their usual smoking pattern, with the heavy smokers tending to persist in their stereotyped patterns while the lighter smokers will compensate. Further tests with finer analyses will be necessary to reveal whether such differences do in fact take place.

Guillerm and Radziszewski used a miniature flowmeter actually incorporated into the cigarette to analyse smoking pattern when a milder cigarette was substituted for the usual one. The experimental cigarette was 20% lower in nicotine, 50% lower in tar, and very much lower in acrolein and phenols. They found that their subjects increased their inhalation coefficients and thereby their carboxyhaemoglobin levels when smoking milder cigarettes. It is evident that the smokers did tend to compensate for the dilution of one or more components from their usual cigarettes.

The three papers by Schachter, Armitage and Kumar and their collaborators dealt with the possible role that nicotine might play in maintaining the smoking habit. It has been surprisingly difficult to demonstrate the apparently obvious fact that people smoke in order to obtain nicotine. Schachter showed, as did Finnegan, Larson and Haag (1945); Russell et al, (1975), Jarvik (1977), and others, that switching smokers to a low nicotine cigarette resulted in what appeared to be imperfect and sometimes no compensatory increase in number of cigarettes smoked. Obviously, there are more variables than nicotine controlling smoking behaviour. Schachter proposed that urinary pH is one of these. As with other alkaloids, the lower the pH, the more nicotine is excreted. Furthermore, Schachter demonstrated that stress could decrease the pH, and that the smoker's response is to smoke more to compensate for the increased excretion of nicotine. Schachter made the provocative point that the heavy smoker gets nothing out of smoking – that smoking merely keeps him at the level of a non-smoker in subjective feeling. In other words, a smoker smokes only to prevent withdrawal. One of the dysphoric symptoms of withdrawal is high irritability and annoyance with minor discomforts. This is similar to Wikler's theory of why a heroin addict sticks to his drug or relapses so easily (Wikler, 1977).

Armitage reviewed some of his very basic work explaining why cigarette smoking has become so popular. At the turn of the century, pipe and cigar smoking were relatively more popular, and snuff and chewing tobacco were used a good deal more than they are now. The development of flue-cured tobacco with a low pH for cigarettes made it possible for the first time to inhale the smoke and greatly enhanced its absorption. He has been able to study the absorption and fate of nicotine in animal preparations and also in humans, using radioactive nicotine. It is evident that there is still much to be learned about the absorption, fate and excretion of nicotine.

Kumar and his colleagues described their very interesting and important study of the effects of intravenous nicotine. In contrast with the only other carefully controlled study of intravenous nicotine by Lucchesi, Schuster and Emley (1967), Kumar et al, found no effect of this mode of administration upon simultaneous cigarette smoking rate. This was in contrast to the effect of preloading by cigarette smoking, which had a very definite inhibitory action on subsequent smoking. This study would tend to cast doubt upon the role of nicotine in smoking. However, I believe that the levels of nicotine administered may have been too low. It would be important to monitor blood levels of nicotine to see that they are comparable with the levels obtained from smoking. Also, different results might be obtained if subjects were allowed to self-administer the nicotine to determine whether a subjectively satisfying effect might be obtained. Clearly, more work must be done with the intravenous route of administration of nicotine.

Sutton and his colleagues indicated that although some degree of compensation occurred when filters of different air dilution were used, the compensation was far from perfect. In other words, diluting the smoke resulted in a lower level of nicotine in the blood of the individual. The carefully done study of Professor Thompson's group with two-third length cigarettes, indicates again only a partial compensation for the diminished length of the cigarette. It is obvious that factors other than nicotine control smoking behaviour in all of the experiments in which titration has been attempted (e.g. Gritz, Baer-Weiss and Jarvik, 1976; Finnegan, Larsen and Haag, 1945). What the factors other than nicotine might be have not been defined or measured as yet. Whenever smokers are asked to rate the satisfaction, however, as in the Finnegan, Larsen and Haag experiment, they are pretty accurate in estimating that the low nicotine cigarettes are less satisfying even though many of them continue to smoke them in the same way as their regular cigarettes. Sutton et al, suggest that there are regulators and non-regulators or compensators and non-compensators. Whether this is a reliable trait, of course, is difficult to determine. They indicate that some people take longer to compensate for low nicotine than others, but that ultimately all smokers probably would compensate.

Russell has summarised the beautiful studies done at the Maudsley Addiction Research Unit. These are attempts to determine whether smokers will work to keep their intake of nicotine relatively constant. Logically enough, the experimental manipulations vary along a continuum from nicotine-free cigarettes at one end to cigarette-free nicotine at the other end. Most investigators of the titration phenomenon, including us, agree with Russell and his colleagues that titration is imperfect and sometimes lacking altogether, and these findings pose some difficulties for the nicotine reinforcement theory of cigarette smoking. However, we believe there are loopholes for the theory which can accomodate lack of titration and still support nicotine reinforcement as the major source of reinforcement in cigarettes.

Russell describes several titration studies. In the first, subjects were given high and low nicotine cigarettes. It is not clear whether other constituents of the smoke, such as tar, were kept constant. Subjects compensated with the high but not with the low nicotine cigarettes. Russell points out that it is easier to cut down than to smoke more. However, I should have thought that subjects could easily have increased to much more than 12.5 cigarettes in five hours from their usual 10.7. What kept them from increasing (and I realise there is a touch of tautology here) was probably behavioural inertia or stereotypy. Furthermore, as Finnegan et al showed in 1945, low nicotine cigarettes produce dissatisfaction but are innocuous enough to smoke. High nicotine cigarettes, on the other hand, are markedly aversive as they produce symptoms of nicotine toxicity. Further experiments should be designed to disentangle the different reinforcement mechanisms involved: behavioural stereotypy, need for satisfaction, and avoidance of toxic effects such as throat irritation and nausea.

The second study showed that nicotine chewing gum could depress smoking. However, placebo gum also depressed smoking, though a little less than the nicotine gum. The plasma nicotine peaks indicated that there was some regulation, but the fall produced by placebo gum showed that chewing interferes with smoking. It is well known that eating food also depresses smoking even in chain smokers. We have found evidence that the nicotine gum provides satisfaction to selected subjects (Schneider et al,1977).

In the third study, Russell found that shortening cigarettes resulted in a significant increase in consumption of cigarettes, but 'no evidence whatsoever of compensation in the plasma nicotine levels'. This conclusion is somewhat surprising, and we must agree with Russell that the role of nicotine is still not clear, though on balance it seems to have a great deal to do with the control of smoking. One of the greatest drawbacks of the experiments done in his laboratory and in ours is that for the most part they are acute studies done in the course of a few days. One of our earliest studies (Goldfarb, Jarvik and Glick, 1970) was an attempt to study the long-term effects varying the nicotine content in lettuce cigarettes. With great difficulty, we succeeded in getting subjects to smoke experimental cigarettes over a three week period and we took measurements for five weeks. There was surprisingly little effect from adding or subtracting nicotine from these cigarettes, and we assumed that any possible effects were blocked by the aversiveness of the cigarettes. However, in retrospect, this explanation is inadequate since subjects smoked these cigarettes at a fairly high rate (15.0 cigarettes per day), though significantly lower than their normal rate (21.7 cigarettes per day). In the fifth week of the study, when subjects returned to their own cigarettes, they smoked them at a considerably lower rate. In retrospect, this was probably due to loss of tolerance from lowered nicotine intake over the previous three weeks. That they smoked nicotine-free cigarettes at all can only be ascribed to behavioural stereotypy or high resistance to extinction. In the marketplace, smokers extinguished rather completely with these same lettuce cigarettes since the company went out of business due to lack of sales.

At this stage, we hypothesise that nicotine (possible interacting with tar) is the main reinforcing agent in cigarettes. However, the smoking habit is so overlearned that extinction may take months. At present there are no meaningful long-term studies of extinction. Friedman and Fletcher (1976) reduced the nicotine yield from 1.4 to 1.0 mg with cellulose filler, a clearly inadequate reduction. Indeed, long-term studies are extremely difficult, if not impossible to design because nicotine and tobacco must be made unavailable to the subjects over several months.

By the same token, nicotine alone may not be as reinforcing as cigarettes to practiced smokers because of the acquisition of secondary reinforcement over years of smoking. Part of the reinforcing property of smoking is the ability of the smoker to adjust the intake of nicotine and studies should be done which enable the subject to do this.

In summary, the papers in this volume confirm the fact that smoking is a very strong habit, easy to start and hard to stop, and that it is a source of much pleasure to an enormous number of people. Personality, especially extroversion, may determine a predisposition to start and stop the habit. People may smoke for relaxation or stimulation and maybe for other reasons, and the same people may smoke for different reasons at different times.

Nicotine probably plays a role in reinforcement, though the evidence is conflicting. Pure nicotine alone has rarely been shown to be reinforcing and, conversely, large reductions in the nicotine yields of cigarettes do not necessarily proportionately reduce smoking behaviour. Although it is obvious that secondary reinforcement plays a strong role in maintaining the habit, there has been little systematic analysis of such stimuli (Jaffe and Jarvik, 1978). More work needs to be done on drug reinforcement mechanisms in the brain to throw light on nicotine action (Stein, 1974).

Improvements in technology will certainly facilitate smoking research in the future. The puff duplicators described in this volume constitute a formidable advance for our understanding of smoking patterns. Improved chemical analytical technology will enable us to trace nicotine and other smoke constituents in body fluids and correlate these with subjective effects. Only by discovering the real physiological reasons why people smoke will we be able to make smoking a safer and saner habit.

References

Andersson, K. (1975) Effects of cigarette smoking on learning and retention *Psychopharmacologia*, **41**, 1-5.

Finnegan, J.K., Larson, P.S. & Haag, H.B. (1945) The role of nicotine in the cigarette habit. *Science,* **102,** 94-96.

Friedman, S. & Fletcher, C.M. (1976) Changes in smoking habits and cough in men smoking cigarettes with 30% NSM tobacco substitute. *British Medical Journal,* **1,** 1427-1430.

Fuxe, K., Agnati, L., Eneroth, P., Gustafsson, J.A., Hokfelt, T., Lofstrom, A., Skett, B. & Skett, P. (1977) The effect of nicotine on central catecholamine neurons and gonadotropin secretion. I. Studies in the male rat. *Medical Biology,* **55,** 148-157.

Goldfarb, T.L., Jarvik, M.E. & Glick, S.D. (1970) Cigarette nicotine content as a determinant of human smoking behaviour. *Psychopharmacologia,* **17,** 89-93.

Griffiths, R.R., Bigelow, G.E. & Liebson, I. (1976) Facilitation of human tobacco self-administration by ethanol: a behavioural analysis. *Journal of the Experimental Analysis of Behaviour,* **25,** 279-292.

Gritz, E.R., Baer-Weiss, V. & Jarvik, M.E. (1976) Titration of nicotine intake with full-length and half-length cigarettes. *Clinical Pharmacology and Therapeutics,* **20,** 552-556.

Jaffe, J.H. & Jarvik, M.E. (1978) Tobacco Use and Tobacco Use Disorder. In *Psychopharmacology: A generation of progress.* ed. Lipton, M.A., DiMascio, A. & Killam, K.E., pp. 1665-1676. New York: Raven Press.

Jarvik, M.E. (1977)   Biological Factors Underlying the Smoking Habit. In *Research on Smoking Behaviour.* ed. Jarvik, M.E., Cullen, J.W., Gritz, E.R., Vogt, T.M. & West, L.J., pp. 122-146. NIDA Research Monograph 17, DHEW USPHS, Alcohol, Drug Abuse, and Mental Health Administration, Rockville.

Lucchesi, B.R., Schuster, C.R. & Emley, G.S. (1967) The role of nicotine as a determinant of cigarette smoking frequency in man with observations of certain cardiovascular effects associated with the tobacco alkaloid. *Clinical Pharmacology and Therapeutics,* **8,** 789-796.

Nelsen, J.M., Pelley, K. & Goldstein, L. (1975) Protection by nicotine from behavioural disruption caused by reticular formation stimulation in the rat. *Pharmacology Biochemistry & Behaviour,* **3,** 749-754.

Russell, M.A.H., Wilson, C., Patel, U.A., Feyerabend, C. & Cole, P.V. (1975) Plasma nicotine levels after smoking cigarettes with high, medium and low nicotine yields. *British Medical Journal,* **2,** 414-416.

Schneider, N.G., Popek, P., Jarvik, M.E. & Gritz, E.R. (1977) The use of nicotine gum during cessation of smoking. *American Journal of Psychiatry,* **134,** 439-440.

Stein, L. (1974) Norepinephrine reward pathways: Role of self-stimulation, memory consolidation and schizophrenia. *Nebraska Symposium on Motivation.*

Walter, W.G., Cooper, R., Aldridge, V.J., McCallum, W.C. & Winter, A.L. (1964) Contingent negative variation: An electric sign of sensorimotor association and expectancy in the human brain. *Nature, London,* **203,** 380-384.

Wikler, A. (1977) Characteristics of Opioid Addiction. In *Psychopharmacology in the practice of medicine,* ed. Jarvik, M.E., pp. 419-432. New York: Appleton-Century-Crofts.

Index

Index

Printed in Great Britain by Bell and Bain Ltd.,
Glasgow